DATE		

2d edition

DIMENSIONS in PROFESSIONAL DEVELOPMENT

Caroline Reynolds
Texas Christian University
Fort Worth, Texas

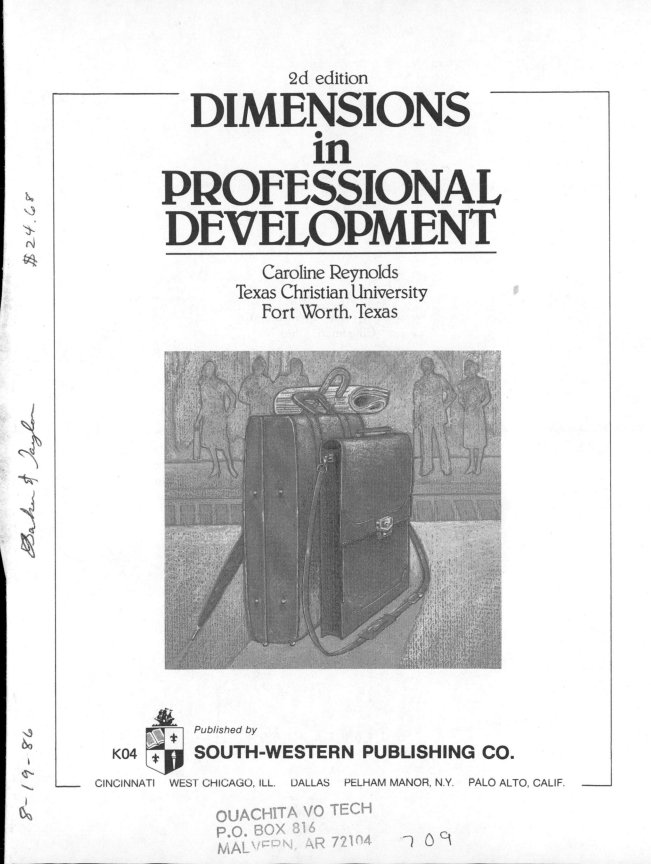

Published by

K04 **SOUTH-WESTERN PUBLISHING CO.**

CINCINNATI   WEST CHICAGO, ILL.   DALLAS   PELHAM MANOR, N.Y.   PALO ALTO, CALIF.

ISBN: 0-538-11040-6

Library of Congress
Catalog Card Number: 82-60582

2 3 4 5 6 7 K 8 7 6 5 4
Printed in the United States of America

PREFACE

Learning a skill that will enable us to make a life that is fulfilling is what we strive for in early adult life. We hope that we can be measured by our efforts and our accomplishments in our chosen jobs and be rewarded accordingly.

Doing a good job, of course, is necessary to success; however, unless we are the best in our fields, much more is expected of us. Most jobs are in a social atmosphere rather than in a solitary one. The people involved in such an atmosphere make doing an effective job dependent upon relating cordially with colleagues. To see that people relate more easily to those whose behavior and appearance they understand is easy. To see that difficulties arise when behavior and/or appearance indicate disagreement is apparent, too.

Most organizations will recognize and reward you according to the success you have in developing yourself, presenting yourself, and functioning in the social arena. Business stresses work performance but evaluates people on the personal impression they make more often than on the quality of the job done. Schools concentrate on skill development but studies show that teachers are influenced in evaluations by the personal qualities of the student. You have the opportunity to prepare for success through study. Success rarely just happens. It is achieved through development of ability *and* development of the person with ability.

Making adjustments in oneself usually is more difficult than making adjustments in areas of life outside oneself. Think of the adjustments you discover you need to make as growing in your efforts to achieve success. Observe the reaction of others to you as you achieve the "norm" for people working in your field. You should find that less effort is needed to convince people of your competence and more effort can be used in your achievements than that needed by people who try to function outside the acceptable modes of behavior and appearance.

The effort in this book centers on making clear what business has come to accept and appreciate in its employees. The purpose is to enable you to recognize in yourself the strengths you have already developed and to develop new areas you can nurture. Further, you will learn how to present yourself so that you can demonstrate in a receptive climate who you are and what you can do.

Many people and organizations have cooperated to make this book an effective one. Their contributions are acknowledged. In addition to recognition, I extend my appreciation. Without both the people who worked directly with this book and the people who offered encouragement and suggestions, many without recognition, my job would have been much more difficult. I am grateful to them.

To the students who learn from these efforts, I hope you achieve a measure of fulfillment and success that enables you to know the joy of such sharing as I have had in preparing *Dimensions* for you.

Caroline Reynolds

CONTENTS

Part Two: *Professional Image*

Part Three: Individual Matters

ACKNOWLEDGMENTS

For permission to reproduce the photographs on the pages indicated, acknowledgment is made to the following:

Chapter 3

p. 40 (Illus. 3-2): Courtesy of the Greyhound Corporation

Chapter 4

p. 50 (Illus. 4-1): Reprinted with permission from Westvaco Corporation

p. 52 (Illus. 4-2): Walgreen Company

p. 57 (Illus. 4-4): Seagram

p. 59 (Illus. 4-5): Burlington Industries

p. 60 (Illus. 4-6): American Express Company

Chapter 5

p. 73 (Illus. 5-9): IBM Corporation

p. 81 (Illus. 5-12): AMF Incorporated

Chapter 6

p. 86 (Illus. 6-1): Hart Schaffner & Marx

p. 87 (Illus. 6-3): McAlpins

p. 88 (Illus. 6-4, left): Simplicity Pattern Company

(Illus. 6-4, right): Photo courtesy of Butterick Fashion Marketing Co.

p. 92 (Illus. 6-7): McAlpins

Chapter 8

p. 123 (Illus. 8-3): Wrangler Activewear

pp. 133, 134, & 135 (Illus. 8-9, 8-10, & 8-11): Courtesy SELF. Copyright © 1981 by The Condé Nast Publications Inc.

Chapter 9

p. 140 (Illus. 9-2): Hair Surgeon Designers

(Illus. 9-3): McAlpins

p. 141 (Illus. 9-4): Hair Surgeon Designers

p. 142 (Illus. 9-5): Hairstyle by Kenneth Battelle

p. 143 (Illus. 9-6): Hair Surgeon Designers

p. 144 (Illus. 9-8): Hair by Glemby International

(Illus. 9-9): Hair Surgeon Designers

p. 146 (Illus. 9-12): The Van Heusen Corporate Markets Company

Chapter 12

p. 176 (Illus. 12-1): AMF Incorporated

p. 181 (Illus. 12-4): Exercise Bicycle courtesy of Huffy Corporation

p. 182 (Illus. 12-5): Photo Courtesy of PepsiCo, Inc.

p. 184 (Illus. 12-6): Charter Medical Company

p. 186 (Illus. 12-8): Photograph Rudy Molacek. Copyright © 1981 by G. Q. Magazine Inc.

Chapter 14

p. 210 (Illus. 14-1): Johnson & Johnson

Chapter 15

p. 233 (Illus. 15-7): Courtesy of Norton Simon Inc.

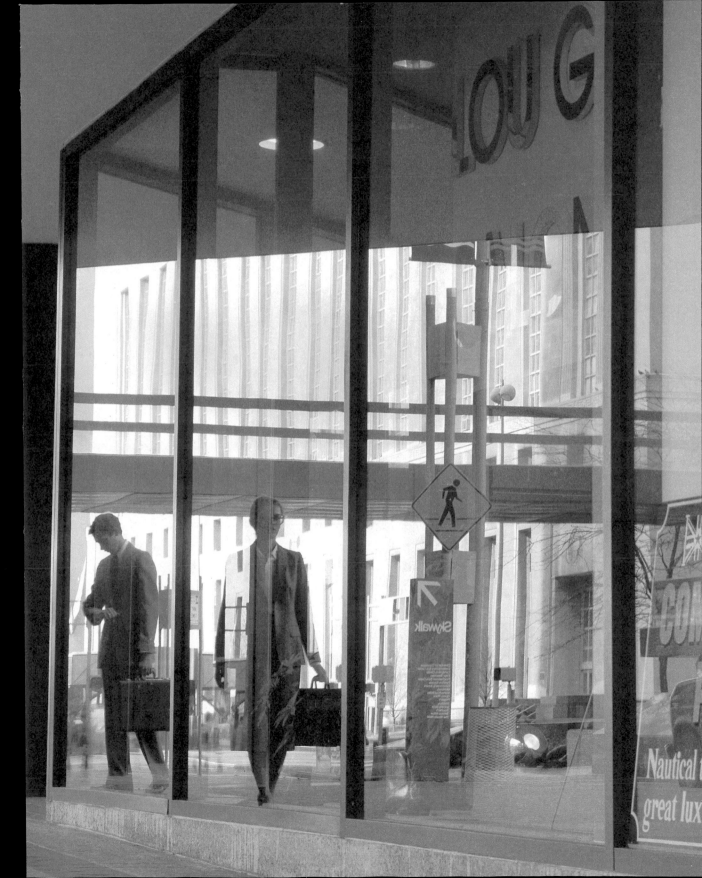

PART ONE: *Professional Strategy*

Part Objectives

After studying this part, you should be able to:

1. *Secure a job that meets your needs.*

2. *Adjust easily to the people and situations at your job.*

3. *Evaluate your needs for growth, plan procedures for growth, and execute your plans.*

4. *Maintain the image you desire at your job.*

5. *Effectively manage your money.*

6. *Efficiently manage your time on and off the job.*

Chapter 1

Securing a Job

Chapter Objectives

After studying this chapter, you should be able to:

1. *Determine who can help you get a job and how they can help you.*
2. *Determine what you can do for yourself in seeking a job and how you should do it.*
3. *Prepare yourself for the questions you are likely to be asked during a job interview.*
4. *Prepare questions you want to ask during an interview.*
5. *Write a resume.*
6. *Write a cover letter.*
7. *Write a thank-you letter.*

A job has a major impact on the quality of your life for a very long time. The most obvious impact is that of providing money for you to live in this free enterprise economy. Your job will also influence your satisfaction with yourself throughout your life. You want a job that utilizes your abilities, that allows, even encourages, growth, and that gives you a feeling of accomplishment.

Getting the right job, one that utilizes your abilities and gives you satisfaction as well as money, is as important as any consideration you have. Since finding a job — the best job for you — is so very important, how will you go about it?

———— *The Job Market* ————

There is no magic place where jobs are located. They are everywhere and sometimes nowhere. Part of the job-finding process is to locate jobs. The national job market is not organized. You won't find a list of all jobs available at any given time, and you won't find a person who knows where all the jobs are. How then do you find that important place where you can use your abilities, gain satisfaction in your performance, and earn money to live on?

Being Creative and Resourceful

The disorganization of the information about where jobs are leaves it to you to organize the job hunt. The bewildered feeling a first-time job seeker experiences can be overcome with some careful thought.

The job search is often undertaken with great expectations. After a few days or weeks, enthusiasm wanes and often depression sets in. If you are aware of that pattern, you can guard against it. The best ways to avoid depression are to keep busy looking for a job and to avoid talking about your failures. The perfect job for you exists; all you have to do is keep looking for it until you find it. Thinking about your failures won't help; neither will talking about them. Very few people want to be around job seekers who are depressed — interviewers included. Keep your chin up and stay busy looking for that job.

Looking for a job should be a full-time job if you are not currently employed. Because there is no magic source of job information, you will have a full-time job just making sense of what is available. It will be tempting to schedule an interview now and then and take the afternoon off for a visit with friends or a movie. Don't be tempted. Schedule productive efforts in your job campaign to occupy you all day, five days a week, until you find that perfect job. What kind of productive efforts yield best results?

Getting Help

The nature of job hunting assures that only productive people get jobs because the job hunter does most of the work. You have to be a productive person merely to find a good job.

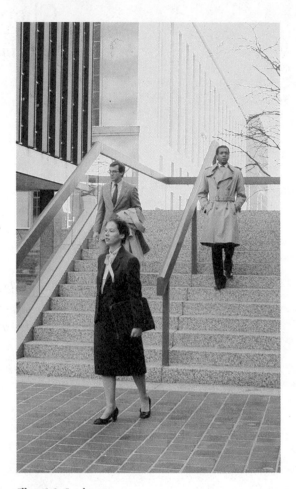

Illus. 1-1. Looking for a job should be a full-time job if you are not currently employed.

Being productive, however, doesn't mean that you find a job without help. You find a job through your own efforts but with the help of others. The others who can help are found in a variety of places. The most obvious are:

1. Private employment agencies which charge a fee.
2. Public employment agencies which don't charge a fee.

3. Help-wanted ads.
4. School placement services.

Studies show, however, that of people who currently are working, those sources helped only 15 percent of them find their jobs. The Manpower Administration of the U.S. Department of Labor published a study in 1970 that showed methods used to find current jobs. The breakdown is:

One percent found employment through private employment agencies.
Three percent used public employment agencies.
Five percent used help-wanted ads.
Six percent used school placement services.

That means that 85 percent of the people working used other methods to locate their jobs. The study also showed that:

Twenty-four percent *contacted potential employers directly.*
Forty-eight percent *found their jobs through friends or relatives.*
Thirteen percent used a combination of methods and techniques.

It is easy to see that you increase your opportunities vastly by letting everyone know you are looking for a job — almost half the people working today used just that method. It is important to note that almost one fourth of the people working used *their own initiative* in contacting companies directly to land just that job they wanted.

Because your chances are three out of four that you will find a job through your own efforts, most of your energy should be centered around your own efforts. However, because this is so important a campaign, leave no resource out:

Illus. 1-2. How People Find Jobs

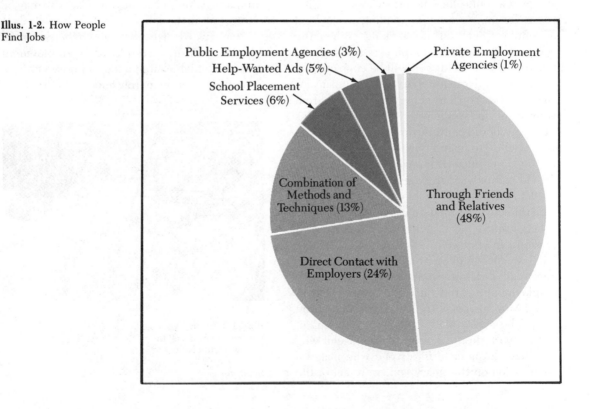

Public Employment Agencies (3%)
Help-Wanted Ads (5%)
School Placement Services (6%)
Private Employment Agencies (1%)
Combination of Methods and Techniques (13%)
Through Friends and Relatives (48%)
Direct Contact with Employers (24%)

Register with those free agencies who might help; follow up ads that may yield a job; and by all means register with your school placement service if you have one. The benefits from exposure to these people who regularly deal with job seekers will be a learning process in itself. You will get used to answering questions and filling out forms and will thereby gain poise in dealing with interviewers. Who knows, you may be the one in four who actually finds a job with one of these methods.

Registering at an Employment Agency

Whether you use a fee-charging private employment agency or not is up to you. Public agencies provided by your tax money are available without a fee, and they have a better record according to the Manpower study. For both agencies the formats are similar. You will be assigned a counselor who interviews you. That counselor may test you depending on the kind of employment you are seeking. When the counselor is called by employers seeking employees in your field, you will be contacted by the agency and told to report to the company for an interview. You may get several referrals from your agency or you may get none. During this time you should continue looking for a job. You cannot afford to sit and wait for an agency to call. If you don't hear from your counselor, you should call or visit the agency at least once a week to keep your counselor informed that you are still actively pursuing a job. Ask about recent vacancies, and generally keep yourself foremost in your counselor's mind.

Use good judgment and be conscientious about all dealings concerning your future employment — the quality of your life is at stake. Most agencies are honest; however, you should be aware of the possible problems in dealing with them. Beware of a counselor who may have a quota to fill or one who makes a commission on the salary you are to get or the

number of people placed; such counselors may have you interview for jobs unsuitable for you or for jobs you do not want.

Using the Help-Wanted Ads

Research shows that only one of every five jobs is advertised. You should, however, check the help-wanted ads because it takes so little effort and expense to pursue this 20-percent chance. During your job campaign, check the ads every day, but particularly on Sunday. If you see a job that looks like what you want, use the most direct method available to contact the employer: Go to the office at opening time on Monday morning if the address is listed; call at opening time on Monday if only a phone number is listed; if a P.O. Box number is listed (known as a blind ad), mail your letter and resume Sunday so that your letter gets to the company before that of anyone else who may be interested in the job.

One word of caution about help-wanted ads. Many of them are placed by employment agencies which charge a fee to find you a job. Sometimes, the ad merely endeavors to get you

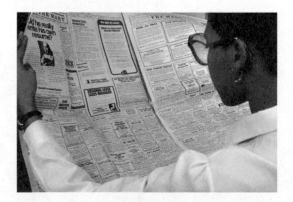

Illus. 1-3. During your job campaign, check the help-wanted ads every day, particularly on Sunday.

to the agent's offices so that the agent can sign you up as a client rather than to provide a job opening. If you are not sure about whether the listing is from such an agency, check for the name in the yellow pages of your phone book under employment agencies. If no name is given, you will have a chance to check after they respond to you.

Contacting Companies Yourself

Study the business community in which you want to work. Identify those companies that employ people in jobs like the one you want. When you find a company that is a potential employer, make a study of it. Read the business pages of the newspaper of the community to learn about the current activities of the company. Check with the local librarian for reference books that will tell you about the company. Most companies are affiliated with some registry that is maintained at the library. Often you can learn about products, the number of employees, and the locations of various offices through these registries. You can learn whether the company is growing or not. Very often the names of the current officers are listed. You can learn how the company compares to others in its field. By calling or writing the company headquarters, you may be able to get an annual report of operations published by the company which will give you a good overview of the company. In short, learn everything about the company you can before you set up an interview.

Try to learn the name of the supervisor of the people in your job category that work in the company you have selected. Try to interview with that person first. Your friends and acquaintances may be able to help. Sometimes, however, you simply may not be able to identify that particular person. If not, you will be forced to go through the personnel department for an interview. Your approach will not be "do you have any openings?" It will be "let me show you that I can be a good employee for the time when you do have openings." Employee turnover in organizations is much higher than normally assumed, especially at the entry level.

The turnover resulting from one person who terminates employment can be great. For example, if an executive secretary in Office A terminates to move to another city, the secretary just down the hall in Office B may apply for the executive secretary job, leaving the Office B secretary job vacant which may be pursued by the typist from the word processing center in Office C. A mail clerk from Office D then applies for the upcoming vacancy in Office C, leaving the mail clerk job open. During this process, four vacancies have occurred from one termination. You might have entered at any level depending on your skills and the impact you made on the supervisor you contacted.

Telling Your Friends and Relatives

If only one of five jobs is advertised, four of five are not. How, then, do employers find employees? They ask their own employees and their friends and relatives. They deal with people they know. You can enhance your chances by the same methods. Let everyone you know, especially anyone you know who may work for a company that employs people in your field, that you are looking for a job. Let them know that you are looking full-time and that you can go for an interview on very short notice if necessary. Be industrious about pursuing leads they may give you, and follow up by letting them know how you fared in pursuing the lead.

Your Tools

Before you actually talk to an employer, you need to prepare some tools to use in your job hunt. One of these is known as a resume (res-oo-may), vita, data sheet, or qualifications brief. Regardless of the name, it is a list of your qualifications and can take many forms, depending upon your purpose. The next tool is a cover letter for your resume that introduces you to the potential employer who may not let you in the office to introduce yourself personally or to an employer in another city. You also will need to think about some questions you may be asked which typically require some thinking before being answered. A thank-you letter that follows your interview should be written so that you can send it immediately after the interview.

Constructing a Resume

Your list of qualifications will be the only thing many potential employers will have by which to evaluate you. You give it to your employment counselor, your school placement office, people whose names you have used as a reference, your friends and relatives who may be helping you find a job, and to supervisors and employment offices of companies where you want to work. Ideally, you hand it to the person who is interviewing you when you interview. Interviewers get a chance to see you in person and to see your qualifications listed while they talk to you about the job.

Because it may be the only criterion a person has who is considering interviewing you for a job, the resume must be constructed very carefully. Such things as one misspelled word have eliminated people from interviews. One study showed that the main reason resumes and cover letters are discarded are spelling, punctuation, and sloppiness. Employers get so many resumes they need a way to reduce the stack to a manageable size and may use various criteria to accomplish the size reduction. Your resume must be perfect — giving an employer no reason not to interview you. Other than getting the spelling correct, what are some other things you should know about a resume?

Including All Pertinent Data

Employers expect to see certain data in a resume. At the top, they expect to see your name, address, and a telephone number where you can be reached. After that, you usually describe the kind of job you are looking for. Your education and experience are next. The one you choose to describe first should be the one that is *most likely* to make you appear to be the best person for the job. The last section probably will be "other qualifications" that may show something about you that experience and education do not include. Finally, you can include your birth date, your marital status, and other personal information if you wish. You should not include your race or religion. The last section, if you have room, is a list of three references with complete mailing addresses and phone numbers of people who know you as a good citizen but who are not related to you.

Just being sure that you have all the expected information is not enough to make your resume one that an employer keeps. You need to make the resume interesting enough to make you sound like a person who can and will do the job. For example, when you describe the job for which you are looking, you add a phrase that indicates that you can be relied upon to do a good job: Secretary in an office where efficiency and cheerfulness are needed; or Accountant who is good working both with figures and with people. When you describe your education, describe any special successes or activities you had that show that you worked harder than you had to: Earned 30 percent of college expenses while a full-time student; or President of Student Council two years. Describe your education in terms of the courses you did well in. Employers are more interested in what you *did* than where you were. Talk about what you accomplished first and where you accomplished it second. Your work experience should be described in terms of your abilities and what you accomplished: Worked as a part-time sales-person winning top sales awards twice in four months; or developed improved inventory control procedures while working as a stock clerk during summers. Tell what you accomplished before you describe where and when you accomplished it.

Your references may be listed on your resume. They should be respected and well-known people in the community if possible. You must, however, ask permission of people *before* you use their names as references. The reference listing should include complete mailing addresses and phone numbers.

Creating a Favorable Impression

Employer time spent looking for good employees is time the employer would rather have spent being productive in the business — it is time that costs business money. If your resume shows you to be a person who understands what the employer wants and who wants to do the job, you will be well received. Several things can be done to create this favorable impression.

Just having a resume puts you ahead of the crowd. It shows that you are industrious and organized enough to have prepared a list of your qualifications. Having a resume that is attractively placed on the page, carefully and professionally typed on quality paper, shows something about your thorough approach to doing a job well. Statements about your abilities rather than statements about where you spent time show that you learn from your experiences rather than simply accumulate them.

By stressing your strongest abilities in terms of what you can do for the company (not what you want the company to do for you) and emphasizing successes you have had in the past, you can often impress the employer. Because most people describe the job wanted, for example, by saying what they expect from the company (sales position offering opportunity for promotion to management) and by describing how they have spent their time (19– to 19–, Worked as Sales Clerk) rather than the success they may have had in the job, they limit themselves. In fact, one study showed that simply telling where they were rather than what they accomplished was the third most frequent reason applicants were denied interviews.

You will create a favorable impression by keeping your resume brief. One page is the best length for a resume. That length requires you to use phrases rather than complete sentences and to choose your words carefully. Some of the things you can leave out of your resume that will help you keep the length down are: vague summaries about your experiences, reasons for leaving previous jobs, pay (both what you have earned and what you expect), date of availability, location preference, social security number. Some starters for phrases that help keep your resume brief are: conceived, directed, managed, accomplished, developed, achieved, and saved.

Beginners often have a hard time saying nice things about themselves. You cannot afford to be modest when you prepare your resume. However, you can describe yourself in terms of what others have said about you: Voted Most Likely to Succeed; often praised for efficiency on the job; was asked to return the following summer; People often comment on my ability to perform under stressful situations.

Using strategy in organizing your resume can help create a favorable impression. Choose what you think the employer is most interested in or will value the most to place first in your resume. In some cases that may be your education; in others, your experience.

Individually typed resumes on good quality paper are the most impressive. However,

Joan (or Joseph) Job Seeker

1409 Inverness Avenue
Fort Worth, Texas 76132-6295

817-555-1032

Objective: ASSISTANT TO EXECUTIVE where communication skill and
a pleasant manner in dealing with people are needed.

Experience: Assisted professor of management in developing
research in management communication problems while
I was a student at Texas Business School, 19-- to
19--. Developed interview techniques that yielded
unbiased information ready to be processed by com-
puter. Professor's comments: "Joan (or Joseph)
showed unusual skill in organizing data and in handling people and played an important role in developing the research project that qualified for a
$50,000 grant."

Helped people locate information in a scholastic setting while working as assistant to the librarian at
Texas High School, 19-- to 19--. Especially liked
helping students define problems to be solved and
aiding in organizing the search for answers.

Education: Completed requirements for Associate of Arts degree
in Business Communications at Texas Business School,
19--, graduating in upper ten percent of class.
Maintained 3.4 average overall and all A's in Management and Communications courses while earning 75 percent of my educational expenses on scholarship. Included office administration training as electives
and learned to appreciate importance of accuracy and
attention to detail in business.

Special: Worked as a volunteer at the local hospital where I
served as assistant to admitting clerk in the emergency room during summers, 19-- to 19--. I learned
to put people at ease while questioning them closely,
gaining the most information in the shortest time
under stressful situations. Learned to maintain confidence of patient's family during long, tedious waiting periods.

Personal: Born January 20, 19--, single, in good health. Find
tennis and racquetball relaxing leisure-time activities. I enjoy organizing and leading community activities such as softball and basketball leagues.

Illus. 1-4. Resume of
a Person with No Paid
Job Experience

Sam (or Sue) Job Hunter

222 West Street
Dallas, TX 75333-3894

214-555-7569

Objective

Product Manager for food manufacturing concern where creative
          ideas and knowledge of consumer preferences are
          important.

Education

Marketing Major with a Bachelor of Business Administration
          Degree from Texas Business University (19--) where
          I combined accounting, finance, and management with
          marketing concentration to gain understanding of the
          whole picture of business. Excelled in sales and
          display techniques graduating with honors. I served
          as President of the Marketing Club three of my four
          years increasing membership by 100 percent in first
          two years.

Experience

Developed display and marketing techniques while working as a
          stock clerk and checker at Good Food Grocery during
          summers 19-- to 19--. Was asked to return full-time
          after graduation as Assistant Manager.

Developed telephone survey techniques raising response levels
          from 30 to 60 percent while asking about consumer
          preferences for packaging of certain grocery items
          for Food's Incorporated Research Firm, part-time to
          earn 30 percent of educational expenses while in
          college.

Coordinated high school "supply store" at Dallas High School dur-
          ing junior and senior years building from a 20-item
          inventory to over 100 items and increasing profits
          by 140 percent during those two years.

Personal

Born April 10, 19--, single, good health, enjoy meeting people
and selling.

References

Professor J. S. Lee   Ms. Sarah Davids, Director
Texas Business University   School Concessions
Fort Worth, TX 76111-1021   Dallas, TX 75212-2437
817-555-9435   214-555-4044

Illus. 1-5. Resume for
a Job Requiring a College
Degree

unless you are an expert typist with a lot of time to type resumes, you will need to use some means of reproducing your resume after you have one perfect copy prepared. If you are applying for a job lower than supervisor, you can use xerography that is clean. Jobs at higher levels usually require resumes that are reproduced by offset methods. About 25 copies are appropriate for your first resume when you are letting everyone know you are looking for a job.

The most favorable impression is created by tailoring your resume for a specific job and typing it individually. Don't overlook this fact if you know of *a specific job* you want in a specific company and if you have time to tailor your resume. For example, you might entitle your resume: Qualifications of (Your Name) for the Position of Secretary to Personnel Director of Ace Company. You may also need to rearrange the order of experience and education items to give a stronger impression of yourself for the specific job, especially if you have training and experience in the area (personnel in this case) as well as in your field (secretarial in this case). You, of course, will need only one original copy of this resume. You should, however, always keep a copy (carbon or photocopy) of your resume for your file.

Keeping a file of your resumes and records of letters you write both asking for and thanking for interviews is a good idea. You can also keep lists of names of people you know in the company and of names of those you encounter during interviews for future reference in this file.

Writing a Cover Letter

If you cannot set up interviews by visiting the company itself, through friends and relatives, or by telephone, you will need to write a letter that will get you an interview.

The goal of your letter is to get you an interview for a job. Your approach should be to show how you can help the employer by doing a job well — better than anyone else. Before you can describe how well you can do a job you have to know some things about the company and its needs. Use the local newspaper business page, your local library reference room, and the company's annual report if you can get it.

The letter itself should be addressed to the person you want to work for if you can learn that person's name. If you can't, address your letter to the president of the firm. Do not address your letter to the Personnel Director, Personnel Department, Dear Sir, Gentlemen, or Ladies unless you want to fall in with the large group of people applying for a job and risk having your letter and resume thrown out. By learning the name of the person for whom you want to work and addressing your letter to that person, you get ahead of those whose letters must go through the personnel department. If you address your letter to the president, your letter will be sent by the president's office to the personnel office, but it will carry more impact by coming from that direction than by coming by way of the mailroom. Personnel departments rarely throw out anything coming from the president's office.

Make your letter one page if you can. Stress abilities and accomplishments rather than biographical data. Boring letters are those that list how you have spent your time. Anyone can do that. Interesting letters show how your abilities are used and can be used to accomplish the firm's purpose and further its goals. Companies are interested in people who know how to use their abilities and who are interested in using them to help the company become more successful. Describe yourself that way, and you are likely to generate interest in your employment.

Ask directly for an interview. Do not leave it to the employer to call you to set up a time. Saying that you will call in a few days to make

1409 Inverness Avenue
Fort Worth, TX 76132-6295
(Today's date)

Mr. A. L. Ray
Ray Public Relations, Inc.
424 Calgary
Arlington, TX 76020-4290

Dear Mr. Ray:

In view of your company's growth in the past few years, it is
reasonable to believe that you have a place for me.

Ever since I watched your management of the public relations
of our mayor during his election campaign, I have wanted to
become part of your dynamic team. Studying and participating
in communication problem solving where working with people to
achieve mutual goals provided growth in both areas uniquely
prepared me to work in your company.

Could we talk about my working for you after you read my attached resume? I'll call you later this week for an appointment for an interview.

Sincerely,

J. J. Seeker

J. J. Seeker

Enclosure

Illus. 1-6. Cover Letter

222 West Street
Dallas, TX 75333-3894
(Today's date)

Mrs. S. M. Way
Vice-President, Marketing
Procter and Gamble, Inc.
Cincinnati, OH 45202-1228

Dear Mrs. Way:

Procter and Gamble's innovative methods of introducing new products have tremendously impressed me. My growing interest and
enthusiasm for your marketing procedures have convinced me that
I want to be a part of your team.

My marketing studies at Texas Business University combined with
my day-to-day development of display and marketing strategy in
foods on the job give me a balance between theory and practice
that I think sets me apart from others.

Can we discuss the possibility of my working for Procter and
Gamble? Will you please review my enclosed resume and give me
an interview when I call you in a few days?

Sincerely,

S. J. Hunter

S. J. Hunter

Enclosure

Illus. 1-7. Cover Letter

an appointment for an interview keeps your letter and resume on top of the desk rather than in a file drawer where it must be retrieved when you call. If you are sending out many letters and resumes to cities where your call would be long distance, you may ask the employer to respond by calling you collect. The risk is that the employer can simply ignore you knowing that you will not have to be dealt with personally or by phone. Saying that you will call, and doing so, gets you more attention.

Do not let the fact that no openings exist deter you from interviewing. You can persuade the employer that you should be the first hired when an opening does occur. More often than you think, employers create openings for people who appear so eager and capable that they shouldn't be let go. Even if you do not land a job, you can get advice from the interviewer about seeking a job that will help you, especially if the interviewer is impressed with you.

Neatness counts. Remember that resumes can be thrown out because of one misspelled word. So can letters. Be sure that your letter is perfect. Use good quality, plain white paper and a typewriter with clean keys. If you cannot type a good letter yourself, have someone type for you. Do not send copies of your letter. Send originals only. Post your letter to arrive on any day but Monday (unless you are responding to a blind ad). Tuesday through Thursday are lighter mail days, and you are likely to get more attention on those days. Try to call the employer within two days of the receipt of your letter. That gives the employer time to think about your letter but not time enough to forget about it.

The Interview

After you get an appointment for an interview, you have some preparation to do. You need to learn as much as you can about the company and its concerns. You need to formulate answers to questions you may be asked about yourself. And you need to prepare yourself mentally and physically for a good first impression.

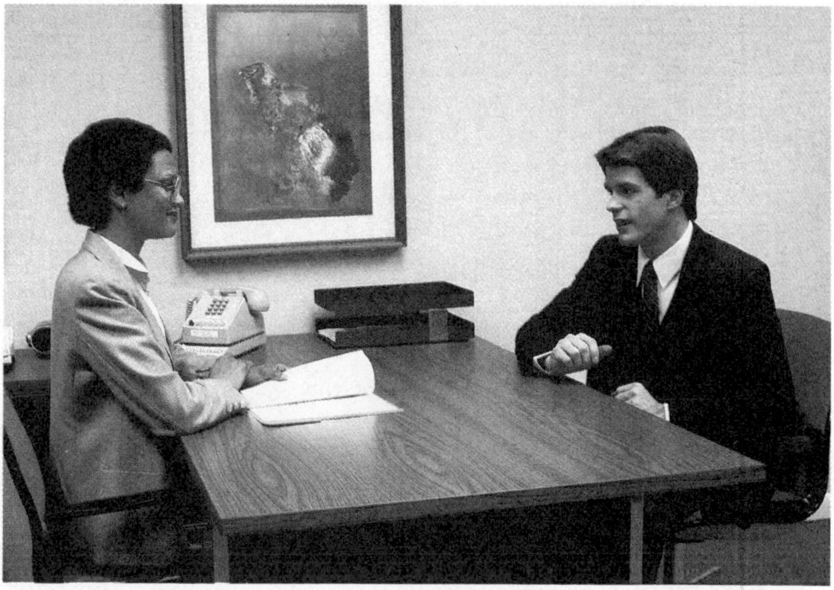

Illus. 1-8. Prepare mentally and physically to make a good first impression in your interview.

Thinking About Questions

You already know how to learn about a company using the newspaper, library, and your friends. You may develop some questions from your research. Plan to ask them at your interview.

During the interview, the employer will ask you questions. Sometimes these questions are open-ended and intended to get you to talk. Sometimes they are designed to get information. You need to know what some typical ones are and think about how you will answer them during the interview. Employers also expect you to ask questions. Keep in mind that you are examining the job while you are being examined for the job. You need to think about the things you want to know about a job and formulate questions that will give you that information. Some typical questions are:

Questions from the Employer —

- What can I do for you? (You can give me a chance to [say what you can do for the company].)
- Why are you interested in working for us? (Talk about using your abilities to advance the company's purpose.)
- What attracts you to us? (Use what you found out in your research to describe specific areas that interest you about the company.)
- Tell me about your experience. (Talk about accomplishments rather than how and where you have spent your time.)
- Why do you want to change jobs? (Be honest and describe your reasons in terms of what you want to achieve instead of what you want to get away from.)
- What is the ideal job for you? (Describe the job in terms of meeting the company's needs rather than yours.)
- Describe your education for me. (Talk about your best subjects and educational accomplishments rather than listing schools and degrees alone.)

- What kind of grades did you make? (Be honest. Talk about the courses you did best in. Do not downgrade teachers or others for any failures you might have had. In fact, don't mention failures at all unless you are asked.)
- Who has exercised the greatest influence on you and how? (Talk about those who inspired and motivated you to become your best.)
- Have you ever been fired or asked to resign? (Be honest. Explain the situation but do not downgrade others.)
- Why did you leave your previous job? (Talk about where you wanted to go, not what you wanted to leave if possible.)
- Describe your health for me. (Talk about good attendance records and active hobbies you have in this discussion.)

Questions for the Employer —

- Did my resume raise any questions I can clarify?
- Would you describe the duties of the job for me, please?
- Was the person who previously held this job promoted?
- What is the largest single problem facing your staff now?
- Could you tell me about the people I will be working with?
- From what I've told you, don't you think I could do a good job for you?
- Could you tell me about the benefits program of the company? (Ask *after* the employer has indicated interest in hiring you.)

If, during the interview, the interviewer seems restless while you are talking, it probably means that you are talking too much. If the interviewer says you are not right for the job, ask if others in the organization might be interested in your qualifications and experience. If the interviewer is undecided, ask if you can check on a later day (specify) that week.

If the interviewer asks about the pay you require, be prepared. You should have a figure in mind. That figure should be within the range of what people in your field are making. In order to learn what that amount is, you may have to do some research. There are salary surveys published for the members of the College Placement Council. See if your school counselor has one. Also you can check the *Occupational Outlook Handbook* in your local library. These sources will give you a range for the position you seek. Aim 10 percent above the absolute minimum you can accept, but always state your needs in terms of a range.

Preparing Mentally

Keep in mind that the employer needs good employees and that you are a potential one. The employer wants to find those people quickly and get back to work. The more you are able to help in that process, the more likely you are to be hired. Good tools like a resume and ready answers to questions in terms of what the employer needs help in that process. A genuine interest in the employer's needs, interests, and operations helps in achieving the "good employee" tag. Showing pride in your own past performance is not considered boastful but indicative of a person who cares about and who takes pride in doing a job well. Displaying sound ideas about the job and the employer's concerns shows that you've done your homework about the company and the job. Being able to take control of the interview if the employer is distracted or just plain tired of interviewing can make the difference between you and someone else who may want the job but who waits for the interviewer to come up with thought-provoking questions. Carrying extra copies of your resume is a good idea in case you are asked to talk with other members of the firm and in case your original one was mislaid.

Some of the characteristics employers describe as being important have nothing to do with your job skills. In one study of 225 firms, 215 said they considered primarily the personal qualifications of the individual. That means that your maturity, initiative, enthusiasm, poise, appearance, and your ability to get along with people are more likely to get you a job than being the best in your field.

Some of the things that employers list as keeping you from getting the job you want are not skill related. Talking too much, impatience, disorganization, being late to the interview, overplaying "hard to get," inability to communicate your abilities, poor preparation for the interview, lack of knowledge of the company, failure to ask good questions, poor judgment about social situations, and dishonesty during the interview are factors that are often listed as deterrents to employability.

Honesty is important if you have had problems in other jobs or at school. Prepare honest answers that explain the situation but that present you at your best. If your attendance and punctuality are poor, you will probably be asked about the reasons. If you have had frequent job changes, you will be asked why. If you have had periods of unemployment (other than when you were a full-time student), you will be asked why. If you have ever been fired, you should be able to discuss it. Explain situations without blaming others. Talk about the problem in terms of how you solved it — by growing in maturity, by learning to avoid hasty decisions and perhaps other ways.

Preparing Physically

People expect you to dress well for an interview. They think you are wearing what you consider your most appropriate clothing for the particular job. If you wear wrinkled, soiled, or unsuitable clothes for the interview, the interviewer usually assumes your appearance will not be any better and probably will be worse after you are hired. Appearance counts. A recent haircut for men and clean hair for both men and women is noticed in the interview. Small things like clean, neat fingernails, shined shoes, clean teeth, and a firm handshake can make the difference between a good first impression and a poor one.

Many interviewers stress good posture as you enter the room. A firm handshake (with a dry, not sweaty, palm) is expected. They like for you to sit in an alert but not strained position. They want you to refrain from smoking and chewing gum — *always* — even though they may offer you a cigarette and may be smoking themselves. They want you to be energetic but not nervous. They notice if you have nervous gestures such as stroking your hair, twisting your ring, or drumming your fingers on the chair. They want you to look them in the eye when you speak, to listen carefully to what they say, and to smile when appropriate. They want you to respect their territory by sitting where they indicate, in an alert, upright position. Place your briefcase beside you rather than on a desk, and be alert to when the interviewer wants to terminate the interview. They want you to be prepared with information such as references' names, phone numbers, and addresses in case they are needed; your social security number; extra copies of your resume; a pen and pencil; and any other information you may have that is pertinent to your job hunt.

The day before the interview, call and confirm the time, place, and name of the person for the interview. Plan to arrive a few minutes early for your interview. Tense muscles and fast breathing caused by hurrying can make you seem more nervous than you should be. Be ahead of time so that you can sit down in the waiting room, take two or three deep breaths, and concentrate on relaxing.

Some of the physical aspects employers describe as keeping a person from getting a job have little to do with physical ability to do the job. Such appearance factors as a beard on a man have kept applicants from getting jobs in a company that is accustomed to seeing its employees clean-shaven. A sport coat or blazer on a man or woman interviewing at a conservative company may count against the applicant. Heavy perfume or body odor offends employers. Hair that is longer (on men or women) than that of people the company usually employs can keep you from getting a job. Employers explain these physical biases by explaining that they try to hire people who look like they will fit into the organization with a minimum of adjustment. New jobs are stressful just because they are new — no need to add the stress of personal adjustment problems by hiring people who may not fit in personally. People who show up for the interview with personal eccentricities such as unusual clothing, hair, or mannerisms are perceived as people who will require more training before becoming productive members of the team than those who already look the part.

Evaluating Your Interview

When you get home from the interview, carefully evaluate your performance.

- Were you on time?
- Did you use the information you had gathered about the company to further your cause?
- Did you interview with the person who will supervise your work if you get the job?
- Were you dressed and groomed like people who already work for the company?
- Did you show energy and self-confidence to the interviewer?
- Did you describe yourself as a "doer" rather than a "be-er" — in terms of your accomplishments instead of where you spent time?
- Did you have everything the interviewer wanted to see (your resume, references' names and addresses, and other such information) with you?

- Did you recognize when the interviewer wanted to end the interview?
- Did you seek permission to call later about the decision on the job?
- Did you get a job offer?

Writing a Thank-You Letter

Within two days after an interview send a thank-you letter to the people who talked with you. If you interviewed with several people in a company send each one a thank-you letter. Use the letter to let them know you are interested in the job. Use it to emphasize something you want them to recall about you. Such a letter labels you as a person who is thoughtful, thorough in completing a project, and just a cut above the average applicant. A thank-you letter also gets your name in front of the employer one more time.

```
                                1409 Inverness Avenue
                                Fort Worth, TX  76132-6295
                                (Today's date)


    Mr. A. L. Ray
    Ray Public Relations, Inc.
    424 Calgary
    Arlington, TX  76020-4290

    Dear Mr. Ray:

    Thank you for showing me around your offices and for giving me
    time to tell you about myself.

    The job we discussed is just what I hoped for, and I look for-
    ward to joining the "Ray Team" as soon as I hear from you.

                                Sincerely,

                                J. J. Seeker

                                J. J. Seeker
```

Illus. 1-9. Thank-You Letter

```
                                        222 West Street
                                        Dallas, TX  75333-3894
                                        (Today's date) .


        Mrs. S. M. Way
        Vice-President, Marketing
        Procter and Gamble, Inc.
        Cincinnati, OH  45202-1228

        Dear Mrs. Way:

        Thank you for taking time to talk with me yesterday about work-
        ing for Procter and Gamble.

        Your description of P&G's plans are precisely what I want to be-
        come a part of.  I look forward to the challenges you described
        and to hearing from you soon about your decision to hire me.

                                        Sincerely,

                                        S.J. Hunter

                                        S. J. Hunter
```

Illus. 1-10. Thank-You Letter

Questions for Chapter 1

1. What help is available to you in locating a job?
2. Which source is most likely to help you in securing a job?
3. What preparation should you make before you contact a company yourself?
4. Why should you tell your friends and relatives that you are looking for a job?

5. Who needs a resume? Why?
6. What do employers expect to see in a resume?
7. How can you create a favorable impression in your resume?
8. What is the purpose of a cover letter? What do you ask for?
9. What can you do to prepare for an interview?

10. What mental preparation can you make for an interview?

11. What physical preparation can you make for the interview?

12. What is the difference between a "be-er" and a "doer"?

13. Why should you write a thank-you letter?

Chapter 2

Adjusting on the Job

Chapter Objectives

After studying this chapter, you should be able to:

1. *Anticipate the behavior and attitudes of the people you encounter at your job.*
2. *Decide what to discuss and what not to discuss at work.*
3. *Weigh carefully your criticisms and phrase them in a way that will improve the situation.*
4. *Take criticism.*
5. *Handle unjust criticism.*
6. *Work with your peers and subordinates as well as with your superiors.*
7. *Function within or outside the political sphere, according to your preference.*

Every organization of people of which you become a part has a code of behavior. You may not have thought about it or observed it, but chances are that you have practiced an informal code of behavior if you have gotten along in organizations before. Business has an unspoken, unwritten code of behavior that varies little from office to office. Carefully observing the behavior of people and learning what to look for will be your best source of information. This chapter will help you identify those areas you will want to scrutinize.

Learning your job, of course, is the first order of business. You can expect to expend a great deal of energy and devote almost all of your attention to it at first. All the while, people will be observing you and your behavior. The sooner you learn what is expected of you and make the adjustment to the organization's way of doing things, the sooner you can relax and enjoy your job.

Making the adjustment does not mean going along with behavior you have moral objections to. It means adjusting your routines so that you fit easily in the routine of the organization. If you encounter situations so counter to your beliefs that you cannot tolerate them, you are in the wrong organization. Your choice is clear: If you cannot change your beliefs, you may have to change your job.

Every generation has its differences in codes of behavior. Most of the adjustments you will make will be to accommodate the differences between your own generation and those of the generation in power in the organization you join. One is not right and the other wrong; they are just different. Until you become the powerful influence in the organization, you will be expected to be the one to adapt. The powerful figures will not adapt to you. They have earned the right to their preferences. You will have to earn the right to exercise your own by becoming important in the organization. Because business has a main purpose of earning a profit, it has neither tolerance, time, nor resources for social rebellion. It is easy to suppose that no one needs to adapt; that differences can coexist. Unfortunately, much time is wasted if everyone marches to a different drummer. Businesses waste money when they waste time. They lose money when they lose faith with customers and clients. Change comes slowly. For you to go in expecting to change the tastes, procedures, or organization is a mistake. They will not risk changing to your unproved ways — money and clients are at stake. They have practiced their ways for a number of years and have done quite well, thank you.

As a young person, you no doubt will find many areas that can be improved with change. Don't be discouraged when you can't implement your ideas. Keep them "on file" in your mind or on paper if you wish. When you have proven yourself in other ways, you may get an opportunity to effect changes that will help. Until then, learn to adjust.

People

Beginners in a job usually think that learning the job itself is the major undertaking. It is important. But just as important is working with the people that are part of the organization. You will need to know what status people around you have, what treatment by others they expect, and where you fit into the organization.

You need to know who works for whom and who reports to whom in the organization. Get a copy of the organization chart if one is available. If not, ask your boss to outline the formal structure of the company for you.

Illus. 2-1. In a job, you will need to know what status people around you have, what treatment by others they expect, and where you fit into the organization.

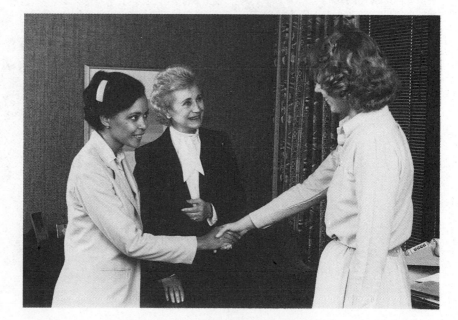

A good source of information about the informal structure of the organization is old-timers in your department who may be willing to help you understand the organization. You will learn not only who reports to whom but which departments have the power, who the prospective leaders are, who is expected to emerge as a leader, and who will probably replace whom from such a source. The organizational chart is the formal structure; the personalities of the people themselves carve out the informal structure.

If you phrase your questions properly, you can usually ask the boss when you want to know something about the relationship of your department to others in the informal structure. Simply to say "Who are the power people around here?" is poor taste. A better approach is to ask the boss which executive in the organization is the most interested in the department or makes the best use of the reports your department generates.

Your Superiors

Remember that you work *with*, not against, your superiors. When you start a new job, you are entering the boss's realm; let the boss establish the working relationship that will prevail. The boss probably already knows what works well in the specific environment and company in which you both work. Let the boss decide how formal or informal the situation will be. The boss, for example, may choose to call you by your given name, but that does not indicate that you may call your boss by a given name. Use the title and surname until you are told you can use another name.

Respect your boss's time. Make a list of points you want to discuss and questions you want to ask. Choose a time when the boss is not engrossed in work to ask for a moment to talk. If no time appears to be available for such discussions and they can't wait, write a memo. One advantage of a memo is that the executive can

Illus. 2-2. When you start a job, let the boss establish the working relationship that will prevail.

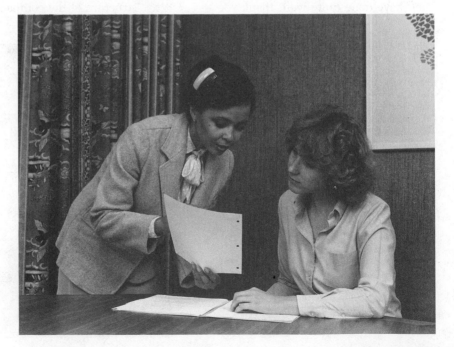

think about questions or requests you may express. Memos are especially appreciated if the executive does not know the answer right away about something you need to know.

Observe strictly the chain of command. Even if you think your boss will not be able to answer the question or solve the problem, you use good manners when you approach your boss before going beyond that level for help. Besides observing good manners, you serve to notify your boss of a problem or question that may not have been obvious or recognized before. Your boss may then join you in quest of the solution or answer, giving you aid as you reach to higher levels for solutions.

If your boss gives you an unacceptable answer or solution, you may respectfully disagree, but you take a chance of alienation if you do not carefully handle your pursuit of the solution or answer. If you and the boss reach an impasse on a problem that is critical, one which you cannot ignore, ask your boss for permission to have someone above you both arbitrate the matter. If possible, when permission is received, use a memo to explain the situation; and by all means send a copy to your boss so that the higher-up understands that you have not violated the chain of command.

You may have to earn superiors' confidence. You earn confidence by doing your work well. More than that, though, you earn confidence by learning about the informal structure of the organization. Supervisors will notice when you perceive situations and relationships beyond what you are told and adjust your behavior accordingly. They will notice when you avoid pitfalls and unpleasant situations by proceeding with care in relating to others in the organization. They will know they can trust you to do the right thing regarding your work *and your behavior* by observing you doing the right thing day after day, in situation after situation.

An impression is conveyed by your manner. Your manner can help you or hurt you. If you give the appearance of confidence, people will believe that you are confident, no matter how many doubts you have. If you look disheveled, people will believe you lack confidence, no matter how much confidence you have. If your voice is excitable, your face red, your movements erratic, you will not inspire confidence. If, however, your voice is calm, your appearance neat, and your movements graceful and measured, people are more likely to believe in your ability. In short, you must look and act the part you want to play.

There is a difference between being impertinent and being strong; a difference between showing respect for differences and being servile. No one expects you to be a robot who does as told without question. People do expect you to use good judgement and manners in expressing your concerns and differences. Learning tactful behavior in situations that are vital to you and the functioning of your department requires careful thought and planning.

Choosing words that are not inflammatory, choosing a time that is appropriate, choosing the right person to talk to, and carefully examining your own motives before you speak are some of the elements of tactfully presenting your differences. You will not gain much agreement or sympathy if you rush in, blurt out something, and nag forever after about a subject.

Your best plan is to decide what will correct a situation, not what is wrong with a situation. That makes your point of view a positive one, rather than a negative one. People are more receptive to positive suggestions than to negative complaints.

When you are criticized by your boss for a mistake you've made, remember that it is your mistake that is being criticized — not you. Don't take it personally. The criticism is intended to keep the department running smoothly, not to hurt your feelings. Keep your personal feelings out of it.

Use your energy instead to correct the mistake and to plan to avoid mistakes in the future. No one has time to indulge sulking in the office — it is a waste of your time and energy. Take criticism graciously; you will stand out. Concentrate on the problem, not yourself, during the exchange. Ask questions about the problem rather than defending your mistake. Propose solutions to correct the mistake rather than alibi for making the mistake. After all, the damage has been done. After it has been brought to your attention, you can use your time and energy to correct it. No need to waste time and energy thinking about how bad you feel about it.

If you are criticized for someone else's mistake, use all the restraint you have to keep from blurting out that it was someone else's fault. Tactfully, ask questions about the situation until the boss realizes that you are not involved and have no responsibility for the error. If you blame others, you will simply be marked as a tattletale, giving yourself a bad reputation with both your boss and the person whose fault the mistake was.

If you and your boss disagree on issues, don't bring the matter up repeatedly and don't harp on the subject to others. There are some issues on which you will be overruled by rank. Your best revenge is simply to work your way up the ladder until you are not outranked; then make the decisions you think are best. The only times you can take complaints over your boss's head are:

1. when you know you cannot discuss the subject with your own boss.
2. when you have discussed it with your own boss and discovered that the boss and you cannot solve the problem and have reached an impasse.
3. when you have notified your boss of your intentions to go higher up.
4. when you have invited your boss to be present for the presentation to a higher-up.

Keep your personal life your private affair. The boss is not a person to confide in about your personal life. In fact, no one at work is ideal to confide in because as promotions take place, relationships change, and you could be embarrassed if you have confided in someone who could use the information to gain advantage over you in a competitive situation or if you have confided in someone whom you must now supervise or who must now supervise you. To confide is to compromise your independence and freedom to be observed objectively. Keep your personal life out of the office or business environment. Make confidants people outside work to share your personal concerns with.

Your Peers

Simple good manners will win you many friends among your peers. Some of the things people appreciate are:

1. Your respecting their property and their space. Do not sit on other workers' desks, use their supplies, or otherwise infringe on their personal territory.
2. Your refraining from trying to sell them anything. If you are pushing something, be it life insurance to lottery tickets for charity, people object to your taking advantage of their being colleagues of yours by trying to sell them anything.
3. Your paying your own way. Don't borrow money from your colleagues, not even for lunch.
4. Your getting your work done on time. Usually people depend on you for completion of their own work in an organization. By completing your work on time, you make their lives easier.
5. Observing good personal manners. Don't correct others' mistakes publicly. Don't gossip about people's personal lives. Say please and thank you. Conduct yourself in such a way as to make encounters with people

pleasant and friendly, no matter what the circumstances are.

6. Your refraining from gloating over your own good fortune. Share your happiness only with people outside the business. Gloating over a raise or praise you have gotten at work makes others at work feel less appreciated than you.

Be friendly but not intimate. Discuss common interests but not personal matters with your peers. Don't encourage intimate confidences from your peers. They may be embarrassed later if your relationships within the business change. You may be inclined, yourself, to consider confidential information later when you are in a position to influence the person's future in the company. You can easily lose your objectivity when you know too much about a person's private life, especially if it is troubling.

Never, but never, discuss your superiors with your peers. Such discussions seem always to get to the person being discussed, and you will suffer in the translations.

Carefully avoid discussing business situ-ations with peers who have no need to know about them. Be *very* discreet about the information you have about your part of the company. By nature of organizations, parts of the same company have competitive areas, for example in budgets, and you must keep in mind that you are not to divulge information to others casually which they have no legitimate business reason for knowing.

If you are asked under the guise of friendship a business question that you consider improper, be noncommittal and tactful in avoiding answering the question. Do not reprimand. The questioner knows the question was improper; you do not need to be discourteous in responding. You can protect information about which you are asked by saying you need to consult your boss before you release the information or by saying you will ask the secretary to get you the materials later so that you can review them, bringing yourself up to date before discussing them.

If you are working on confidential material, keep your work in a folder. When others enter your office, casually close the folder to protect the information. Information about salaries and

Illus. 2-3. Conduct yourself so that your encounters with people are pleasant and friendly.

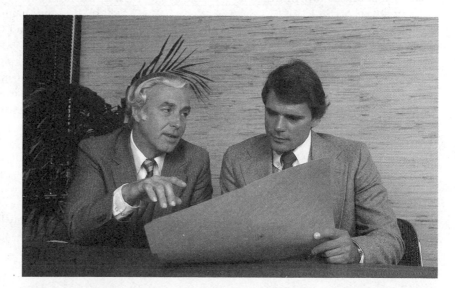

bids are examples of confidential information. Closing a folder is much easier and less obvious than frantically gathering up information and shoving it into a drawer or under a cover on your desk.

Adjusting to the peer group at work can be the most difficult job you have. Some peer groups are cutthroat, constantly competing, and unpleasant. Because all of you want to progress in the business, you all are somewhat naturally competitive. Being cutthroat and unpleasant is not necessary. Intelligence and industry, however, are not the only means to placing yourself in a position to advance in business.

As discussed in other parts of this book, people are judged by appearance. Your physical appearance will make you a keener competitor without alienating others. If you dress for the part you want, you are more easily visualized for the part when promotion time comes.

Manners and personal conduct are also important to placing yourself in a position for advancement. Superiors in a business want people who will fit well in the group in which they must function. Violating any of the codes of behavior will hurt your chances of joining a group.

While you are learning your job and preparing yourself for more responsibility and status, however, you want to enjoy your co-workers. Careful conduct on your part is necessary so that you can relate well at work and maintain long-term, productive camaraderie. Avoiding political games can win you many friends among your peers because they will trust you to put the good of the group ahead of the personal goals you may have. People who trust you with their welfare will support you when you need it. They will cover your duties when you are out because of illness and shield you from unnecessary unpleasantness if possible.

Your Subordinates

Subordinates who work with you often influence how well you do on your job. They deserve your utmost consideration and your best manners. Don't make changes unexpectedly that cause them to repeat work they have completed. Don't make arbitrary decisions about their working conditions without investigating the impact on their lives. When they make mistakes, don't explode; carefully examine the situation yourself and talk to them privately about the mistake. Remember to praise them for their work and to show genuine appreciation for times they go out of their way to help you. Simple day-to-day courtesies that subordinates appreciate are:

- A pleasant greeting in the morning and a pleasant good-night in the evening.
- Saying thank you and please when appropriate.
- Criticizing *only* in private and *only* when necessary.
- Following protocol regarding people's names within the company.
- Introducing people who work with and for you by their full names rather than by their titles (Mr. Edmond Giles instead of my assistant, Giles).
- Refraining from asking others to do personal errands for you during their free time.
- Buffering criticism from superiors when they attack people who work for you. Taking the "heat" yourself for your department when you head it.
- Alerting people who work for you as soon as you know about possible overtime work or exceptionally heavy or rushed work loads.
- Refraining from cross-examining people about what they may have heard in the business cafeteria or through the informal office "grapevine."

Visitors from Outside the Organization

When you are expecting visitors in your office from outside your company, be sure that you have seating for them, a place for their hats and coats if necessary, and that you put on your jacket before greeting them if you are a shirt-sleeve worker. (Some companies prefer to be known as "shirt-sleeve" companies and do not put on jackets before greeting outside guests.)

Make a decision about whether people will be invited to smoke in your office. If so, provide ashtrays. If not, be sure no ashtrays are around. A simple sign saying "thank you for not smoking" is sometimes placed on the desk or table in a room where no smoking is allowed.

If your expected guest has an appointment, you will be rude if you keep the guest waiting. If something unexpected occurs that prevents you from greeting a guest with an appointment on time, ask someone to greet your guest and explain the delay. It is good practice to offer a waiting guest coffee or a magazine to make the wait more pleasant. When you do greet the waiting guest, apologize for the delay.

When a guest enters your office or approaches your desk, stand and offer to shake hands, giving a warm greeting of welcome. Refrain from talking on the phone when someone is visiting at your desk. Explain that you have a visitor. Ask callers to leave a number and allow you to call back.

If your visitor turns out to be long-winded and takes more of your time than you have to give, find a place in the conversation where you can stand, extend your hand, and thank the visitor for coming to see you. That is the most direct way to let the person know you have to continue with other business. Sometimes, you can have a prearranged signal with someone in the office to remind you of an appointment that will alert your visitor that time has run out. Remember to warmly shake hands as you say good-bye.

In-house Visitors

When people who work in the same company as you drop by your desk to discuss business with you, treat them with usual courtesy by giving them your attention. Refrain from taking phone calls other than very brief ones. You simply tell callers that you have a visitor and that you will return the call later, unless, of course, the caller is someone who cannot be put off; then, you make the call as brief as possible to keep your visitor from waiting.

Telephone "Visitors"

The most important thing to remember about telephone calls is that they take a backseat to personal callers. When people take the time to visit you personally, they take precedence over someone who telephones you. Ask your telephone caller to let you call back after your visitor is gone.

Answer your telephone promptly. Ringing telephones are irritating to people. Identify yourself at once. Usually all that is necessary is to say your name and department. If you work closely with someone whose calls you answer, answer with that person's name and your own name, Sarah James' office, Jane Moore.

Even if you are interrupted, keep your voice pleasant on the telephone. Friendliness on the phone usually works in your favor even if the caller is an irate customer. When you are called on the telephone, usually you let the caller terminate the call. If you are terribly pressured for time and you think the caller has completed the business of the call but shows no sign of terminating it, you can say something like "Is there anything else we need to discuss?" or "Is there anything else you want me to do?" or "Is there anything else I can do for you?" to show that you need to terminate the call. Hang up gently. Slamming a telephone receiver down is rude and genuinely produces discomfort in the other person's ear.

Illus. 2-4. Even if you are interrupted, keep your voice pleasant on the telephone.

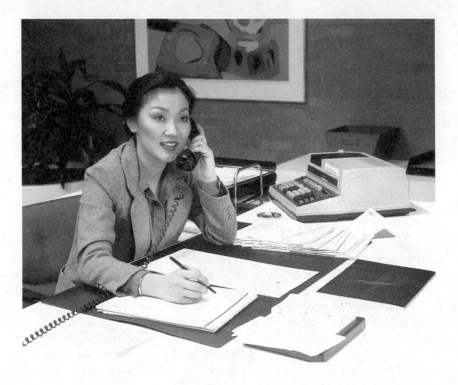

When you call someone else, announce who you are at once. Guessing games are not appropriate on the telephone — not at home and not at work. If the person answering is not likely to know the nature of your business, briefly identify your reason for calling immediately after you identify yourself. Keep business calls as brief as possible. Take care of business and hang up. People will appreciate your courtesy about taking their time.

Office Politics

There is a vague, elusive force in organizations known as office politics. It evolves because people want to protect themselves and their positions and to gain power. Through "politicking" they keep others from threatening themselves and their jobs.

Sometimes politicking for this power is done by people who hold jobs for which results are difficult to measure and who, therefore, cannot gain status through outstanding performance. Sometimes because people themselves are not sure they are "up to the job" and want to prevent others from finding out, they use office politics to fortify their positions. People know that status attracts people to them, especially people who want status themselves, and they gain acceptance as they gain power. This explanation of political motivation reveals why many things done and said at work are not in the main interest of getting the company's work done. They are instead done and said in the interest of helping an individual.

It will be impossible for you to avoid the political arena. It is not necessary for you to actively participate for your own benefit if you choose not to, but you will not be able to avoid being judged alongside those who do choose to participate.

Some characteristics of the political system surprisingly are good even if you are not looking for power. These are quasi-political ideas concerning getting to know your boss. You are, after all, a part of a team. If you are to play a vital part on the team, you need to know something about the leader:

1. What is the mission of your boss? What is the boss trying to accomplish?
2. What irritates the boss? Do subordinates have practices or do things that irritate the boss?
3. Does the boss want to be recognized by subordinates for a job well done? Does the boss want to be complimented?
4. Who are the boss's friends and enemies in the company? Who can your boss depend upon for help outside your department? Who can your boss beware of outside your department?
5. What is the most important problem facing the boss and the department?
6. What are personal qualities of the boss? Does the boss play golf or tennis? Does the boss collect stamps? These personal qualities can tell you something about the boss's value systems and something about the way you will be evaluated.
7. How does the boss measure performance? The boss's value system will be imposed on you when your performance is measured. If you are able to demonstrate ability in terms the boss uses, you are more likely to get favorable evaluations than if the boss has to adjust to your standards of performance.
8. Is your boss in a power struggle? Is the boss playing politics for some reason? If so, what is the reason?
9. Does your boss like to confer with subordinates? Does the boss like to hear what

those who work in the department are thinking, what they hear, what they propose?
10. Does the boss have "better times than others" for conferring? Is the boss subject to moods? If so, what are they? How can you know the best and worst times for conferring with the boss?

Your future in an organization will depend a great deal on what your superiors think of you. The image you project is up to you. You need to put some thought into how to project the image you want. Most people want simply to do a good job and be judged accordingly. Unfortunately, unless everyone else is doing a miserable job, a good job alone is not enough to make you stand out. You, the person, rather than your work will make the difference.

Your own code of ethics will govern how you will conduct yourself in various situations. You may think that the end justifies the means and therefore set for yourself a different set of procedures for reaching your goals than your neighbor sets. You may, on the other hand, think that the means are the end in themselves and concentrate on developing a set of procedures that themselves satisfy your ethical needs. Your own ideals and personal evaluation of yourself as you conduct your business should be the guidelines you follow for setting up your procedures for ethical conduct in your job. Some decisions you may have to make are suggested so that you can think about them before the time comes to act on them. The right or wrong depends upon your own values. Expect yours to be different from your neighbors' at least some of the time; at most, all of the time.

• I will develop the same interests and hobbies as my boss to fortify my position if possible.
• I will ask my boss's opinion on things that the boss has an interest in even though I don't need advice.
• I will dress according to business standards

Illus. 2-5. The image you project is up to you.

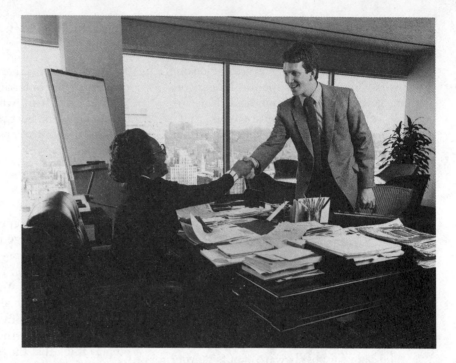

to further my career even though I prefer other clothing.

- I will go out of my way to be nice to important people even though I don't personally like them.
- I will keep careful mental notes about who has helped me along the way and about who has hurt me along the way.
- When possible I will seek assignments that will make me look good and avoid if I can those that gain me no attention.
- I will avoid being the person who has to give negative opinions or bad news to the boss.
- I will not blindly trust people's work that may reflect on me. I will carefully check work that others do for which I am responsible.
- I will not discuss anything at work that may later be used against me as perhaps a flaw in my character.
- I will carefully select subordinates who know how to make the boss look good.
- I will always appear calm and cool even though I am upset and angry.
- I will think about how my actions will be interpreted by superiors before I take action.
- I will attend company social functions even though I prefer to do other things.
- I will compete only if I know I can do well.
- If the truth will hurt someone and a "white" lie won't, I'll tell the lie.
- I will try to have lunch with people who can help me get ahead.
- I will let my rivals make a mistake rather than warn them.
- I will learn what is wanted in a report before I complete it for my boss.
- I will come early and stay late to impress my boss.
- I will not participate in a cooperative venture if it means that I lose personal advantage.

- I will carefully avoid discussing political preferences that I know conflict with the boss's views.
- If apple-polishing helps me get ahead, I'll polish apples.

Overcoming Office Politics

There are some ways to overcome office politics. When you are working for someone who uses politics to manipulate people, you are limited in what you can do about it. If you can handle it well and survive to outrank the political game player, then you can have a significant impact on the games that are petty.

Because people tend to engage in politically unproductive behavior when they cannot achieve recognition through their work (because it is not measurable), one way to reduce the need for politics is to set definable tasks for people. Be sure you know what is expected of you and what you expect of others if you are responsible for their work. Let people know that you think that their work is important and makes a significant contribution to the progress of the organization.

Every organization has tasks that are not challenging and interesting but that must be done. Try to spread these tasks around so that no one person or group is burdened with all the unpleasant but necessary tasks. People who are stimulated by their jobs are less likely to spend time in politicking. Reward people both with money and with praise for the work they do. People who feel they are treated fairly are less likely to spend time "jockeying" for better spots within the department.

When you are in a position to manage other people's work, keep in mind that they notice whether or not the manager plays politics. Avoid manipulating people, discrediting opponents, and deceiving others. Set a good example of how employees are to conduct themselves, and you will have fewer problems with political games among those whose work you supervise. A climate of openness and trust among those in a group disarms most political games. When people believe they can tell you the truth about what is going on in the organization without repercussions to themselves, they are less likely to cover unproductive behavior or to participate in it.

Stop gossip by either ignoring it or challenging it. The gossiper runs out of listeners when people ignore gossip. The gossiper then is left to more productive work. A challenge to gossip puts the gossiper on the spot, making gossip more trouble than work. The gossiper is more likely to choose the route of less trouble — work.

If you think either praise or criticism of yourself or of others is politically motivated, check it out. You want to find whether or not it is factually based. If it isn't, don't be naive. Discount it.

When people try to involve you in politically unproductive games, you can innocently ask, "Why are you telling me about this?" or "Why are you behaving toward me in that manner?" Be ready for a blank look at such a confrontation, and be ready to hear an answer that probably doesn't ring true. Few people want to admit that they have ulterior motives.

Keep yourself invulnerable to coercion by staying away from shady practices yourself. Refrain from setting others up for failure. Avoid doing favors which make people indebted to you. Do your work honestly and conscientiously. Confront problems and solve them; don't bury them or put them off on others. When you are good at your job, competent, and confident, you are less likely to become vulnerable to office political behavior. Those who are less able probably will not want to tangle with you.

Staying Neutral

If you find yourself in an organization where two or more factions seem to be constantly at odds with each other, your best policy if you are to work among all of them is to stay as neutral as possible. Listen to everyone, but do not counsel. Remain placid and do not comment on the propriety of a situation described to you that denounces someone else in the business. Be courteous to everyone and be calm and collected in your manner. Be concerned as a friend to everyone. Be sure that no one reads hostility or animosity in your manner. Refrain from being a messenger to any part of the parley; just don't repeat what you hear about someone else. Concentrate on your job performing your duties as best you can under the circumstances.

Learning Not to Be Defensive

Defensiveness can take many forms. It may surface as an explanation. When you are asked if you did something you have not done but should have, you probably will go into a lengthy explanation if you are defensive about not completing the work. Usually the questioner only wants to know whether or not the work was done and not why it was or was not done. When you are unprepared for something such as a meeting, you may be tempted to go into an explanation defending yourself for not being prepared. People need to know only whether you are ready, not why you are not. If you are asked why after you answer the question, then you can explain. Don't explain until you are asked.

Defensiveness also takes the form of rationalization. We figure out how something unpleasant really was beyond our control, how we had nothing to do with it, instead of using the thought and energy to resolve the situation. We spend effort justifying why it happened — wasted effort. People who mention the situation become our enemies because we are touchy about it. All we really need to do is make a mental note not to get into the same situation again, whatever the cause.

Learning Not to Be Critical

Criticism often takes the form of questioning someone. We ask a question "to get information" but really intend to point out a weakness in the other person. These questions put other people on the defensive. They know they are being attacked rather than being asked for information, and they respond accordingly.

Sometimes criticism takes the form of a statement such as "That idea is irrelevant," meaning that the person offering the idea is not held in high esteem. "This work is not organized" indicates that the worker is disorganized. What you want are better ideas and better organized work. Instead of attacking the person with the ideas and the work, make suggestions for improving the situation, such as "Could you clarify that idea for me?" or "Show me how it helps the situation," or "Could you devise a plan for improving the flow of work in this department?" or "Could you reorganize the files?"

Self-criticism also is not productive. To condemn yourself for something is different from analyzing how you can do better in the future. If you want to grow, observe and analyze your own actions; don't judge them to be "bad" or "good." Select the ones you want to repeat. Don't brood over past mistakes. Seek a better way and don't second-guess yourself. It is wasted time and energy.

Dealing with People Who Are Critical

When you are with people who are arguing, criticizing, and complaining, stay alert to the conversation. Instead of commiserating with them, ask thought-provoking questions to change the tide of the conversation. If someone attacks you, ask questions on how to improve the situation rather than listening to the attack.

Questions for Chapter 2

1. Why is the new employee expected to adjust rather than have the organization change to suit the new employee?
2. What do you need to know about the people who are part of the organization?
3. What is a good source of information about the formal structure of the organization?
4. What is a good source of information about the informal structure of the organization?
5. Who establishes the relationship parameters between the boss and new employee?
6. How can you respectfully disagree with your boss?
7. What constitutes a look of confidence?
8. When you are criticized for a mistake you made, what should you do?
9. When you are criticized for a mistake someone else made, what should you do?
10. When can you take complaints over your boss's head?
11. Why should you keep your personal life private?
12. What are some ways you can win friends among your peers?
13. How can you protect business information when you are asked improper questions about it?
14. What are some day-to-day courtesies subordinates appreciate?
15. How can you tactfully let guests know they have stayed too long?
16. Can you avoid all political behavior at work?
17. Will "just doing a good job" help you get ahead in an organization?
18. How can you disarm destructive political maneuvers at work?

Chapter 3

Growing on the Job

Chapter Objectives

After studying this chapter, you should be able to:

1. *Accurately assess your own desire to grow on the job.*
2. *View your chances for growth and conduct yourself in a way that provides for growth if that is your choice.*
3. *Determine what behavior deters growth on the job and what behavior promotes it.*
4. *Identify those people who can help you and deal with those who won't.*
5. *Handle failure and deal with success for a happier working life.*

If you think you want to move up in your job, remember that more responsibility and influence often carry with them the obligation of more time and energy. Consider the effect that a more responsible job will have on other aspects of your life when you are thinking about moving up.

——— *The Decision to Grow* ———

Growing is more than higher pay and more prestige. It affects your relationship with your friends and family. It takes time from the activities you currently enjoy with friends and family. You may "outrank" your friends economically and incur jealous reactions.

You may forfeit independence. Organizations require a great deal of their leaders and managers. Secretaries and clerks usually are through with work at the end of the day. Managers rarely are. During crises, even on weekends, managers may be called in to work. Lower level workers rarely are. Are you willing to make yourself available for such additional work?

If mobility is required, you may be asked to leave your present work place to move to another, and adjust your family obligations to a different city, state, or country.

The financial burden may be higher as you move to higher levels within your organization. The financial rewards will be higher, but sometimes the burden, such as social obligations, transportation, and personal needs, changes in such a way as to make the financial situation less desirable on balance. Moving up within your organization may be expensive.

Illus. 3-1. The Decision to Grow – Advantages and Disadvantages of Promotion

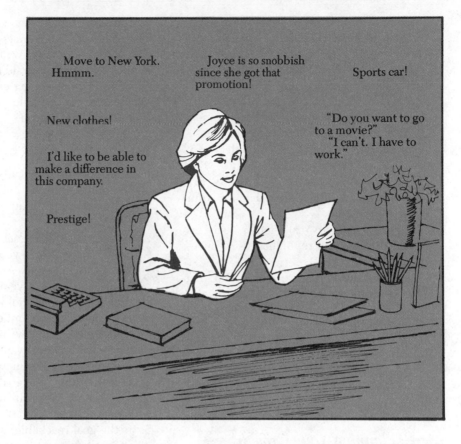

Considering changes in your relationship to friends and family, your independence, mobility, and financial status, will the prestige, achievement, and self-fulfillment be rewards enough for the change you are seeking?

Ask yourself some other important questions when you consider whether you want to grow on your job.

1. Do you like the idea of deciding what to do, telling other people how to do it, and being responsible for the way they do it? Or, do you prefer being told what to do after a decision is made and being responsible only for what you do yourself?
2. Are you willing to make the adjustments that show that you are in the job force for the long haul, that you are serious about your career, that you will make sacrifices in other areas of your life if necessary to have a successful career? Or, do you feel that your work is simply a means to a better life outside work and that when it comes to a showdown between your job and something else important to you, your job will suffer.
3. Are you willing to compete with people who may have advantages over you, who may have contacts you don't have, who may have more experience, more ability? Or, do you wish to be passively evaluated on your performance alone, refusing to develop contacts who may help, to compensate for lack of experience or ability?

4. Are you willing to be criticized by subordinates who formerly were your peers?

5. Are you willing to stay late and work on weekends if necessary to keep things going smoothly?

6. Are you willing to risk the relationships with your friends, family, and professional colleagues by changing your level of job?

7. Can you fire a person who is ineffective if you rise to a level of management?

8. Can you take being judged by organizational results rather than by your own efforts?

9. Are you willing to make tough decisions jeopardizing your reputation as a "nice" person?

10. Can you admit you are wrong and that others on the staff may have the answers?

11. Can you adjust to moving at the rate of your slowest subordinate?

12. Can you put organizational goals before your personal needs at work?

13. Can you lead others rather than manipulate them?

——— *Planning Your Growth* ———

Despite drawbacks, most people are not satisfied with the status quo, and they want to move up. If you decide that you want to climb the ladder in your career, make some plans. Set some goals, prepare yourself, and evaluate your chances.

Setting Goals

To grow on a job, you must know how you want to grow. Do you want, for example, to be the best at the job you start in; or do you want to supervise the department you start in; or do you want to supervise the entire organization? Defining how you want to grow helps you to set

intermediate goals that you can accomplish along the way. As you accomplish your intermediate goals you may want to revise your ultimate goal. Don't be afraid to. Many of the jobs of the future don't even exist today. You may decide you want to hold one of those when it becomes visible to you.

Some decisions you want to consider when you are setting growth goals are:

1. Is the goal one you really want to accomplish or reach? Is it something you want for yourself or is it something someone else wants you to reach?

2. Will reaching that goal make your life richer? Some goals lead you to jobs that conflict with your life-style. Are you willing to adjust, maybe even give up, your current life-style to reach and hold the goal?

3. How much can you influence your reaching of the goal and how much help must you have? Is that help available? Does reaching the goal depend somewhat on chance?

4. Can you define the goal specifically enough to make actual plans and to take action to accomplish it?

5. Is the goal reachable? Can you realistically expect to reach the goal?

6. Is the goal worth reaching? When you reach it, will the costs to you have been worth it or will you regret what you have had to give up to reach the goal?

Preparing for Growth

Learn everything about the job you want that you can. Make yourself known to those people making the promotion decision by asking what skills or qualities are needed by the person expected to fill the job.

When you identify a job you want, prepare for it. Begin to look like the person needed to fill the job. Show characteristics of a person who can handle the job, and if the job is soon to be available, make it known to the decision makers that you are interested in having it.

Associate yourself with people who are growing. Learn from them. Listen to their experiences and observe their behavior and attitudes.

Professional Support Groups

One way to grow in your career is to associate yourself with others who are in your field. Professional organizations serve a vital purpose in helping people to develop professionally. Members meet periodically to share experiences and resources useful to their profession. From them you probably will learn about developments in your field, creation of new jobs in your area, new approaches to old problems, and the attitude of the group to the community and vice versa. Involving yourself in your professional organization is an excellent way to grow in your field.

Personal Support Groups

Your friends probably will constitute your personal support group. These people may not help you with career matters, but they can help you adjust personally when career matters are tense. It is important to have friends who are supportive, who listen to give you feedback honestly, and who care how you get along.

There are also organized support groups you may find beneficial. They usually are people who share some common interest like symphony support or park improvement. These groups can be of help in your personal life. Join them if you need to share your everyday concerns and if you are unable to make compatible friends outside such organized groups. You may find your life easier to organize and run if you hear how others are doing it in your community.

Conditioning Yourself

You can condition yourself for growth by expanding your sensitivity now. There are several areas where you can invest and be rewarded with personal growth. One of these is to expose yourself to new ideas and new sensations. New ideas are found in books, by listening to people describe their ideas and experiences, and by formulating new methods and principles. New sensations are found in new sights, sounds, tastes, and feelings. You can go to new places, eat new foods, listen to unfamiliar music, study new art forms, meet new people. As you explore, you train your mind to grow. As your capacity grows, you will experience widening opportunities for growth.

Another way to grow is to invest your energy in training yourself. Because discipline is demanded when you are training yourself, you can gain immense satisfaction from the process itself as a result of the changes that take place in your life.

Learning to conform to the ground rules of your group will help you to grow, interestingly enough. The reason is that conforming to ground rules takes less effort than not conforming when you are an adult. Save your energy for causes that are important instead of flying into the face of social amenities. Continue to evaluate what you do as it relates to your growth. To conform blindly to everything is unproductive because you lose your ability to control your own time. You stagnate. Selectively conform to those activities and mores that make life at work go smoothly for you.

Many opportunities for growing lie in the unfamiliar. When you are faced with unfamiliar people, products, and methods, study them carefully. Relate the observations to what you already know and stretch your imagination. As you figure them out, integrate the ideas into your own.

Illus. 3-2. Expand
your sensitivities with
new sights.

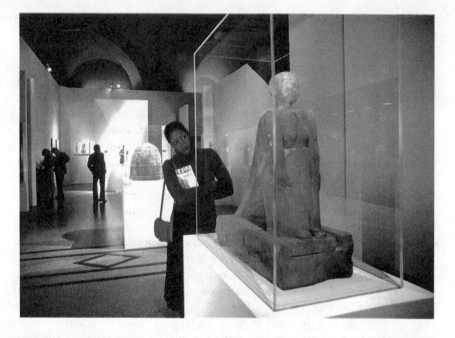

Deterrents to Growth

Organizations carefully watch those who show potential ability for promotion. Many things you say and do will be noticed and evaluated in light of a future decision about your role in the organization. Be aware of some of the things that can hurt you.

A blabbermouth is not promotion material. Carefully avoid telling things that you should not — personal things and business things. A loose tongue loses you trust. You may think that telling just one person something is OK because that person will tell no one else. You may be right; that person may not tell anyone else. That person will, however, remember that you told something you should not have told and will classify you as one who cannot be trusted to keep a secret.

Refrain from harshly criticizing your own organization and people in it. If you have legitimate criticism, phrase it carefully and constructively, saying to an appropriate person what you think should be done rather than what you think is wrong and berating the person responsible. An acid tongue will win you no friends and probably will keep you from rising to a position where you can have real impact on making changes in the organization.

Refrain from criticizing your own organization and people in it to people outside even when you use carefully chosen phrases and positive constructions. You will appear to be disloyal both to those who hear you and to your own company when it gets back to them, as it surely will. When you find things wrong in your organization, figure out ways to make them right and suggest to the appropriate people the appropriate action in an appropriate format at an appropriate time. Avoid being labeled a critical person.

Refrain from being part of a clique. Clique members typically are perceived to be poor risks for promotion because they aren't team players. Their loyalties seem to be to each other rather than to the organization or their jobs. If one member of a clique is promoted, the others may gain favors from the promoted one leaving people outside the clique with poor morale. Try to be friendly with more than just a few of the people in the office or organization. Have lunch with a variety of people. Don't confide in anyone at work, but be pleasant to everyone if you want to be promoted.

Other "friendships" that may hinder your moving up in your organization are those that make you look like you are teamed up with someone everyone else is alienated from. The outcast may try to get close to you as soon as you join the organization simply because you are the only one who will respond — everyone else has been alienated. Be friendly, but keep your distance. Don't team up with one person or with one group too soon.

Avoid being caught up in the "everyone else is doing it" syndrome. You may see others taking advantage of lunch hours, office supplies, and such for personal use. You may cynically think that you are a fool not to join in. Refrain from joining in. Maintain your individual integrity in small matters, and you will be perceived to have integrity in the big things. To behave like the masses may mean that you will be treated like the masses — and not promoted. Set yourself apart from unethical practices if you can no matter how minor they seem. Avoid becoming cynical about others' lack of ethics. Most people prefer to be led by ethical persons, and you are more likely to be selected to lead and to get support in a leadership role if you keep your integrity.

If you want to grow, do not be insensitive to organizational politics. Organizations are political, and you have to deal with the practices effectively if you want to grow. To be passive or resentful will hinder your progress. Political relationships in the organization form the power coalitions necessary to make and carry out decisions. The alternative is an autocratic or a purely democratic organization which rarely works well. Most organizations work on coalitions of groups joined by shared interests. You are best equipped to work within the political system if you treat people as individuals, trying to understand their motivation and their goals. People are not objects to be manipulated. They have personal sensitivities bearing on their actions. Keep those sensitivities in mind as you work with them.

Evaluating Your Chances

Once you decide you want to be promoted, you must look around your organization to determine on what basis people are promoted. Usually it will be one of two ways. Either people will be promoted based on their accomplishments at a previous level or they will be promoted because they are perceived to have skills useful at the next level. Ideally, people are promoted for both reasons.

When people are promoted simply because they are doing their present jobs very well, mistakes are often made. Just because a person performs well at one job does not mean that person will perform well at another job. Nevertheless, evaluations of you in your present job often will be at least one of the criteria that are considered when you are looking for promotion.

Qualities that are perceived as needed for leadership and managerial roles are observable and are considered by organizations concerned with effective leadership. Some of them are: communication skills, human relation skills, counselling skills, supervision ability, knowledge of human behavior and motivation, decision making and judgment skills, and planning skills. You can exhibit skill in all these areas at your current level and show yourself to be managerial material if you work at it.

Loyalty is expected in organizations. Sometimes it means one thing, sometimes another. Some of its meanings are:

1. Obedience to the needs of the organization or to the superior.
2. Protection of the organization or superior.
3. Hard work.
4. Succeeding in spite of difficulties.
5. Honesty, no matter what.

Excesses, however, in any area may make you poor material for promotion. Obedience at all costs may turn you into a "yes" man or woman. Honesty, no matter what, may make you tactless. Protection of the organization or superior who is in the wrong may label you as having poor judgment. Hard work meaning Saturdays and Sundays even when you don't make a contribution on those days but simply are seen puts your practicality in question. Succeeding in spite of difficulties may mean you disregard other people and their values to get what you want.

Loyalty to the organization should be practiced with selectivity. You must monitor its effect on you and on others. Blind loyalty without evaluation may work against you.

If you aspire to a role of leadership in your organization, you will have to do more than your job well. You will have to fit in with those in leadership roles. Be alert to circumstances out of your control which prevent you from fitting in. In some companies, things which you cannot change may affect your acceptance in a role of leadership. Age, education, race, sex, ethnic background, major personality characteristics, or your area of expertise sometimes influences whether or not you will rise to a position of leadership. If you find yourself with such liabilities in an organization, you may have to consider changing jobs to rise to higher levels in your career. You can learn about such prejudices by carefully observing those in leadership positions and noting whether or not they have similarities that are not coincidental in any of these critical areas.

Making Your Move

When you are firmly committed to growing, make your move.

1. At whatever level in the organization you are, "package" yourself as an executive. Look like you belong one step higher on the ladder making yourself as presentable as you can without overspending.
2. In the great scheme of things you may think that such a thing as making appearance important is picayune. Don't be tempted to defy this and other management prejudices. To do so will win you no promotions, no salary increases, and little job satisfaction. All you may get is the feeling you have sacrificed a great deal for a picayune matter.
3. Cultivate a presence that denotes success. Be open and approachable, but not insensitive. Be tall and thin, even if you are not, by bearing yourself as if you were.

Other people will, of course, play a vital role in your moving up. You will find people who will help and people who will hinder. You should know how to deal with both.

Carefully plan your strategy even if you are seeking only a raise. Some considerations that may make it easier are:

1. Try to take the emotional responses out of your evaluation of yourself and your job. Define your rationale.
2. Determine whether or not there are organizational guidelines to help you in determining your worth — a schedule of raises, promotions, and time periods.
3. Evaluate ways you have made money for or saved money for the organization —perhaps in terms of how your job has expanded, how you have found more efficient ways to do your job, or ideas you have suggested and implemented.

4. Make a written list of reasons why you deserve a raise or promotion for yourself. It is a good psychological booster. Refrain from listing need as a reason.

5. Investigate the financial position of your company. Time your request at a time other than budget tightening time or when business is unusually slow. Try to time the request when you have been recognized for doing a particularly good job on something.

6. Make your presentation logically and diplomatically. Carefully avoid sounding defensive about not already getting a raise or a promotion. Arousing guilt in your superior may hurt your case. Logical persuasion with a sound case for a raise is a better strategy. Especially avoid threats and ultimatums. They usually make people defensive and rarely get you support.

7. Carefully practice your presentation before you actually make it to your superior.

8. Have a salary amount in mind. You may need to investigate what others are getting, and that information may be carefully guarded. As a last resource, the Department of Labor keeps statistics on salaries for various regions of the country that may help you. Their figures are usually in the local public library.

9. Tactfully mention the amount you have in mind if you are not asked. You could say "I believe that $1,000 is standard for people who have been here a year, but $2,000 is appropriate for me because" and list your reasons.

10. Remember to thank the person who is successful in getting you a raise or promotion.

11. If you don't get what you asked for, ask what you could have done differently to obtain it. Be diplomatic, not offensive. If you don't get as much money as you think you deserve, ask how you can qualify for the higher amount in the future. Avoid making demands and allow time for the superior to investigate the matter for the answers.

12. Carefully prepare your questions about money by saying "What can a person do to earn more money here?" Don't badger, but be sincere about your interest.

Mentors

After you have worked on your job awhile, you probably will have made friends with people at work. One or more of these friends may have assumed a role of informal advisor about your career. Very often this person is one who admires your potential, is older, and has been with the organization longer than you have. This person assumes the role of guiding you through the maze and up the ladder in the organization. The name for this advisor in business is "mentor."

People have not talked about mentors very much in business but they have existed since Odysseus left Troy. The benefit accruing to you as a result of this relationship is that you will receive useful information and encouragement. Your mentor may inspire you to greater things in the organization and may make suggestions on how to attain your goals. The mentor gets the satisfaction of teaching, leading, and helping someone else. It is much like a parent-child relationship. The mentor helps someone as the mentor was helped during earlier times.

The advice you get may be about useful courses to take, people to meet, and experiences that will enhance your professional success. If your mentor is also a supervisor, you may be "groomed" for the supervisor's job as the mentor moves on. This nurturing helps you to grow and to avoid mistakes that might hinder your career.

There are some problems with a mentor relationship. Sometimes the protege outgrows the mentor and achieves promotion beyond the

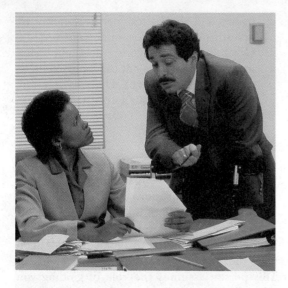

Illus. 3-3. A mentor assumes the role of guiding you through the maze and up the ladder in the organization.

mentor. That may terminate the relationship and may do so negatively. If a sexual relationship grows out of the mentor relationship, your career will probably suffer. The complications of a sexual relationship with someone at work are usually insurmountable, and one or the other of the parties usually has to leave the organization. If you are the younger one with less power, it will be you.

Another problem can arise if the mentor and you do not perceive each other's role in the same ways. If you seek approval and the mentor is critical, even constructively so, you will have problems.

The mentor relationship usually "just happens." It is informal and usually not openly acknowledged. If one does not "just happen" for you, you may be able to develop one if you want it. Identify someone you admire who can guide you through the maze of pitfalls and opportuni-

ties in your organization. Before you talk to that person, thoroughly examine:

1. What you want from the relationship. Doors opened, introductions, advice?
2. What you are willing to give to the mentor in return. Free labor, loyalty?
3. How long do you expect to need the mentor?
4. Will you be willing to help someone else when you can become a mentor?

When you are comfortable with what you have in mind, ask to talk informally with the person you have identified. People of the same sex usually will understand your needs better than those of the opposite sex. Women, however, may find it difficult to find women at this time who are able to help them in this way.

You probably will be surprised by the response you get to your conversation with your chosen mentor. Many people are flattered to think that you will seek their help, and they accept readily. If you are unable to secure the chosen person as your advisor, don't despair. You probably will find someone else. Business has functioned in this way for centuries and will continue to.

Defeats

As you try to grow on your job you are likely to have a few setbacks. These may take the form of criticism, refusals, and dismissals. To grow in your career you must be prepared to deal with all these eventualities.

First of all, remember that no one wins all the time. Trying to do only things that you are sure you can do means that you don't stretch yourself enough. You are probably not asking enough of yourself to find out how much you can really do. Taking a risk and going for something you may not be able to accomplish takes courage and an attitude that you will survive even if you fail at the immediate venture.

Being criticized for something you have not done well or for something you tried that does not materialize is the easiest setback to take after you have overcome your own disappointment of failing in your venture. Someone else's evaluation (criticism) of your failing effort can confirm your poor opinion of yourself if you let it. A better way to handle criticism in this matter is to direct it to the act which failed and away from the person who tried. Don't take it personally. Criticize your efforts, your strategy, your procedures, your goals, or whatever, but don't criticize yourself as a person and don't accept other people's criticism as being of yourself but of your activities.

You can disarm criticizers by partially agreeing with them. That shows that you can be objective in evaluating a failure and that you probably will learn from it rather than merely suffer from it. It shows that you have nothing about which to feel guilty or defensive. After all, you made an effort and failed. That is more to be admired than not making an effort at all.

One of the most productive activities resulting from defeats is a careful analysis of the reasons for the defeat. It is easy to rationalize and to blame others for your defeats — it is also unproductive and you set yourself up to fail again. Realizing what kept you from succeeding — what you could have done differently, anticipated, planned for, reacted to, or judged more accurately — may help you discover why you failed at a venture. Knowing the truth can help you avoid failing later. Rationalizing or blaming others will do nothing but give you temporary relief from feeling bad.

As far as you can, continue to conduct business as usual after a defeat. Get on with your usual routine, cooly and calmly relating to others, even those who may have succeeded where you failed. To do anything else makes a greater issue of your failure and defeat than it should be. If anything, perform your routine with more vigor, efficiency, and enthusiasm than ever.

Immerse yourself in regaining the self-respect you had prior to your defeat through the same kind of performance you had prior to trying something new. By doing so, you will also regain the respect of others who may be waivering in light of your failure.

When you try and are refused, cooperate with the person refusing you. Holding a grudge will get you nothing and may worsen your situation. The "uncooperative" label once achieved is hard to remove and may follow you for a long time. Taking refusals graciously is appreciated by people who want to grant what you ask but cannot. It disarms people who refuse you unjustly. Both ways you look better.

You may at sometime in your career lose your job. First of all, begin immediately to look for another job. If you see the dismissal coming, begin looking for a job before you are dismissed. The tempting reaction to dismissal is to gain sympathy from your friends and family — to sit in the corner and lick your wounds. Don't do it.

After you have begun your job search, carefully analyze why you were dismissed. Remember, the most unproductive activity is to blame others for your misfortune. If, for example, your dismissal came about because you could not get along with the boss, don't blame the boss for being someone you don't like. Examine yourself to learn how you can get along with someone like the boss if the situation demands it (at least until you find a better situation). Figure out where and when you went wrong in the relationship and what you can do in the future to avoid a situation where someone fires you. Learn to be on the lookout for signs of unresolvable problems in relationships, and plan to take action on your own to resolve the situation rather than waiting to be forced through dismissal to take action. Look at yourself carefully to see if you are inflexible in accommodating other people's idiosyncrasies, their procedures which appear less efficient than yours, their attitudes which are different from yours. Don't blame yourself for shortcomings you may find. Resolve to expand your thinking, to grow through exposure to differences in people, and to anticipate better in the future when a situation is deteriorating to the point of dismissal.

After any defeat, be alert for positive signs. People subtly respond to those in need, sometimes unconsciously. If you conduct yourself with grace and strength, people will respond to your defeat with small favors, sometimes no more than a warm smile, sometimes with an invitation to lunch. Be alert to signs such as these that show support for a person who tries but fails. After all, you probably will succeed next time.

———— Growing Gracefully ————

As you grow on your job, achieving promotions and raises, remember not to flaunt it. Don't make drastic changes that attract attention to your success. Subtly make any changes that are necessary, and people will not become jealous of you. Remember that you are a member of a team and that you need support from all the members. If you lose support because of jealousy, your position is weakened, and your performance may be threatened by those on whom you must depend.

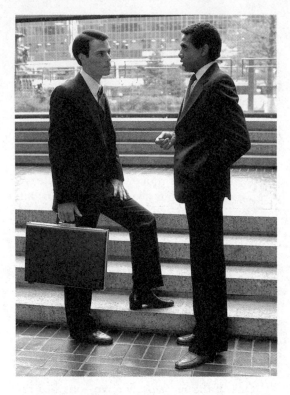

Illus. 3-4. If you conduct yourself with grace and strength, people will respond to your defeat with small favors, sometimes no more than a warm smile, sometimes an invitation to lunch.

Questions for Chapter 3

1. What are some considerations that are involved in growth on the job?
2. How can you evaluate your growth goals?
3. What are some ways to prepare yourself for growth?
4. What does condition yourself for growth mean?
5. What are deterrents to growth?
6. What are the qualities perceived as needed for leadership and managerial roles?
7. Can you be excessively loyal?
8. What do you have to do besides do your job well to reach a leadership position in most organizations?
9. What are the strategic considerations for making your move?
10. Are you likely to want or need a mentor in an organization?

11. How can a mentor help you?
12. Can you expect to have some defeats on the job?
13. How can you respond to criticism of a failure you have had?
14. What can be one of the most productive responses to defeat?
15. How should you conduct yourself after a defeat?
16. If you lose your job, what should you do first?
17. What should you do after you begin your job search?
18. Why should you refrain from flaunting your successes?

Chapter 4

Visibility

Chapter Objectives

After studying this chapter, you should be able to:

1. *Identify the characteristics associated with successful people in business and describe how those characteristics are shown.*
2. *Be assertively productive, innovative, and persuasive without alienating co-workers.*
3. *Improve communication skills that enable you to read between the lines of what people say and write to you.*
4. *Polish your speech by adjusting your language and timing to those of business.*
5. *Avoid unacceptable comments by learning the subtleties of business that keep up morale.*
6. *Handle destructive practices in a positive and productive way.*
7. *Handle sex in business.*
8. *Conform to the etiquette of business.*

In business people rarely get to know you very well, partly because you consciously keep your personal life to yourself, and partly because the work place does not allow for your complete personality to emerge. You are judged mainly on what people do see of you, and that depends on what you allow them to see of you, your visibility.

As a part of the team in an organization, you will fill a spot. Whether you are effective and contribute to the overall good of the organization depends upon the skills you have. Whether you are judged effective and productive depends upon *how others perceive you*.

They make those judgements based on how you appear physically and how you sound when you speak. They will listen to your expression of thoughts to judge your ability to think and organize. They will watch you respond to feedback.

If you wish to be effective in an organization, you must be able to give and take feedback effectively. Feedback may be neutral, negative, or positive. It plays a very powerful role in the functioning of the organization.

Neutral feedback generally carries no ulterior motives and messages. However, sometimes negative feedback is disguised as neutral and does carry ulterior messages. Be aware of your response to what people say to you in response to your actions and your ideas. Set yourself a range by which you can measure your comfort and discomfort from the feedback you get from people and analyze what causes you to feel the level of comfort or discomfort you experience. Most of the time, discomfort comes not because people disagree with our ideas or put them down but because we interpret the disagreement and criticism as rejection of ourselves rather than of our ideas. Negative feedback is easier to handle if you take it as it relates to things — not yourself. When you are the one responding to others, keep in mind how you react to negative feedback. If you have to criticize someone's actions or ideas, be sure you make it clear what you object to. Let the person know that it is the action or idea, not the person, you are critical of.

Develop the ability to use negative feedback to your advantage. Often you get it because people do not like the *way* you have presented an idea or action rather than because of the idea or action itself. You can figure out what you might have done differently if that is the case.

Positive feedback takes the form of compliments. Concentrate on graciously accepting positive appraisal of your work and sharing credit with those who have helped you with it. Develop ways to praise others who do good work so that you show sincerity rather than flattery.

Certain characteristics are associated with people who are believed to be successful in business. Most of us have these characteristics along with many which are perceived to be associated with people who are not successful. It is important to be aware of the impression you give at work if you are to influence people and work effectively. Most people want to be associated with successful people and want to avoid those who are not perceived to be successful.

By cultivating characteristics that help you appear successful in business, you make success easier for yourself. People tend to treat those they perceive as successful with confidence and respect. More importantly, we react more often than not according to the way we are treated — with confidence and integrity — regardless of our own perception of ourselves. Therefore, if we look and act successful, we will be treated as such and will react as such. Try it; it is worth the effort.

– Qualities Associated with Success –

Many of the qualities associated with successful people are those that you would expect to accompany success. You must do more than develop these qualities, though; you must learn to function with them in business and to communicate them effectively.

The Qualities

Determination is one quality that is believed to be associated with success. Few people succeed with a lackadaisical attitude. The urges to compete, to get things done, to make a difference, to see results, and to overcome obstacles all show determination and are important to succeeding in business.

Intelligence is another quality most successful people exhibit. Intelligence in sizing up situations, analyzing results, choosing correctly among alternatives, handling sensitive situations, and dealing rationally with panic situations is usually shown most effectively by a calm, cool approach to situations accompanied by clear thinking in evaluating them.

Physical *energy* usually accompanies success. Laziness rarely achieves. Energy when it is intelligently directed rarely fails to achieve. People who take care of themselves physically usually show energy others do not.

Tactful human relationships are important to success. Success rarely is achieved without help, and abrasiveness clearly alienates people who can aid in achieving success. *Tact* is shown by courtesy and consideration for others. It often means controlling one's tongue to keep from blurting out thoughts that would complicate the situation. It means pointing out corrective procedures rather than problems, saying what can be done, not what cannot be done. In short, it means dealing positively with people rather than negatively and keeping people's feelings in mind.

Leadership in the form of persuading people to perform rather than coercing them to perform is characteristic of people who are successful. The ability to convince people that they want to do whatever you need gains friends, provides for pride in accomplishment, and usually yields a better overall job than does force.

Humor is characteristic of people who succeed. The stern, solemn person who sees no humor in him- or herself or surrounding situations usually cannot attract others who can support and help in achieving success. Humor takes the burden of work and makes it enjoyable — it lightens the load most successful people carry and makes being associated with them enjoyable.

Courage is necessary to succeed because risk is involved in success. If nothing but a sure thing is ever tried, few major successes are usually within reach. Usually, successful people show courage in trying new things that are worth the risk. They tackle obstacles with the sureness of people expecting to succeed but prepare to go on if they fail. They are able to wander out of the comfort of a sure thing and try the unknown but worthwhile atmosphere of new situations.

Illus. 4-1. The qualities associated with successful people include energy, leadership, optimism, and creativity.

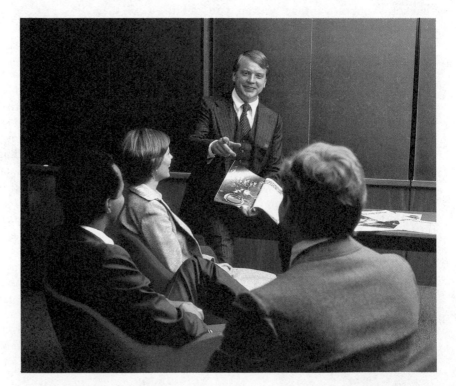

Successful people usually show *optimism*. They expect to succeed. They evaluate, plan, and try, fully expecting to accomplish whatever they want. Rather than dreading new situations and challenges, they look forward to opportunities to work in new situations and meet new challenges. They are expectant and sure, not full of dread and tentative.

Creativity marks most successful people. They are able to work with others and to see situations from various points of view. They see things others don't see. They make connections between seemingly unrelated situations and facts. They perceive new relationships. Their minds are neither tied to the past nor ignorant of it. They appreciate what went before, learn from it, and use it to make the present and future better.

The Person

It is not enough to know about the qualities expected of a person who is successful; you need to know how those qualities are applied and interpreted in business situations. It is one thing, for example, to be intelligent and another to act intelligently in business situations. Your daily behavior is the acid test of how people will perceive you in the business situation. Some suggestions to get you started and help you avoid pitfalls include use of assertiveness, company resources, criticism, innovation, enthusiasm, persuasion, and discussion.

Being assertive about your rights can be a virtue. Nagging people day after day over small matters that gain you very little, however, labels you as a pest. If you experience violation of your rights, carefully evaluate the situation to determine what you can gain and how you can gain it by asserting yourself. Plunging blindly into a situation when you are feeling deprived probably will get you nothing but a bad reputation for dealing with adversity. Constructing a plan to right a wrong and presenting it well are more likely to get you what you want than constant complaining or an outrageous outburst.

Be scrupulously *honest* with company resources. Nothing marks you as poor promotion material more than dishonesty. If you use company expense accounts, be honest; if you use the company vehicles, be honest; if you make purchases for the company, be honest. Keep good records and don't cheat yourself; no one expects you to subsidize the organization with your own funds. They do expect you to be conscientious with the business's money and to ask for only what you are entitled to.

Refrain from "badmouthing" former bosses. Complaints about previous bosses threaten your present boss, who expects the same kind of treatment after you move on. The present boss's only protection will be to keep you from moving on, and perhaps the best course of action is simply to move you out — out of the organization entirely.

Innovation and *enthusiasm* are appreciated in an organization. Haphazard changes for the sake of change and unbridled charging into a situation without proper investigation are not appreciated. Organizations usually have customary ways of handling change. You will fare better if you observe such customs when you are proposing changes. Your changes will be better received, too, if you carefully investigate the effect they will have on people and prepare for those effects. Surprises can be very unpleasant for people safely situated in their jobs. Proper preparation will gain you cooperation and favor.

There is a difference between *persuasion* and *coercion*. Learn to examine your case before you present it so that you can pick out all the reasons it is good and spot its weaknesses. Disarm weaknesses by evaluating them and balancing them against strengths. Then, present your case with all its points. That is the heart of persuasion. You show people what will help,

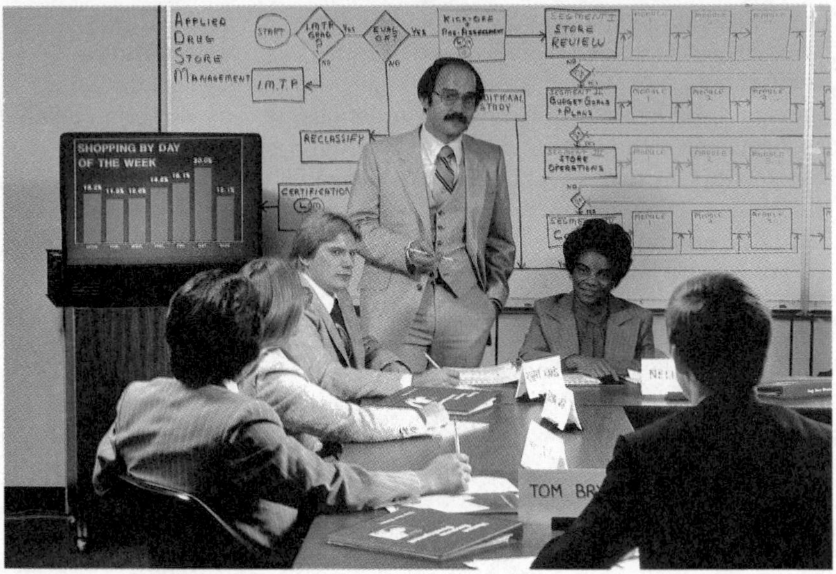

Illus. 4-2. Use the merits of the case rather than a threat to get people to agree with you.

will work, will benefit them, and you relieve their fears about disadvantages.

Coercion, on the other hand, usually has little to do with the real case. You coerce people when you threaten unrelated action if acceptance is withheld. You coerce people when you force them to accept what you offer without complete knowledge. Coercion is rarely either forgotten or forgiven. Learn to do your homework when you are presenting a case for change. Use the merits of the case rather than a threat to get people to agree with you. You will win not only their agreement but also their admiration for a job well done.

There is a difference between *arguing* a point and *discussing* a problem. It is normal to formulate a solution when you see a problem. Remember, though, that the solution you see may not be the best one. When you see a problem, formulate a solution, and another, and another, and another until you have exhausted your imagination. Then discuss the problem and the many possible solutions you can see with the people who can help you solve the problem. By examining all possibilities, you are

more likely to discuss than argue. Because you have not committed yourself to a single solution, you have no stand to protect. You may think one solution is better than the rest, but by presenting all possibilities, you give yourself and others space to examine alternatives. People won't feel that you are forcing something on them.

Once you take a stand, you probably will find yourself arguing rather than discussing. At that time you must begin negotiating, giving in to others' demands in order to get a solution, and it probably won't be the solution you want but a variation of the solution you want. Discussions, on the other hand, can yield just the solution you want if you examine and present alternatives well. Remember, problems are to be discussed, not argued.

—— Successful Communication ——

If you are unable to communicate your qualities and strengths to people, you will be perceived as unsuccessful by people. Time spent on refining your communication skills may yield more benefits than any other skill development.

Communication means more than talking. Some of the components of inter-personal communicating are listening, speaking, writing, and reading. The components of organizational communication you may not have a chance to develop until you reach a higher level in an organization. They concern the abilities to disseminate information among workers, to develop systems of information dissemination and informal networks, to set policy and to establish formal communication systems, and to meet with visitors and colleagues in conferences.

By developing your interpersonal communication skills now, you can prepare for times when you will have the opportunity to become involved in organizational communications.

Listening

Few of us learn to listen. We listen only to enough to know how we will respond. Teach yourself to listen in a new and complete way. First of all, give your full attention to people

speaking. That means that while the other person is talking, you cannot worry about getting your turn to speak. It means that you cannot be formulating your response while the other person is talking. It means that you must hear and concentrate on the message of the sender. Listen to the words, look at the face if possible, observe the mannerisms. Interpret all the signals of the sender of the message. Listening completely will be easier if you select a place that is quiet enough and comfortable enough to avoid distraction.

When the speaker is through, don't assume that what you heard is what was said. It rarely is. Clarify what you think you heard. Paraphrasing what you think was said is one way to check whether or not you got the message that was sent. If you learn you are wrong, ask questions to clarify the message. Observe the speaker carefully to learn if there are underlying feelings that are obscuring the message both to you and to the speaker. Be as perceptive as you can in interpreting the underlying feelings that may be influencing both the speaker and you. One way to get to underlying feelings without offending or threatening the speaker is to say

Illus. 4-3. To listen, you must hear and concentrate on the message of the speaker.

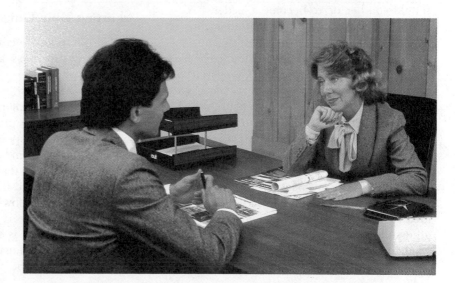

"Do I hear you saying . . .?" The speaker may then recognize for the first time what message is really intended and be relieved that you have really listened. Some of the things that people want to tell you but don't want to say are that they are:

1. frustrated by circumstances beyond their control in doing their jobs.
2. angry because a faith or trust was betrayed and the job was bungled.
3. confused because they are getting conflicting messages from various levels of management.
4. overwhelmed by the work piling up which requires action by others before completion.

By listening for underlying feelings in messages, you may more astutely discern the content. You learn about your speaker by considering both the feeling (response) about the situation and the content of the verbal description of it. You may learn that the speaker responds with anger, frustration, confusion, or dismay in various situations. That knowledge will give you vital clues in working with people so that you avoid negative feelings on their parts should you decide to become a leader.

Remember that part of communicating is silence. You make a statement by not responding and by "holding your tongue" when prudent. Silence is necessary on your part if you are to listen to others. Silence is also necessary if you are to think and allow others to think. In business, remember that disturbing others' peace during work is rarely appreciated.

Conversations should be an exchange. Don't mistake a monologue of your thoughts for a conversation. Few people want to witness your thought process as you crystallize your ideas. Do your crystallizing silently, and allow others the same privilege. Converse when you want to participate in an exchange, not when you want to perform.

Carefully avoid presenting problems and ideas to people who are already worried. Anything that can wait, should, when as a bearer of bad news you must approach someone who is in a worried or otherwise harried mood.

Avoid talking when you don't know what you are talking about. It is better to be silent than to show your ignorance. Ignorance is boring and can make you a laughingstock. Silence is better. At least when you are silent, people must speculate on your intelligence and knowledge; you are not confirming or denying it.

Speaking

Most people have been speaking since they were very small children. So, what is there to learn about speaking now? People in leadership roles speak for many purposes. They must first of all be understood; therefore, they must speak clearly. They must be persuasive; therefore, they must know language that persuades and incentives that motivate. And they must command attention when they speak; therefore, they must know what speech elicits the attention of others.

Adjusting Your Language

Corporations have some contradictions. In many ways business and industry adopt a space-age philosophy toward action. In some ways they are the last to change. Although millions are spent to explore and develop modern systems and update procedures, human conduct, appearance, speech, and behavior are very slow to change in business. Standards and formalities are those that have been around for a very long time, and those that have changed have done so very slowly and at great peril to the changers.

Proper English is required in speech as well as writing. Fashionable "jargon, idiom, and culturalisms" will be viewed as inadequate speech in the business world. Words and phrases that are appropriate with your friends during your leisure time may not be appropriate in business situations. You don't "freak out," for example; you are surprised. You don't "tune in"; you agree.

If you choose your words carefully, avoiding fad phrases, local dialects, and technical terms when possible, you are more likely to be understood, appreciated, and admired by your listeners. Short, simple words that convey the message are preferred to those that are longer and less familiar to listeners. If, however, a long, unfamiliar word more precisely conveys the meaning of what you want to say, use it. A good vocabulary is noticed and appreciated. It marks you as a person who puts effort into communicating well by learning the language well.

There is a quality in people called presence — the manner of carrying oneself — that has an important influence on how they are treated and perceived by others. Concentrate on appearing important when you have something important to say. The bearing which usually works best for those growing in their careers is one of cool and calm awareness, a tall, thin body structure (even when they are only five feet tall), and conservative behavior.

Timing and Place

Be sure you consider the appropriate time when you are speaking. To say to someone else, "I like your work," tossing it over your shoulder while rushing out a door, does not have nearly the impact of sitting face to face quietly in an office. Environment can have almost as much impact as the words themselves. You can fortify your message by providing the best environment in terms of placement and timing. On the other hand, you can destroy your message by ignoring the importance of placement and timing.

Distortion

Because we all have different experiences (frames of reference), we all interpret different things from what is said. Keep this principle in mind when you are speaking. What you say is interpreted somewhat differently by everyone listening to you. What you hear someone saying may not be exactly what that person means. The only way you can clear up distortions in communication is to ask questions.

Many problems that can be solved with discussion arise from distortions. You can solve some of these problems by keeping in mind that *based on what you heard or read*, you may disagree and see no acceptable line of action. If you ask others for their interpretations, new ideas for lines of action may open to you because you get different perceptions of what occurred. Your skill in communicating grows as you learn to integrate perceptions different from yours into your interpretations.

Planning

The impression you make when you speak depends upon more than your voice and your vocabulary. Your ability to think and organize is reflected in your speech. At least as much effort should go into your preparation for speaking as in the speaking itself.

Often you will be asked questions on which you have opinions and knowledge but on which you have not organized your thoughts. Don't be tempted to flounder as you try to answer. Stall for time while you organize before speaking. One way to organize is to ask if the questioner can be more specific. You then gain time to mentally organize your answer. Speaking slowly in such a situation allows you time to choose wisely your words and to organize mentally your next sentence and idea. A low-pitched voice, too, carries more authority and gets more trust than a high-pitched one.

If you are to make a presentation which you have time to plan, plan well. Make an outline; or write out the presentation completely if necessary and then outline it with key words designated. Never, never read a presentation. Doing so makes you appear unable to organize your thoughts while you are speaking — it makes you appear less able than those who make presentations without reading.

When you are planning presentations, use audio and video equipment that is available to you for practice. If you have a video tape recorder, tape your presentation so that you can see how you look as well as hear how you sound. You may be surprised to see gestures you didn't know you had. You may be surprised at the sound of your voice. If video equipment is not available, use a tape recorder to listen to yourself. Try to listen for:

1. The rate at which you speak. Is it too fast or too slow (few are too slow)?
2. The variation of pitch. Monotones are boring. Some enthusiasm for what you are saying should be reflected in varying pitch.
3. Your choice of words. You appear less intelligent when your vocabulary is weak and you use slang than when you use standard English.

Plan the content of your presentation so that you have a beginning, a middle, and an end. The beginning should introduce your subject and tell the listeners what you plan to talk about and perhaps the order of the presentation. The middle should be the heart of the matter. And the end should tie the points together, draw conclusions, or review the important points you want your listeners to remember or to act on.

Listen to yourself as you practice to see if you can discern between the three parts of the presentation. Ask someone else to listen to your tape and to repeat what they remember of it to you. You will learn whether or not your points are being made.

Listen to your pronunciation. Use standard pronunciation, and use a dictionary if you are unsure of words. Practice words and combinations of words that are difficult for you to say.

Subtleties and Practices in the Business Environment

Like people who have self-confidence, organizations which have self-confidence perform with greater assurance than those which are tentative because of lack of self-confidence. Because of this situation, certain "beliefs" are professed which often are unsubstantiated and probably unsupportable. It is not necessary for you to espouse these beliefs; it is necessary that you not challenge or deny them without very good reason and without consideration for the consequences to both the morale of the people in the organization and to yourself.

The Best

Most organizations like to believe they are the best in their field. Often they find a "best" area, such as largest, fastest growing, fastest gaining, most efficient, best return on investment, or other descriptions on which to base this "best in the field" claim. If you wish to grow in your career in the organization, you will do better not to ask for an analysis of the basis for the comparison when the claim is made to keep confidence in the company and to boost morale. If you see that the claim gets in the way of seeing real deficiencies that need to be corrected in the organization you should, of course, seek ways to correct the deficiencies with as little loss of faith and face as possible among those who hold the belief.

Leadership

Organizations close ranks behind their own leadership claiming it to be strong and able.

Those at the top are claimed to be wiser and stronger than those on the way up. The belief that people who do the best job are the ones chosen to lead the organization is espoused. That often is not the case. Many times, people who lead others to believe that they are leadership material regardless of the job they do are the ones promoted to leadership roles. You will do well, however, not to challenge openly the capabilities of those in leadership roles of your organization. Do your own job well and convince others that you are well able to lead, and you may make the belief come true at least in your own case.

People Who Leave

People who leave an organization are people the organization says it wants to leave. Organizations rarely admit that better opportunities exist outside for their good people. They like to believe that the organization itself offers the best opportunities for talented people that can be found. You will do well neither to criticize nor to compliment those who leave the organization for better positions. The best description is one which says "That person felt it was time to move on." There is no need to speculate on the reason.

The Competition

Companies like to believe that they are doing things the best way. Organizations that do things differently are perceived as following fads or embracing procedures likely to fail soon. Your job here is delicate. Often you may see others getting ahead of your firm with innovative ideas. You must find a way to help your own organization innovate without challenging the belief that the procedures of the competition are inferior. Try to suggest a variation of a new procedure that your competition has

instituted. A variation that is an improvement is best, so that you can help your own organization keep up. To openly admire the competition's procedures will not gain you favor. To beat the competition at its own game will.

Administrative Versus Technical Ability

Many companies believe that administrative ability is more valued than technical ability. A slanderous remark is one which calls someone a "good technician" because the implication is that the person has no administrative ability and will never rise to levels of management. Technical ability often is the source of satisfying work and gets people started in organizations. It can even gain one a good source of income. Administrative ability, being able to manage people and resources, however,

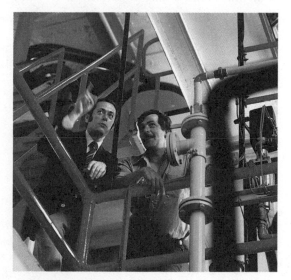

Illus. 4-4. Administrative ability, being able to manage people and resources, is the quality that gains one recognition in an organization.

is the quality that gains one recognition in an organization. To criticize one for lack of technical ability, especially when that person is in an administrative position, is to risk alienating administrators throughout the organization.

Fair and Equal Treatment

Companies like to believe that they treat everyone fairly. They want to believe that discrimination, if it exists, is based on real evidence of inferiority and superiority of persons. To blatantly challenge treatment you think is discriminatory will not win you favor in the organization. To decide where you are cheated and to plan for instituting a change to balance your treatment is the proper procedure for handling discrimination.

Discrimination within the organization and promotions based on job performance rather than on whether a person is male or female or black or white have been discussed and legislated at length. You, regardless of your sex or race, must carefully evaluate how you will approach inequities based on stereotyping. You may feel like nit-picking — pointing out that you do not want men to open doors for you if you are a woman, or pointing out that a woman wants a man to open doors for her if you are a man — when you see larger inequities, for example based on sex. Don't give in to the urge to nit-pick. It gains you nothing but a bad reputation and a "hard-to-get-along-with" label.

If inequities exist that are substantial and that cause you real pain or put you at a disadvantage, select the proper forum, person, and time to discuss the problem. Discuss it constructively in terms of what you would like to have done rather than negatively in terms of what is wrong with the way things are currently done. Be sure you know precisely what you want. If you don't, you are not likely to get it.

Sex in Business

When people work closely together, sex must be dealt with. Man or woman, you must decide that sexual relationships with people at work produce pressure and confusion and more often than not will hurt your career. Decide at the beginning that you will not mix sex with business, and you can curtail most of the temptation and the advances by those who have not so decided.

The environment in which we live is one of sexual permissiveness, and the moral issues regarding sex are confused. You will be better off to handle a first sexual suggestion from someone as a normal reaction to you because you are a person. Gauge your rebuff according to the heavy-handedness with which the advance is made. The stronger the advance, the stronger the rebuff. Most of the time, you can simply say "no thanks" firmly without carrying it further. If "no thanks" does not stem the advance, you will have to resort to stronger rebuffs like explaining that you have other pressures at work or other relationships outside work and you do not wish to add to them with this relationship. If your rebuffs are firm and yet go unheeded, the option to report the advances to a superior is available.

It is important to remember that you must be firm, consistent, definite, and sure. Once you encourage or suggest "maybe" you will have a much harder time changing the tide. More often than not, the person with the least power in a situation that evolves at work loses — either the job, any chances for promotion at work, or other important advantages. If you are firm and consistent, people soon learn that you are not available for sexual relationships and will probably respect your decision. If they don't, don't feel uncomfortable at all about reporting it — it has become sexual harrassment.

Packaging

You may have been taught from childhood that it's only what's inside that counts. Even if that is true (and there are studies that deny it), it is what's outside that shows. If you don't *appear* to fit in, people will assume that you don't.

Most men can walk through an office or business place and learn what is expected of them in terms of appearance. They can see what clothes to wear, how to cut their hair, and how to bear themselves in terms of posture if they are to fit in. Women usually cannot be so confident by observing because not enough women have advanced in jobs to present a unified appearance code.

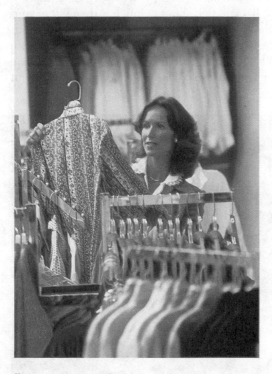

Illus. 4-5. A woman can forfeit growth in her career by dressing inappropriately.

The surest way for a woman to forfeit growth in her career is to offend people with her dress. The offensive clothing in business is that which is *too feminine* and that which is *too masculine*. A middle-of-the-road approach to packaging for women is the safest for those who want to grow. The reason for middle-of-the-road grooming is that people at the top are nervous already about promoting women. Anything that looks extreme or out of place makes them more nervous about promoting a woman. Women who think that this philosophy is unfair should realize that men have "toed the line" for many years, wearing "the business suit" day after day after day, and have risen consistently to leadership positions outranking women financially and authoritatively.

Clothes that are too trendy, sexy, and expensive label a person as frivolous, unrealistic, and not to be trusted with important responsibility. Clothes, too, that are out of date and cheap reflect badly on the company's status and will hold you back. Dress like a junior executive if you aspire to that position. If you are already one, dress like the people on the next rung on the ladder. Wear the best clothes you can buy without looking like you make too much money.

Business Etiquette

Etiquette in business normally is no different from common courtesy you practice every day. Some situations may be different, however. For example, you may be a man in business who is taken to lunch by a woman or a woman who takes men to business lunches. You should know how to react in either case. Introductions are made often in business and you need to be able to make them with confidence. Your visibility in areas you may consider private is scrutinized, and you should know what is expected.

The Business Lunch

Many people consider the business lunch one of the most important functions in advancing a person's career. They consider the business lunch crucial to successful business relationships both within a business and with people outside a business.

You need to be poised both as the host and as the guest. Learn where you can take others to lunch by observing where people are going to lunch together. Observe whether or not reservations are needed and what the best time is for lunch. If you plan to use a credit card or check, call ahead to make sure that the restaurant accepts them. Otherwise, be prepared with cash.

When you are the guest, follow the lead of the host in ordering. If the host has something light, you order something light. Don't drink liquor unless your host does and perhaps not then if you plan to return to work. Pace yourself so that you neither start eating before your host

nor finish long before your host. In conversation, follow the lead of your host. If your host suggests business matters, those are the topics. If not, you may stay with social topics until the host changes the subject.

Review your table manners. Nothing marks you as a loser more quickly than poor table manners. A slob at the table is a slob everywhere in most people's minds and is a person to be avoided. If you are unsure of your table manners, use one of the current etiquette books to study appropriate table manners. Post and Vanderbilt are names that will help you find good etiquette books.

The business lunch often is used to get an appointment with a person that you may not otherwise be able to talk to. When you call and ask a person to lunch, you usually are accepted. What you talk about at lunch is then left to you, the host. It may be business or social. Remember not to expect too much in an informal forum like lunch. You probably only want to come across as a person one wants to know more about

Illus. 4-6. Many people consider the business lunch one of the most important functions in advancing a person's career.

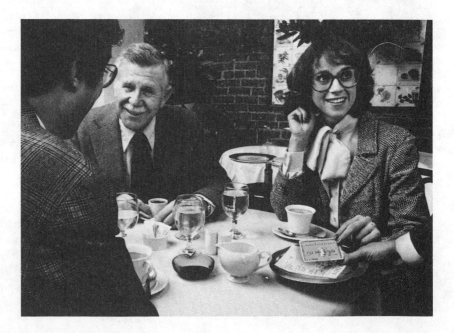

if it is the first meeting.

When you are paying the bill by credit card, you can add the tip (usually 15%) to the total before you sign the charge slip. When you pay by cash, you leave the tip in cash on the table before you leave. If you do not have the correct amount in cash, it is correct to ask the cashier for change as you are leaving, walk back to your table, and leave the tip.

Introducing People

The general rules for introducing people are easy to learn. It is always courteous to introduce people with whom you may be talking if they do not know each other. The generally followed procedures are:

1. A man is presented to a woman: "Mary Adams, I would like you to know John Justin," or "Mary Adams, John Justin."
2. A younger person is presented to an older person when the ages are obviously far apart. This procedure means that a young girl may be presented to an older man (overriding the first rule). "Mr. Jones, I'd like you to meet Mary Adams," or "Mr. Jones, Mary Adams,"
3. Two women or two men who are introduced are presented to each other when they are of equal rank. It makes no difference who is presented to whom. If one is considerably older or is more important within the group, such as the president of the group, the younger or less important one is

Illus. 4-7. The general rules for introducing people are easy to learn.

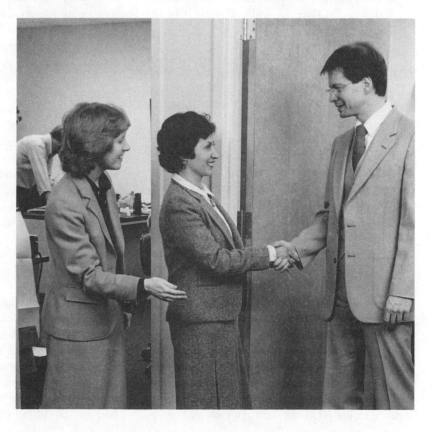

presented to the older or the more important one. "Sue Johnson, this is Alice Hall. Sue is President of our club."

4. When people are introduced in business, they usually shake hands. Be sure your hands are dry and your grasp is firm.

5. Men always stand when they are introduced to other men or to women. Women may remain sitting, unless they are being introduced to a woman who is somewhat older or somewhat more important than they are. Deference is shown to age, and older women are honored by standing for an introduction to them.

6. Deference may also be shown to clergy, governors, mayors, and foreign heads of state, when they are men, by presenting women to them rather than as described in Rule 1. "Mayor Stovall, this is Linda Grimm."

When you are introduced, it is a good idea to repeat the name of the person to whom you are introduced to confirm the name and to say something like, "Mary Adams? Nice to meet you," or, "I'm happy to meet you, Mary," or, "Hello, Mary." It is considered improper to say "Charmed" or "Delighted." Sometimes the person to whom you have been introduced does not hear your name or does not hear it correctly. It is courteous to pronounce it again very clearly if requested so that the other person understands your name correctly.

Addressing People

When you are addressing someone you've just met, either socially or in business, it is usually safer to use a title (Mrs., Ms., Miss, or Mr.) with the surname until you are asked to use a given name. An exception to this general rule is when you are introduced to someone near your own age at a social gathering. Frequently you are expected to call such a person by a given name from the beginning of the acquaintance. In the office and at formal social gatherings, follow the safer tradition of using the title and the last name until you are asked to use the given name.

You may suggest to others that they call you by your given name if you wish. Among colleagues in an office, the use of given names is usually standard procedure. An exception may be between you and your boss.

If You Smoke

Smoking may be very offensive to those who do not smoke. If you are in a closed room such as an office, a restaurant, a theater, an elevator, etc., be most careful. Smoke drifting from your cigarette pollutes the air of those about you, especially if the ventilation is poor.

Smoke clings to other people's hair and clothing long after they have escaped your smoke. It is often an inconvenience and nuisance for nonsmokers to contend with such offensive odors on their person and clothes resulting from your inconsiderate use of smoking. It is as inconsiderate of you to allow your smoke to permeate the hair and clothes of a nonsmoker as it would be of a nonsmoker to spray you with a fragrance you found equally unpleasant.

You should forego smoking and polluting the air of others under such circumstances. Confine your smoking to designated areas so that nonsmokers will not have to tolerate either that smoke drifting from your cigarette or that drifting from your mouth. Both may be most offensive.

If you do smoke, always remain seated or standing in one place until you finish your cigarette. To carry a lighted cigarette in either your hand or your mouth is awkward and dangerous. You may drop unnoticed hot ashes or brush them against someone's clothes as you walk. A cigarette that is hanging from your mouth looks bad and could fall causing fire damage.

Carefully avoid smoking in a windy area since ashes frequently blow from your cigarette onto others who may be downwind. This is especially important when you are traveling in a bus, train, or car with your window open. Very often the person behind you gets hot ashes on clothing or skin if you are inconsiderate.

Before you light a cigarette, be sure that there is an ashtray available to you. If there is not, you should check with the host or hostess to see if smoking is permitted. Many people do not have ashtrays out because they prefer to have no smoking near them. If there are ashtrays out, be sure to use them faithfully. It is rude to drop ashes on the floor or the furniture. Often the ashes are hot and will burn a hole in carpeting and upholstery. You should feel obligated to pay for the repair if you destroy furnishings with your ashes.

If you smoke at your desk at work, keep your ashtray emptied regularly. An ashtray can have an offensive odor with stale cigarette butts in it. Only one or two butts should be allowed to accumulate before the ashtray is emptied. Be very careful about emptying butts into a waste can with papers because you may start a fire with live ashes. Never leave your ashtray full overnight since the stale smoke odor will permeate the entire room before the next day. Leaving your ashtray unattended with a lighted cigarette in it invites disaster. More than once, a cigarette has burned down, fallen out of the tray, and burned the furniture. If you burn someone's furniture, offer to have it repaired.

If You Chew Gum

The chewing gum industry would have you believe that gum chewing is a desirable and acceptable practice anywhere, anytime. It is not. Very few offices approve of chewing gum at your desk especially if customers frequent your office.

Other offices object to chewing gum because the smacking, popping, and constant movement of your mouth are distracting to colleagues. Others disapprove because of the frequency with which the gum seems to end up on floors and shoe soles, under chair seats, and stuck in wastebaskets.

The only proper use of chewing gum is in private, where others will not be subjected to the distractions of it. If you chew it immediately after meals to help clean your teeth or freshen your breath, do so in the restroom. Then throw it away, wrapped in paper so that it won't stick to the waste can, before you return to work.

Toothpicks and other items that are used in your mouth for cleaning food from your teeth and gums should never be used in public. Just as you would not brush your teeth in public, you should not use other methods of cleaning your teeth in public.

If You Use Liquor

Liquor is frequently accepted as part of the social scene in our culture. It is always proper for you to refuse to drink if you prefer not to. No one should ever be offended if you do not wish to drink, and you should never apologize. Most hosts and hostesses provide nonalcoholic beverages for those who do not wish to imbibe.

If you are hosting a gathering yourself, be very alert to the needs of your guests. Provide nonalcoholic beverages along with alcoholic ones, if you desire, and be unobtrusive about it. Never encourage guests to drink liquor if they have indicated a preference for a nonalcoholic beverage. People do not indulge for many reasons. Some people have moral objections to its consumption. Liquor does not mix with certain medications that are commonly used. It cannot be used by people with heart or stomach problems. People who are alcoholic must avoid it completely.

Questions for Chapter 4

1. What are the qualities associated with success? What must you do besides just develop them?
2. What is good strategy when you want to be assertive?
3. Why is it so important to be honest in handling company resources?
4. How can innovation and enthusiasm be threatening?
5. What is the difference between persuasion and coercion?
6. Why are you more likely to get what you want by discussing a problem than by arguing a position you have taken about a solution to a problem?
7. If you listen well, what are you likely to learn about the speaker besides what is being said?
8. Why is silence part of communicating?
9. What adjustments in your language are you likely to have to make for business?
10. What do timing and place have to do with communication?
11. How can you check distortion of your messages?
12. What are some things you can listen for when you practice your speeches?
13. What do organizations profess to believe about themselves compared to other organizations of their kind?
14. What do they believe about their leadership?
15. How should you handle competitive practices that you believe are good?
16. What is the best way to handle unfair or discriminatory practices?
17. What is the best way to handle the question of sex in business?
18. What does "packaging" have to do with the way you are perceived at work?
19. What are your responsibilities as a host at a business lunch?
20. What are your responsibilities as a guest at a business lunch?
21. When you are introduced to someone, what should you say?
22. What are some good practices for people who smoke?
23. Why isn't chewing gum in public a good idea?

Chapter 5

Time and Money Management

Chapter Objectives

After studying this chapter, you should be able to:

1. *Plan your money management.*
2. *Evaluate checking accounts, savings accounts, and banks available to you.*
3. *Keep track of your checks and checkbook.*
4. *Evaluate the use of credit and develop standards for decisions about making purchases on credit.*
5. *Make use of your time according to your priorities and basic biological functioning.*
6. *Organize the time that must be spent in various ways.*

Two of the most valuable resources a person can draw on are time and money. Learning to manage these resources comes easily for some people. For many, time and money management are difficult. Without good management, both resources will slip away from you, decreasing the quality of your life. Good management gives you freedom for the other things in life that make it enjoyable.

Money Management

If you have always had discretionary money of your own, rather than money given to you for specific purposes, you may already have devised a way of managing money so that you have enough for whatever is important to you. If you have not had money to manage in the past, you may need help in arriving at the point where you can have money for whatever is important to you.

A Plan

Planning for managing your money is usually called budgeting, a word that rarely brings pleasant thoughts to people. If you think of it as setting priorities for your money, it may seem more palatable. In constructing a plan for managing your money you can expect to gain at least four benefits:

1. A plan will tell you where your money is coming from and when you can expect it.

2. A plan will provide for the necessities first and the comforts, self-improvements, and luxuries in the order you prioritize them.
3. A plan will give you a means for saving and staying out of debt if that is important to you.
4. A plan will help you build good habits for spending.

To start a money management plan you must first of all construct an outline of where you get money from and when you expect it. A chart with headings such as those in Illustration 5-1 may help. If you prefer a different breakdown, use weeks instead of months. Total each column. List only the net amounts (what you actually get with taxes and other withheld amounts taken out). Include such things as interest income from savings accounts, gifts you may receive from your family, bonuses, and tax refunds.

Using the same headings for the time periods, make a chart that shows your fixed expenses — the "must spend" amounts (see Illustration 5-2). Be sure to include your rent or mortgage, utility bills (telephone, electricity, gas, water), real estate taxes, income taxes that are not withheld on such income as interest, insurance, and medical and dental payments, and include in this list what you think you *must* save each time period to feel secure. If you have installment payments such as for your car, they belong in this "must" list. After you include all your fixed expenses, total each column and subtract the monthly amounts from your monthly income in the first listing you made. That will give you what you have left for comforts, self-improvements, and luxuries — your day-to-day expenses.

Use the same headings for the time periods and make a list that shows your day-to-day expenses (see Illustration 5-3).

If you have a checking account with records of expenses for these items, you have accurate figures to use. If not, you must establish accurate figures by keeping a daily diary for a few weeks. This list should include such items as food, household expenses and repairs, furnishings, clothes, transportation, personal care items, education, recreation, gifts, and contributions. You may think of other items to include in your list.

You may need some guides for this listing. It is tempting to set unreasonable limits on these items. You should use amounts that are realistic. You cannot cut down on food, for example, without specific ideas for cutting down, such as substituting low-cost items you like for the high-cost items you usually buy.

If you want to see how you compare to an "average family" in America, compare your figures to those in Illustration 5-4. By keeping a diary for a while, you can see your spending patterns emerge showing your priorities. By profiling your spending patterns, you learn

WHERE MY MONEY COMES FROM	JAN.	FEB.	MAR.	APR.	MAY	JUNE	JULY	AUG.	SEPT.	OCT.	NOV.	DEC.
1. Salary	___	___	___	___	___	___	___	___	___	___	___	___
2. Gifts	___	___	___	___	___	___	___	___	___	___	___	___

Illus. 5-1. Where Money Comes From

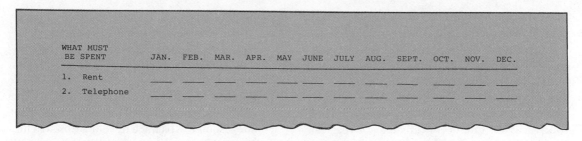

WHAT MUST BE SPENT	JAN.	FEB.	MAR.	APR.	MAY	JUNE	JULY	AUG.	SEPT.	OCT.	NOV.	DEC.
1. Rent	___	___	___	___	___	___	___	___	___	___	___	___
2. Telephone	___	___	___	___	___	___	___	___	___	___	___	___

Illus. 5-2. What Must Be Spent

DAY-TO-DAY LIVING EXPENSES	JAN.	FEB.	MAR.	APR.	MAY	JUNE	JULY	AUG.	SEPT.	OCT.	NOV.	DEC.
1. Food	___	___	___	___	___	___	___	___	___	___	___	___
2. Laundry	___	___	___	___	___	___	___	___	___	___	___	___

Illus. 5-3. Day-to-Day Living Expenses

Illus. 5-4. How the Average Family Spends Its Income

For	Cents of Each Dollar
Food	.223
Housing	.145
Household operation	.144
Transportation	.136
Clothing	.101
Medical care	.077
Recreation	.065
Personal business	.056
Private education	.017
Personal care	.015
Religious and welfare activities	.014
Foreign travel	.007

something about yourself — where you put your money, one of your major resources.

If you are spending more than your income, you will see that quickly too. You will also see places where you can cut to bring expenses in line with income using this planning method. Large expenses, such as a medical checkup and your vacation, that occur only once a year can be anticipated and planned for.

Handling Money

Once you have your income and expenses reasonably managed in terms of amounts, you need to establish a method of day-to-day handling of your money. Your first consideration probably will be safety; the second, accessibility; and the third, rate of return, if any. For most people, a checking account provides the safest and most accessible vehicle for day-to-day management of money. Some checking accounts provide interest on the balance and some do not. Those that do often provide only a minimal interest rate and require that you keep a substantial balance in the account to avoid charges for check writing and servicing. That substantial required balance may earn you more interest in another kind of savings account — more than the charges would be on a non-interest-bearing checking account. You should carefully check the requirements of the checking accounts comparing costs before you select one. Ask if you qualify — as a student, employee of a particular firm, or in some other way — for a special no-charge checking account at the banks available to you. If you do not, you probably will have to select from accounts that:

1. Require a particular balance that exempts you from service charges but pay no interest on that balance.
2. Require no specific balance but charge you a set amount per check.

3. Require a specific balance that allows you a certain number of free checks per time period and set a specific charge for checks above that number during each time period (month, quarter, etc.).
4. Require a substantial balance that allows you a certain number of free checks and pay interest on the balance in your account. This account may or may not return your cancelled checks to you. If it does not, it will provide a listing of your checks cleared for each time period.

Many kinds of accounts are offered because no one kind suits every person's needs. You should decide approximately how many checks you will write per month and figure comparative costs on the kinds of checking accounts available to you. Don't forget to figure the interest you will lose on the required balances as part of the costs for those kinds of checking accounts.

When you are selecting a bank, other considerations are:

1. Savings accounts and rates the banks pay. Are they comparable to other savings institutions in your area?
2. Interest compounding. The more frequently the interest is compounded on savings, the better for you. Make sure your bank is competitive in this area.
3. Availability of your money. Some banks require collection of the money on checks you deposit into your account before they let you write checks on the money. Make sure your money is available to you as quickly as possible and that the bank you select gives you quickest access to your money.
4. Insurance. Banks may or may not be insured federally. If they are not, see what insurance your money has while they handle it.
5. Loans. Check to see if the bank gives you preferential treatment on loans because you also have a checking account there. Many banks do.

6. Safe deposit boxes. If you have documents that must be protected, such as tax returns, deeds, securities, jewelry, or other valuables, you probably will need a safe deposit box. Check on the availability and the cost of the box.
7. Proximity and hours open. Be sure the bank is open when you can do your banking.

In addition, here are some reminders about keeping your checks and checkbook in order:

1. Date each check accurately. Banks can refuse to accept a check which is dated ahead. Number your checks consecutively so that you can keep track of them. Stolen checks with your account number can be cashed and cause you a great deal of trouble.
2. Write your figures as close to the dollar sign as you legibly can. Space left there invites people to add figures to the amount. On the middle line, spell out the amount and draw a line in the unused space to the word *dollars*.
3. Decide on a legible signature and don't vary it with additional initials or with titles. Women, married or not, should use their given names. No Mr., Mrs., or Ms. should be used.
4. If you use checks for less than a dollar amount, use a decimal point before the number between it and the dollar sign and write the word *cents* after it. On the middle line, write "only (the amount) cents" and draw a line through the word *dollars*.
5. Keep a close count on your checks. Professional criminals steal checks from the back of your book so that it takes longer for you to discover the theft. Technically, people who take checks in payment are supposed to get identification from people who sign checks. Professional criminals, however, forge millions of dollars' worth of checks using stolen blank checks every year. Take care of yours; guard them like you guard your money. They almost are money.
6. When you endorse checks others have given to you, you can protect yourself by restricting the endorsement. A nonrestricted (blank) endorsement is simply your name written on the back of the check. That makes the check payable to the bearer just like cash. If you restrict the endorsement by writing "Pay to the order of (name of the person or store)" before you sign your name, the check must be endorsed by the person you named before it can be honored. Endorsing with "For deposit only to the account of (your name)" restricts the check to deposit to your account, and it cannot be cashed by anyone who may intercept it.

Illus. 5-5. A Check for Less than a Dollar

Nov. 12 19-- 92-403
1241
PAY TO THE ORDER OF Mount Cross Company $ .75 cents
Only seventy-five cents DOLLARS
Riverview National Bank
WILLIAMSBURG, IDAHO
FOR C. S. Ruble
⑆124104035⑆ 326⑈08375⑈

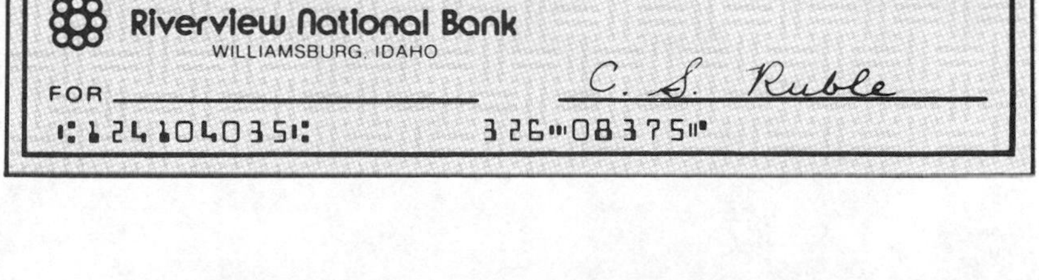

Blank Endorsement

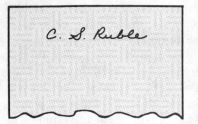

Special Endorsement

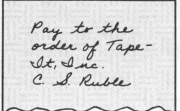

Restrictive Endorsement

Illus. 5-6. Endorsements

7. Deposit checks as soon as you get them. Banks may refuse to honor checks more than three months old.

8. Never write a check to *cash* unless you are standing at the teller's window in your bank. Such checks may be cashed by anyone and used just like cash.

9. Keep accurate records of checks you write. These records may protect you from errors, taxes, and people or organizations that "forget" that you paid your bill.

10. Never, but never, sign a blank check.

11. If you make a mistake on a check you are writing, write VOID across it, put it in your cancelled check file, and start over. Banks can refuse to honor checks with corrections made on them.

12. Always use nonerasable ink on your checks. Using pencil invites people to change the amounts.

13. If you ever lose a single check, notify your bank immediately.

14. If your bank statement is ever mislaid or not received in the mail on time, notify your bank immediately.

15. Reconcile your bank statement within a day or two after you get it. Banks do make mistakes and so do you. You need to check on both of you regularly to keep your records accurate.

16. Destroy old checks and deposit slips if you change addresses or your name. Don't leave your coded number intact with the checks. You invite people to access your account if you do.

Tax Records

Part of good money management is learning to keep good records for tax purposes. The records that you should keep include:

1. A permanent record of your earnings including W-2 forms from your employers, 1099 forms from organizations that pay you interest income, and other kinds of statements showing miscellaneous income. When you make deposits other than your payroll check to your checking account, you should note on the deposit slip where the money came from. If it is ordinary income for tax purposes, you will be taxed on it when you file your tax return. If it is not ordinary income, you need a record so that you can substantiate not paying taxes on it. Income that may be tax exempt includes small cash gifts from family and friends and money you are reimbursed for business expenses.

2. A record of transportation costs (other than commuting to and from work) that are for business purposes. If you use your own car

Illus. 5-7. Part of good money management is learning to keep good records for tax purposes.

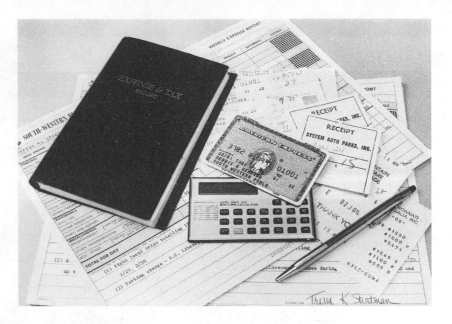

for such transportation, keep a record of the original cost of the car, annual total mileage, business mileage, gasoline and oil, repair costs, garage rent, license and registration fees, tolls, and any other costs that are business related.

3. If you travel out of town for business purposes, keep a diary of all travel expenses involved including hotel bills, transportation costs, taxi fares, meals, tips, telephone charges, stenographer fees, out-of-town clothes cleaning, and anything else you pay for during the travel. Keep receipts, paid bills, and cancelled checks to document travel expenses.

4. If you make charitable or religious contributions, keep a careful list of all of them. If they are other than cash, list the fair market value of the items. Keep account of mileage to and from the place where you make the contribution if you transport it yourself.

5. A record of all medical and dental bills including the mileage to and from the office

of the physician and dentist.

6. A record of all amounts relating to the purchase of a house or apartment including commissions, legal fees, and improvements you make on the property.

7. If you purchase or sell stock, keep complete records of the transactions including date of purchase and sale, commissions, price, and dividends.

Savings Accounts

Most people need at least two months' income saved to feel comfortable. It is not unusual for people to keep six months' income in savings in case of emergencies. Whatever amount you decide to save, you must decide what vehicle you need to keep it in. Savings accounts provide you income in the form of interest. The rate of interest you can earn depends upon how much money you have to deposit and how long you can leave it in the account. The lower the rate of interest, the more accessible your money, generally speaking.

Illus. 5-8. Carefully select a vehicle for your savings.

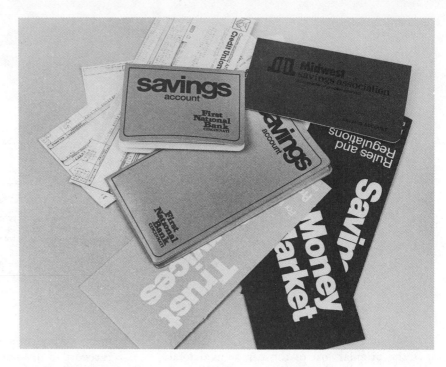

Passbook savings accounts make your money instantly available and usually can be started with as little as $5. The rate of interest on these accounts is the lowest of the accounts offered.

Time deposits are available at higher rates of interest. The length of time varies from institution to institution. If you do not leave your money in the account for the specified time, you usually pay a penalty. Your interest, however, can usually be withdrawn at any time without penalty.

Certificates of deposit usually pay the highest rate of interest, but you incur a penalty if you withdraw the principal before the end of the time period. Often these certificates do not compound the interest like time deposits do. They often require substantial amounts for purchase.

Many other vehicles are available for saving. You should compare their earnings with the ones listed above and select the best rate you can get for the amount of money you have. If you are just starting your savings, you may start with the passbook account. When you accumulate enough to qualify for a higher rate in another kind of account, you can transfer your money to the higher-rate account.

Loans and Credit

Borrowing money is the opposite of saving money. When you save in a passbook account or other vehicle, you are loaning your money to the institution and they pay you for the loan. When you borrow money from one of these institutions, they charge you for the loan. When you buy things on the installment plan, you are borrowing money at an interest rate and getting earlier use of the item than you would get if you saved your money for it. The cost of the interest should be calculated as part of the cost of the item. When you save for an item, the interest you earn will aid you in getting the item sooner than you otherwise would.

Cash buyers pay the least money for items. Cash buyers can shop around for the lowest price and are not tempted to overbuy. Dealers know this and offer "easy credit terms" to encourage noncash buyers who are tempted to overbuy to use their stores.

When you charge or buy things on credit, you have the privilege of enjoying the purchase while you pay for it. You can gain discipline by making regular payments on the price plus interest, but you will pay more than a cash buyer.

Some good times for using credit are:

1. When you are trying to establish your household and you need appliances immediately, such as a refrigerator.
2. When you have a genuine emergency for which you do not have cash.
3. When attractive seasonal sales or specials offer lower prices that make the item comparable to a cash purchase *and* you really need the item.

4. When you are using the money to invest in college or other education. Borrowing money for education usually pays off in increased income for the borrower.
5. When the price of something you need is increasing sharply.

Poor times for buying on credit or borrowing money are:

1. When you don't have a reasonable prospect of repaying the amount.
2. When you are buying something on impulse and the payment terms seem so easy that you think you can make them.
3. When you are buying something to boost your morale.
4. When you are trying to increase your status.
5. When your credit purchases strain your cash reserves and wreck your budget because your payments are so high.
6. When you are purchasing with the expectation of future salary increases.

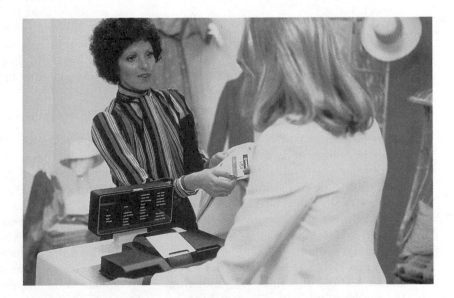

Illus. 5-9. A good time for using credit is when attractive seasonal sales or specials offer lower prices *and* you really need the item.

7. When you are gambling on something risky.
8. When you are using the borrowed money to maintain your daily expenses.
9. When what you are buying will wear out before you make the last payment.

Use everything you know about credit when you are considering using it:

1. Shop around for credit and compare the costs. A credit card account often charges you more interest than a bank would for a loan for the same amount.
2. Keep a close check on your installment loan payments to be sure they don't tax your day-to-day expense budget.
3. Ask lots of questions about the credit deal you are making. The annual percentage rate is the most comparable rate you can use to evaluate various deals. Actual interest over the term of the loan can be compared.
4. To be sure you are not being hooked into an "easy payment plan" by the seller, ask yourself if you would buy the item for cash if you had the cash.
5. Before you sign any contract, study it carefully, and be sure you keep a copy of the contract.
6. Keep copies of your receipts or cancelled checks showing your payments.
7. Stagger your installment debt purchases. Pay off one before you take on another. Don't pile one payment on another.
8. Have the courage to say no if anything looks out of order when you are investigating the deal. Take time to think things over and compare deals. If no time is allowed you for thinking, the deal probably cannot bear the scrutiny you would give it; it has flaws and you should avoid it.
9. Remember that most of the time you cannot cancel the debt by returning the merchandise; you still owe the debt whether you keep the merchandise or not.
10. Never buy anything on credit unless you know the APR (annual percentage rate of interest) and never borrow money from a loan shark. Don't sign a contract for debt that has blank spaces in it, and never co-sign a note for anyone whose debt you are not willing to pay.

Good use of credit can establish you as a good credit risk and allow you to enjoy many things while you pay for them. Poor use of credit can wreck your reputation in your community and make life more difficult for you in many ways. Keep the considerations for the proper use of credit uppermost in your mind when you decide to use it. Misuse of it will follow you for many years hampering your purchase of a home, a car, and many smaller items on credit when you need them.

——————— *Time Management* ———————

If you are achieving what you want in life, you probably already manage time like you want to. If you are rushed, pressed for time, torn in many directions, and always have many things you want to do but can't, you probably cannot manage time to suit yourself.

Poor Time Management

People on their first jobs face demands on their time they have not had before. They think the answer is to work longer and harder. They may temporarily grow under such a burden. Usually, though, they simply become less sensitive to their own needs and more demanding of themselves in terms of time and energy. Such a situation will not allow you to thrive for long. Sooner or later you must learn to manage time.

Some of the symptoms of people who are pressured by time are:

1. They often appear preoccupied.
2. They become irritable.
3. They become critical of others.
4. They look for excuses for what is happening to them.

If you find yourself in these situations, recognize the need to make some changes in the way you handle time.

Your time is one of your most valuable resources. It is in essence your life. You have the opportunity to make of it whatever you want. Take into consideration your personal needs — biological and social ones — and start controlling your time instead of letting it control you.

Personal Considerations

You will have an easier job if you take into consideration your biological preferences when you use your time. Each of us has energy cycles throughout each waking period. We have highs and lows throughout each day. You should make your list of things to do coincide with the lows and highs of your day. For example, if you operate with efficiency during the first few hours of your day, plan your demanding chores for that period. Reserve your less demanding chores for your low periods, which may be late morning and late afternoon. If you find that you have chores scheduled for you that do not correspond with your most productive time, you can boost your energy for that time with a protein snack. Avoid sugar because although it raises energy levels quickly, the aftershock very quickly lowers blood sugar to below where you started. It is a very short-lived energy booster.

Also take into account your tolerance for tasks. Can you complete three demanding tasks consecutively without a break with a less demanding one? If so, you can schedule three in a row. If not, keep in mind that you need a mindless task interspersed among the more demanding ones.

Can you tolerate a closely scheduled day or do you need downtime scheduled? Most people need at least one hour a day for unexpected events and time for themselves. Avoid scheduling yourself so closely that you don't have that time for yourself.

Overscheduling yourself may make you preoccupied most of the time thinking about one thing as you work at another. You may visualize yourself doing something else (daydreaming) and make costly mistakes. Organizing your time requires some self-examination. What are you visualizing most of the time? What are you seeing in your mind's eye? You will act according to the pictures in your mind. To gain greater control of yourself, learn to refine your pictures. That is, picture yourself doing what you want to be doing.

Be more alert to what is going on around you by visualizing it more accurately and by taking it one thing at a time. Usually, too many pictures occur before you get one thing done. You have to slow down the pictures before you can accomplish anything. If not, you will be picturing one thing while you are trying to accomplish something else. Preoccupation! Output is reduced by such distraction.

Such divided attention drains you of energy, too. Thinking about one thing while working at another takes twice the energy that thinking about and performing the single job does. Divided attention causes you to make mistakes also which eventually costs you time by requiring you to correct mistakes.

When you are preoccupied and working with others, you will fail to see when your listeners are confused and when they need help. You will fail to notice when your boss hints to you that you need to make improvements and makes vital points about work. When you are preoccupied you may speak out of turn and destroy relationships that are important to you. So, one key to gaining control of your time is to gain control of your concentration on matters at hand. If you are wondering whether or not you are suffering from preoccupation, some physical clues are:

talking in a monotone
chewing food steadily without change of pace
holding a position for long periods of time without moving
jiggling a foot
rubbing your hands
doodling

Good time management will help you overcome preoccupation because you have time for those things you daydream about. Other activities may be used to help you break the habit of being preoccupied.

Change your routine. If you read the same paper every day, not remembering a single thing when you finish, switch to another paper or to another source for news. If you follow a routine in dressing for work, change it. If you always follow a certain route to work, vary it. By exposing yourself to these simple new environments and procedures you will be forced to give them your attention. You cannot think about something else while you are following new procedures or routes.

At work, change your routines. If you jump into a conversation immediately when someone pauses, practice waiting a few seconds before you reply or raise an issue. Avoid criticizing, making excuses, and disagreeing when you can't offer a better solution. Check what you are hearing in a conversation by asking questions for clarification. Watch speakers to see if their facial expressions and body postures correspond with what they are saying.

As you practice concentrating, check yourself regularly for tenseness. Try to relax while you are in action.

A time-saver you may not think about is exercise. Exercise takes time; how can it save time? Exercise increases your stamina and makes you work more efficiently. As you increase your body strength and endurance, you need less energy to perform routine tasks. That means you have more energy for other tasks and can perform with more efficiency than you can if you are tired.

Another time-saver is good eating habits. Time is wasted when you constantly need a pick-up snack to get you through your next chore. Well-balanced meals, with necessary nutrients, vitamins, minerals, bulk, and so on, approximately three times a day can save you time in snacking that you must do otherwise when you have low blood sugar resulting from lack of appropriate nutrients and poor eating habits.

Scheduling Devices

Besides accommodating your personal needs, the use of scheduling devices and activities can help you to better manage your time.

"To do lists" are the starting place for organizing your time and making sure you know what you want to do with your time. By making lists, you free your mind to concentrate on what you are doing at the time without having to remember what you planned to do next. You have full attention to devote to your current project.

Week-at-a-Glance Book

One of the best organizers you can use is a calendar called a "week-at-a-glance" meaning that the seven days of the week are shown on a single page with places to write beside the days. This book can be your appointment book, your reminder both for business and personal matters, and your record of business and personal activities. The Internal Revenue Service even accepts such a record as a diary of expenses for business purposes when you keep it appropriately.

If you decide to use such a book to keep appointments, both social and business, be sure you write not only the person's name and the appointment time and place, but also the person's telephone number so that if necessary you can call. That phone number usually is easy to get when you make the appointment. It may take a lot of time later if you have to hunt for it in a phone directory. It is just easier, simpler, and more efficient to write the phone number down at the time you record the appointment.

When you get notices to make certain pay-

ments, redeem certain coupons, or you receive other items which must be handled at some future time, use your week-at-a-glance to record the coming event on the appropriate date. At the time you are notified, record all the data you will need and you will not have to find your notice when the time comes to prepare for the action that needs to be taken.

Use your week-at-a-glance to record business activities such as when you asked for something, like a raise, a file, or an answer to a question. Then when you get the answer you

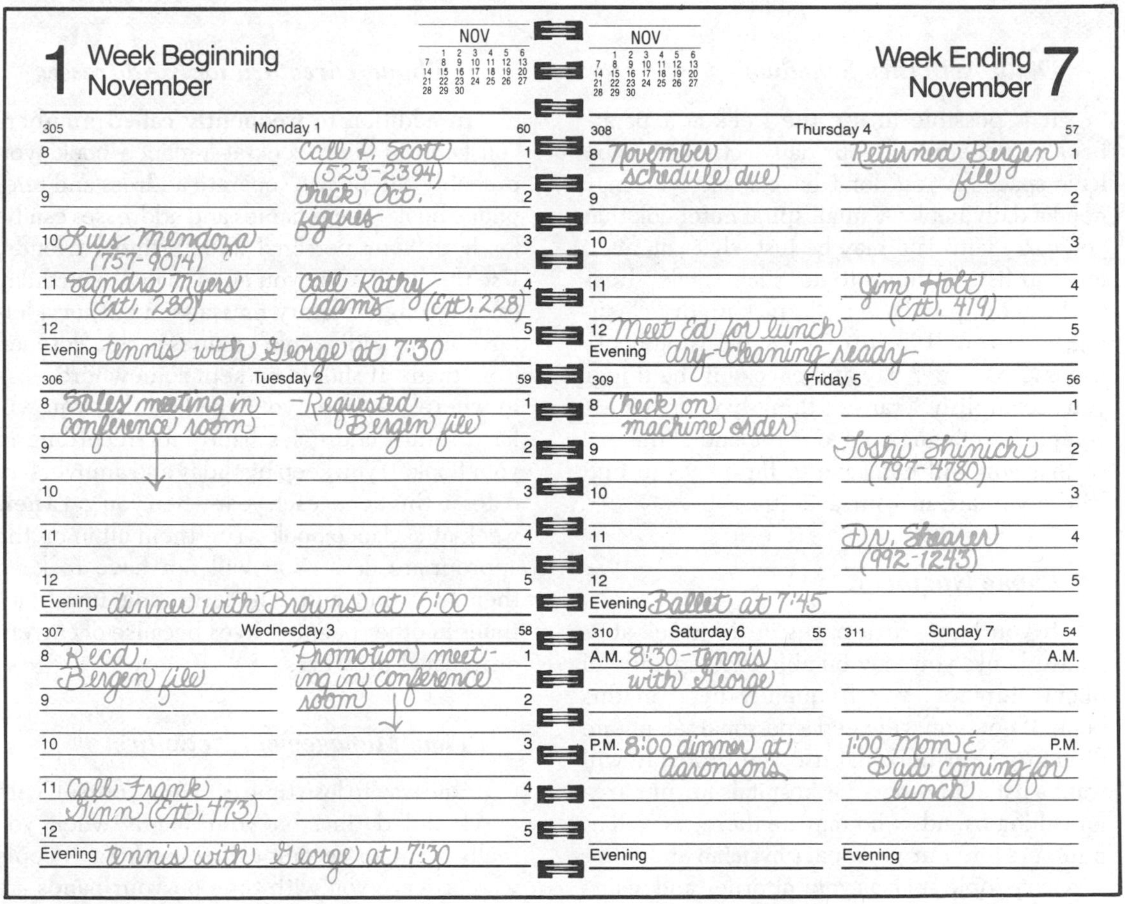

Illus. 5-10. Week-at-a-Glance Book

will have some record of how long things take for future reference. Also, in case someone denies being asked, you will have a definite record of asking. When you request personal things such as a repair, a price on something you wish to buy, or a medical appointment, make a note of the day you called as well as the later date you schedule the activity. You have a reference then for how long it takes to get specific things done. Also, if you have trouble later substantiating when a repair was made or requested, or how much something was supposed to cost, or when you were last ill or had your teeth cleaned, you have a record of it.

Daily Activities Schedule

It is possible to use the week-at-a-glance book for scheduling your daily activities if you have space. If you don't have space, you may need a daily book. A small spiral notebook that you carry with you may be just what you need for your lists of things to do, such as take shoes to the shop, purchase milk, pick up dry cleaning, and so on. If you use such a spiral notebook, use one page per day and check off the things you accomplish. Transfer things you do not accomplish to the next page at the end of the day so that you will not have to flip pages to find where you are in your activities.

Phone Numbers

If you have extra pages in the week-at-a-glance book, you may be able to keep a file of phone numbers you frequently need in this book. If not, you will need a personal telephone directory. For personal use you probably will want a list of numbers for hospitals in your area for calling friends who may be there, as well as numbers for your personal physician and other service people such as your attorney and insurance agent, so that as you need information

quickly from them you don't have to search for their numbers. You may want to include the numbers of your frequent tennis partners, your favorite luncheon partners, the airlines you frequently fly or the train schedule, the office supply store, your bank, and relatives that you call frequently. Emergency numbers, such as those for wreckers, ambulances, and service stations that make road calls, are nice to have in this book. You may find other numbers you need in your week-at-a-glance book. Add them. You can save yourself hours of hunting for phone numbers by keeping this list up to date and complete.

A Phone Directory with Addresses

In addition to frequently called numbers you keep in your week-at-a-glance book, you probably will need a separate address and telephone book. These names and addresses can be for both your personal and business friends. Use this book when you need to mail a birthday card, a congratulatory message, a gift, or a letter. Plan to add people's names as you get mail from them. It should be kept somewhere close to where you open your mail so that you will have return addresses handy for recording in your book. If you keep birthday and anniversary dates in this book, each year when you get a new week-at-a-glance book write them all in on the appropriate days. You will not have to keep them in mind and risk forgetting important times in other people's lives because of current or unusual pressures.

Time Management Activities

One way to lose time is to find yourself with unscheduled time on your hands when you really want to accomplish something. People who observe you with time on your hands are likely to want to help you waste it. If you look busy, people are likely to let you get on with your work. If you don't want to be interrupted, look busy.

Waiting. If you know you will have to wait in a line or for an appointment, take something with you that you've been wanting to read, or use the time to make lists of things you plan to buy or do so that you won't have to keep the list in your head, leaving mental space for other activities. Try to avoid waiting by planning your activities for periods when business is slow.

Long Jobs. When you have a job that you think will take two hours, you probably will look for a two-hour block of time to complete it. Finding such a block of time can take forever and waste a lot of your time. Think of the two-hour job as a series of six twenty-minute tasks.

You are more likely to find twenty minutes six times than you are to find a two-hour period.

Correspondence. At work when you handle correspondence, plan to read it only once. Don't read it now and place it aside for action later — you'll have to read it again. Read it now *and* make notes on it. Jot your reply or action intended on the letter or on a sheet of paper you clip to the letter. Then lay it aside if the time is not right for handling it. The next time you see it you only have to read your notes and follow through. You don't have to read everything twice and make decisions twice. That takes twice as long.

Hunting for Things. Time spent hunting for things you need is time wasted. The way to avoid having to hunt for things is to learn to be

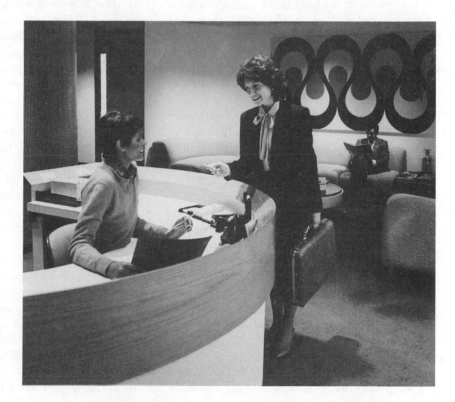

Illus. 5-11. If you know that you will have to wait for an appointment, take something with you that you've been wanting to read, or use the time to make a list of things you plan to do or buy.

consistent. Car and house keys need a particular place in your home and on your person. If the key isn't in the ignition or lock, you should know exactly where it is whether you are at home or out. All you have to do is designate a place and be consistent.

Receipts for coat check, parking, baggage checking, and other such activities should have a particular place. If you always place them there, you won't spend time looking for them. You won't lose them. Be sure you designate a place that is always available. If you place receipts in your wallet, be sure you always carry a wallet. If you select a particular pocket, be sure you always have such a pocket. The key to avoid having to hunt for things is consistency, and you must consistently have a place for those things.

If you do find yourself looking for something that normally has a place, make a note (in your week-at-a-glance book) about where you found it. Then if you ever lose it again, you will have a clue about where you are likely to misplace it. The same is true of files in your business. If you cannot immediately locate a file you need and must search for it, make a note of where you found it when you do. You should keep a running list of such losable files so that you get a clue to how your mind misfunctions in filing when it does.

Dealing with People

If you need to have a meeting with a person at work or during the workday, plan to use your mealtime for business. Ask that person to lunch and spend that time discussing the problem or issue. You will then be using that time for productive work and save office time for completing your own work without waiting for an appointment or a meeting with the person.

When you are planning activities with others, make firm commitments. Try to avoid tentative plans that require follow-up action to confirm them. The tracking down of people to confirm plans that you have can take a lot of time you don't have to spend. Such tracking down and confirming is a waste. Commit firmly to action with an escape plan if either of you must cancel — not confirm.

Learn to control your own time with people instead of letting others control it for you. You can, for example, plan to take and make calls at a particular time of the day and avoid telephone interruptions throughout the day that take you away from your work and slow you down. Set an amount of time you are willing to wait for people with whom you have plans. Let others know that you can wait only a set period of time. They will then know that if for any reason they cannot make it within your waiting period they need not hurry —you will not be there.

Inventory your time spent with people. Do you find that you spend a lot of time with people who aren't very important to you in activities that bore you? Are you keeping up acquaintances with people with whom you have very little in common? If you are, you probably are shortchanging the people who are important to you and with whom you have a lot in common because you have a limited amount of time.

The way to avoid spending time with people who have become habit rather than people you care for is to be firm. You learn to say "no" without being rude. When you are asked to do something, you probably are tempted to say something like "Let me check my calendar and call you back." What you really mean is that you want to think it over and make up a reason for not doing something that you find only marginally interesting or for which you don't have time. Calling someone back with your response takes time as does formulating the response.

You will do better to give a polite no. "I'm sorry. I will decline this time, but thanks for thinking of me. I'll call you when my time pressures ease." That leaves it up to you to resume the relationship if and when you want to. It cuts

Illus. 5-12. Good time management will allow you to spend more time doing things you really want to do.

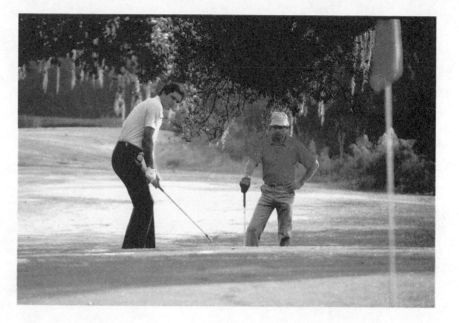

off the mulling over and time wasting you do when you continue marginal activities with people who are not important to you. You will find yourself with more time to spend with those that you do care for, doing things you really want to do.

Questions for Chapter 5

1. What benefits can you expect a money management plan to provide for you?
2. How can you find out what you need for day-to-day expenses?
3. What vehicle do most people use for handling money?
4. What are some features offered in checking accounts?
5. What are some services offered by banks?
6. What are some good rules for writing checks?
7. Why should you reconcile your bank statement?
8. What records are important to keep for tax purposes?
9. What are various features of savings accounts?
10. How is a loan different from a savings account?
11. What are good uses of credit?
12. What are poor uses of credit?
13. What biological tendencies must you consider in planning your time?
14. What is wrong with being preoccupied?
15. How can you overcome preoccupation?
16. What are some good scheduling devices?
17. What can you keep in a week-at-a-glance book?
18. What can you do when you are waiting?
19. How can you schedule a long job?
20. What can you do to help avoid hunting for things?
21. How can you handle your time better in dealing with people?

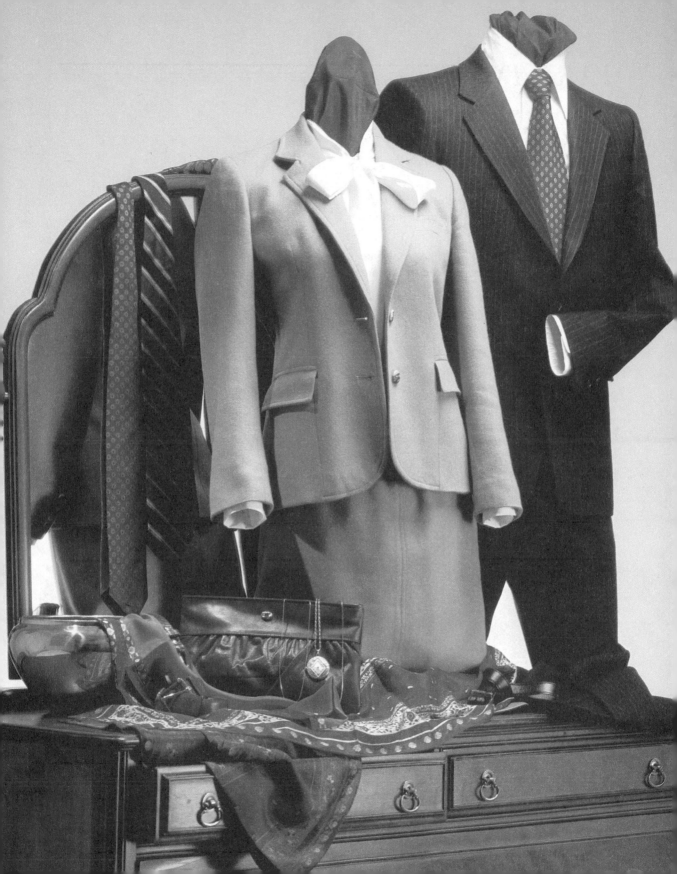

PART TWO: *Professional Image*

Part Objectives

After studying this part, you should be able to:

1. *Assemble a business wardrobe that will make you effective on your first business job.*

2. *Choose among colors and lines that give you the tall, thin look desired in business.*

3. *Groom your face so that your expressions contribute to your effectiveness in business.*

4. *Groom your hair so that it contributes to an appearance that enhances your effectiveness in business.*

5. *Recognize and exhibit postures that are acceptable in business, both aesthetically and communicatively.*

Chapter 6

Dressing for Business

Chapter Objectives

After studying this chapter, you should be able to:

1. *Recognize suitable business clothes.*
2. *Recognize the characteristics of a business suit.*
3. *Recognize the shirts and blouses suitable for business wear.*
4. *Select appropriate accessories for effective business wear.*
5. *Assemble a business wardrobe that will start you on your first business job.*
6. *Shop intelligently for good quality and good prices in business clothes.*
7. *Judge good fit for business clothes.*
8. *Care for your business clothes to protect your investment and keep you well dressed.*

When you enter a job that has an official uniform, you are told about it. When you enter a job that doesn't have an official uniform, you usually have to figure out on your own what you are expected to wear. Unlike police, nurses, and priests, who have official uniforms, business is a profession with an "unofficial uniform."

The unofficial status of the uniform makes it no less important to the wearer than a uniform of official status. Consider the plight of a police officer out of uniform trying to direct traffic. It's possible to do the job out of uniform, but much more difficult. The uniform itself doesn't make the person more capable or more authoritative, but people immediately perceive a *uniformed*

officer to be able and to have authority to direct traffic. You will find that the unofficial business uniform has the same impact in business as the police uniform does on the street — people assume you have the ability and authority to do your job when you are "in uniform."

——— *The Business Uniform* ———

Unlike the police uniform, each person's "business uniform" is *not* identical to the next person's; and no central supplier issues you one. What, then, makes "business uniforms" uniform?

- *Style*. Compared to other clothes, business clothes are conservative in cut, fabric, color, and fit.
- *Selection*. Business "uniforms" are usually suits (men and women) and dresses with jackets (women).

The most often worn business clothes can be described. Some businesses, however, will not be typical, and some people in business will not dress typically. The beginner, however, can observe the general rules of typical business dressing and be assured of being dressed appropriately for business.

The Suit

The item of clothing most conservative (and most reliable for beginners) in business for both men and women is a suit. The business suit has important characteristics:

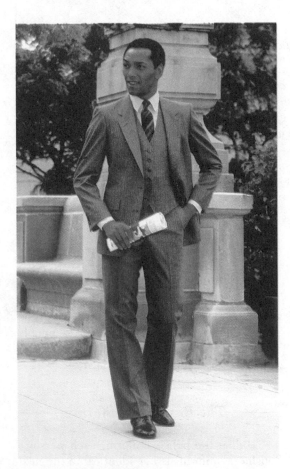

Illus. 6-1. Compared to other clothes, business clothes are conservative in cut, fabric, color, and fit.

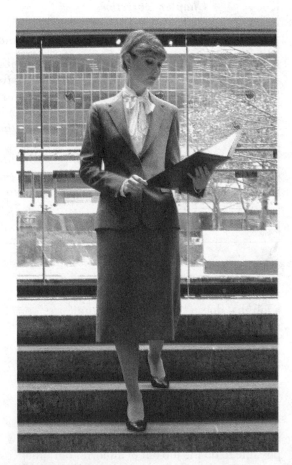

Illus. 6-2. The item of clothing most reliable in business for both men and women is the suit.

1. The jackets are tapered very little at the waist for both men and women.
2. The contours of the body are obscured by the jacket.
3. The woman's skirt is neither too full nor too tight but hangs straight or flares gently, obscuring the contours of the body, and falls within one or two inches below the knee.
4. The pants for both men and women have legs that are neither too narrow nor too flared, having enough room at the hips and thighs to hang from the waist without wrinkling. They are comfortable for standing and sitting, and they fall nicely over the top of the shoe.

Suit Fabrics and Patterns

The best fabrics for business suits are wool, linen, and synthetics that look and feel like wool and linen. Fabrics that do not wrinkle easily are best. For winter, suits are woven in flannel and tweed. Broadcloth, gabardine, and hopsacking weaves are used for year-round wear.

The patterns in fabrics that look most professional are:

• Solids
• Tweeds
• Muted Plaids

Men wear a fourth pattern, the pinstripe, very well. The pinstripe suit, however, usually makes women look masculine.

Suit Colors

Colors found in business suits for both men and women are:

• Dark blue
• Medium, charcoal, or steel gray
• Black
• Camel
• Beige

In addition, women wear dark brown, dark maroon, medium blue, and dark rust. Colors that are not usually worn for business suits are pastels, bright colors, most shades of green, and mustard.

Suit Styles

The style of suit for business may be either single- or double-breasted, although single-breasted styles look better on most people. The coats may have either a center vent or side vents in back. The business suit has no unusual buttons, no unusual stitching, no patches on the sleeves, no belts on the back of the jacket, no yolk, and no leather ornamentation.

Shirts and Blouses

The business suit, of course, is worn with either a shirt or a blouse. Both men and women wear the tailored shirt. Men wear it with a tie; women leave one button open with the collar worn inside the coat collar. Women also wear blouses with a soft bow at the neckline. Blouses with low necklines, ruffles, and other eye-catching treatments are not worn. Sleeves are long enough to show about one-half to one-

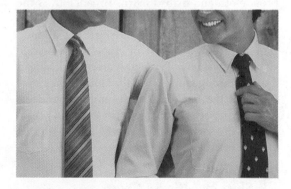

Illus. 6-3. Men wear the tailored shirt with a tie.

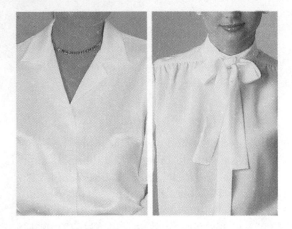

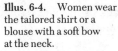

Illus. 6-4. Women wear the tailored shirt or a blouse with a soft bow at the neck.

fourth inch below the suit coat sleeve. The cuff of the shirt or blouse should just cover the wrist bone.

Shirt and Blouse Fabrics and Weaves

The fabrics for tailored shirts are cotton and blends that look like cotton. Blouses are often of somewhat softer fabrics of silk and blends that look like silk. The best weaves for shirts are broadcloth and oxford cloth. Broadcloth is the finer weave; oxford cloth gives a thicker, heavier look because the threads are not as fine. Blouses are often made of crepe de chine and shantung weaves. Typically, crepe de chine is a soft, draping fabric good for blouses that have a bow at the neckline. Shantung is characterized by an occasional thick thread on an otherwise plain surface. If woven of silk, shantung gives a crisp look.

Shirt and Blouse Colors

The most easily matched and therefore most popular blouses and shirts are solid colors.

White and most pastels are the colors for shirts and blouses for business wear with suits. Men's shirts are usually lighter in color than their suits (to avoid the gangster look). Women's blouses and shirts, however, may be either lighter or darker than the suit color.

Shirt and Blouse Patterns

More difficult to coordinate but still good for business wear are shirts that are striped. Dark, thin stripes (pinstripe) on a white background are most often worn. Very simple plaids with very thin lines, both horizontal and vertical, are worn with the business suit. Polka dots, wavy stripes, intricate patterns such as paisleys, and multicolored shirts are not usually worn for business, especially by men. Women who wear them risk being "out of uniform."

Ties

A tie customarily worn by men in business is made of silk or polyester that looks like silk. The ties are either solid colors or have small repeating diagonal stripes or small repeating figures such as dots, shields, animals, diamonds, etc. Ties with large symbols and pictures and ties with patterns hard to look at are not good for business. Neither are bow ties. The usual weaves for tie fabrics are crepe de chine, shantung, batiste, and pongee. Twills, challis, and brocades are also used.

The knot of a business tie should be suited to the shirt collar and bulk of the tie. If the tie is bulky and the collar spread narrow, a small knot such as the four-in-hand knot is used. A wide spread collar and a tie that is not bulky takes a windsor knot. Other shirt collars and ties usually look good with a half-windsor knot. Illustration 6-6 on pages 90 and 91 shows how to tie the knots commonly used.

Ideally, when tied the tips should come to your belt buckle. The width of a tie should be determined by the width of lapel on the suit with which it is worn. Wear wide ties with wide lapels and narrow ties with narrow lapels.

Scarves

Scarves are not necessary for women's business wear like men's ties are, but they are worn frequently with women's business suits and dresses. Scarves are useful to add a contrast for interest to an ensemble much the way a tie does. They can be used to give a completed look to a dress with a plain neckline or a jacket with no collar.

Silk and polyester are the best fabrics for scarves. Solids, stripes, plaids, polka dots, and paisleys are appropriate patterns on scarves for women's business wear. The best weaves are

soft ones such as crepe de chine, batiste, challis, and broadcloth.

Dresses

In addition to business suits, dresses are worn by women in business. The dresses are usually of two styles:

- A shirtwaist dress worn with a blazer.
- A tailored dress worn with a matching jacket.

Solid colors which are the same as for the women's business suit are the colors used for dresses. In addition to solids, women's dresses may be patterned in stripes, paisleys, and checks. Florals and feminine prints are too casual for wear in business. Long sleeves are appropriate for year-round wear and three-

Illus. 6-5. Scarves are worn frequently with women's business suits and dresses.

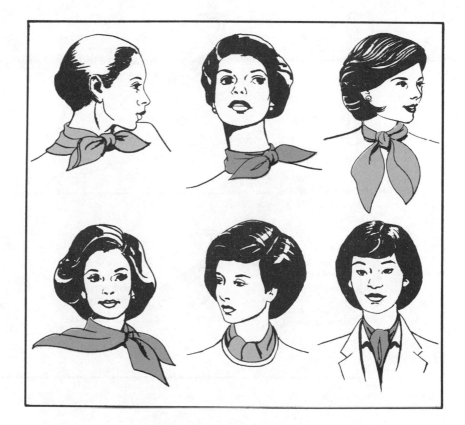

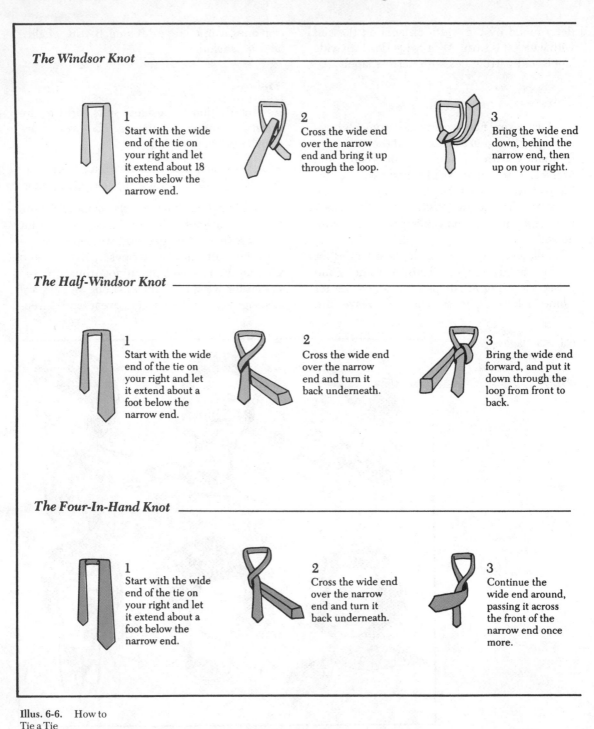

The Windsor Knot

1 Start with the wide end of the tie on your right and let it extend about 18 inches below the narrow end.

2 Cross the wide end over the narrow end and bring it up through the loop.

3 Bring the wide end down, behind the narrow end, then up on your right.

The Half-Windsor Knot

1 Start with the wide end of the tie on your right and let it extend about a foot below the narrow end.

2 Cross the wide end over the narrow end and turn it back underneath.

3 Bring the wide end forward, and put it down through the loop from front to back.

The Four-In-Hand Knot

1 Start with the wide end of the tie on your right and let it extend about a foot below the narrow end.

2 Cross the wide end over the narrow end and turn it back underneath.

3 Continue the wide end around, passing it across the front of the narrow end once more.

Illus. 6-6. How to Tie a Tie

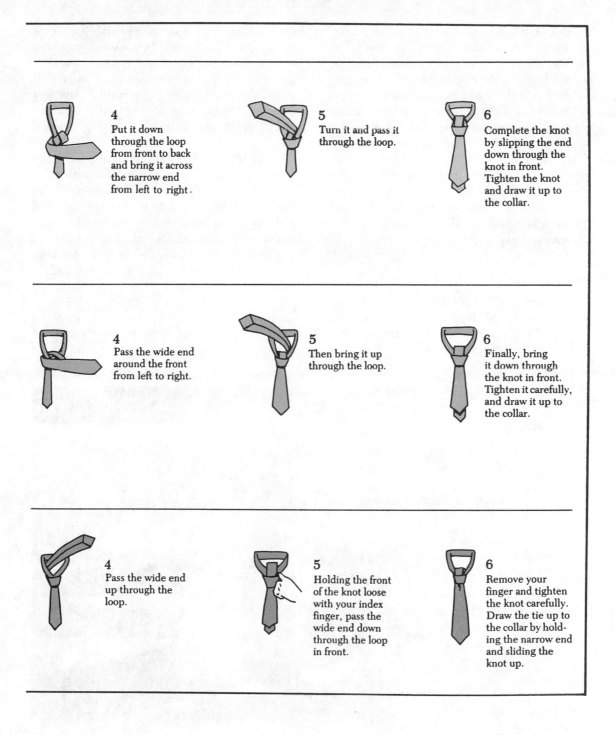

4 Put it down through the loop from front to back and bring it across the narrow end from left to right.

5 Turn it and pass it through the loop.

6 Complete the knot by slipping the end down through the knot in front. Tighten the knot and draw it up to the collar.

4 Pass the wide end around the front from left to right.

5 Then bring it up through the loop.

6 Finally, bring it down through the knot in front. Tighten it carefully, and draw it up to the collar.

4 Pass the wide end up through the loop.

5 Holding the front of the knot loose with your index finger, pass the wide end down through the loop in front.

6 Remove your finger and tighten the knot carefully. Draw the tie up to the collar by holding the narrow end and sliding the knot up.

quarter length sleeves are good for summer.

Fabrics for dresses vary widely. Wool, linen, and fabrics that look like wool and linen are good fabrics for business. Denim, corduroy, clinging, and shiny fabrics usually are not worn for business. Fabrics that hold their shape through many wearings and those that do not wrinkle are the best buys. Broadcloth, oxford cloth, gabardine and challis are the most common dress fabric weaves. Dresses may also be made of lightweight flannel, tweed, and hopsacking weaves. Because crepe de chine and shantung fabrics shine, they are rarely good for a business dress.

Blazers

A blazer is different from a suit coat because it often has metal, leather, or other unusual buttons. The blazer is not considered as conservative as a suit coat. For women, it is worn over a conservative dress acceptably even in conservative businesses. When men or women wear a blazer with contrasting pants or a skirt (for women) the outfit is only marginally suitable for business. In less conservative situations blazer-pants/skirt combinations will be acceptable. In very conservative situations, they will not.

The blazer colors most often worn are navy blue and camel. Navy teams well with rust, camel, beige, and gray. Camel teams well with black, navy blue, and dark brown. Pure wool and wool blended with a synthetic fabric of a year-round weight are the most useful fabrics. The most often worn weaves are flannel in winter and hopsacking or linen for year-round.

Coats

Overcoats usually worn for business are of two types: a raincoat and a winter coat.

Illus. 6-7. Raincoats are usually of a heavy cotton-polyester blend with a zip-out lining.

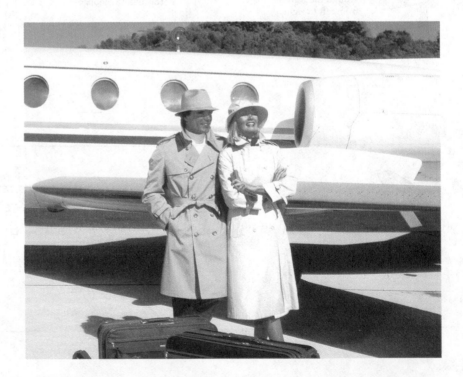

Raincoats are usually of a heavy cotton-polyester blend with a zip-out lining. They are belted and are long enough on women to cover the longest skirt; for men, they fall just below the knee. The colors are beige and navy blue for both men and women. Women also wear black.

Winter coats are of the chesterfield style for both men and women, in the same colors as suits. Women also wear the wrap-around, belted coat in a camel color.

The simpler the detail on an overcoat — no extra buttons, pockets, etc. — the better the coat for business. The winter coat is of a wool fabric or a wool blend. It should be the same length as the raincoat; however, men can wear the shorter coat that falls above the knee.

Shoes

The appropriate shoe for men to wear with a business suit is leather in either the slip-on or lace-up style. Both wing-tip and plain lace-up shoes are appropriate. Slip-ons should not have large buckles or other non-leather trim. Men's shoes are solid black, brown, and cordovan.

Multicolored and patent leather shoes usually are not worn for business.

For women, the business suit usually is worn with a basic plain pump with a heel of about two inches in a solid-color leather. A wider range of colors is worn by women, including navy blue, black, dark brown, gray, cordovan, camel, and beige. Shoes not worn with business clothes are those with platform soles, multicolored shoes, and barefoot sandals.

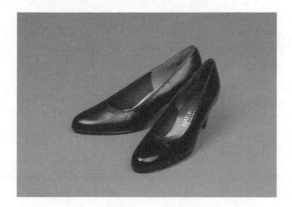

Illus. 6-9 (above). For women, the business suit usually is worn with a basic plain pump.

Illus. 6-10 (below). For women, a heel of about two inches is appropriate in business.

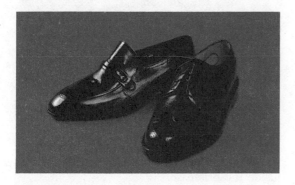

Illus. 6-8. The appropriate shoe for men to wear with a business suit is leather in either the slip-on or lace-up style.

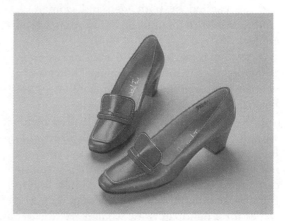

Hosiery

Women wear skin-colored hosiery with business clothes and men wear dark, solid-color, over-the-calf socks. Women's hose are usually made of nylon and are sometimes combined with spandex for support. Hose with reinforced toes and heels wear longer than hose with sheer toes and heels. However, if either your toes or heels show, be sure no reinforcing does.

Men's socks may be made of any number of kinds of fabrics. Cotton and wool are the most absorbent and wash easily. Orlon and other synthetics wash and wear well. Cashmere may need to be hand washed.

Accessories

The accessories you wear with your business clothes are almost as important as the clothes themselves for establishing your credibility.

Leather

Leather and materials that look like leather are used for belts, briefcases, wallets, and handbags. Belts are usually plain with simple buckles. Briefcases are brown and cordovan colors and are carried by both men and women. A simple case with no unusual hardware is a good choice.

A wallet is carried by both men and women. Brown leather is the most popular; however, a woman may carry a wallet that matches either her handbag or her briefcase.

Women may also carry small leather handbags that fit into their briefcases. If you are able to fit your essential items into a wallet, you may not need a handbag. A small leather cosmetic case for a comb, lipstick, keys, etc., may fit into the briefcase and substitute along with the wallet for a handbag. Few women try to carry

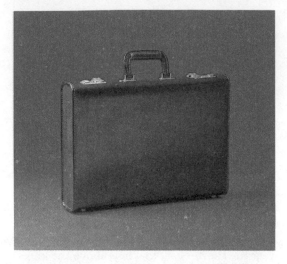

Illus. 6-11 (above). Briefcases are carried by both men and women.

Illus. 6-12 (below). Women may carry small leather handbags that fit into their briefcases.

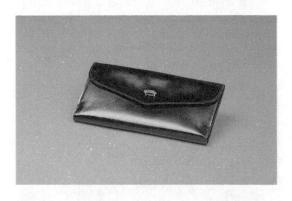

both a handbag and a briefcase. When both are needed, the handbag is usually carried inside the briefcase.

Jewelry

Very little jewelry is worn in business. Collar pins, tie clips, and lapel pins are not necessary and are rarely worn. If a shirt with French

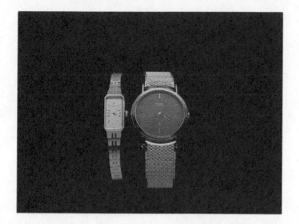

Illus. 6-13. A good watch is worn for business.

cuffs is worn, small cuff links in gold or silver are worn. A good watch with a leather or gold band is worn for business. One ring that is simple and does not bulge is a good choice for business. A wedding ring is appropriate if you are married.

People in business carry a pen and usually a pencil. A good quality gold or silver pen that costs you enough to be important to you is one you will always have with you.

Women in business may wear pendants with gold chains around their necks, but men do not. Women also wear small, not dangling, earrings. Small, simple jewelry is a good choice. Anything that dangles or is noisy is a poor choice.

Handkerchiefs

Handkerchiefs are carried by men in business but are rarely worn in their coat pockets. Handkerchiefs are white and made of linen or cotton. They should always be fresh. Women may carry a white handkerchief but usually find that facial tissues are acceptable for them. Whatever is carried is out of sight, tucked in either a pocket, a handbag, or a briefcase.

Building a Wardrobe

The number of suits, shoes, and other items you need depends on a number of factors. Frequency of cleaning is one factor. Clothes worn next to your body absorb the oil and moisture from it; and, therefore, they need to be washed and cleaned more often than clothes that are separated from your skin by shirts, blouses, and underwear.

Suit coats, pants, and skirts require cleaning when they no longer smell fresh and when they are soiled. Shirts, blouses, socks, hosiery, and underwear require washing every time you wear them; therefore, you will need many more of them.

Variety is another factor. Clothes and shoes need only a day's rest between wearing to regain their shape. Most people, however, tire of alternating between only two suits of clothing day after day and need one or two more ensembles for variety. By changing shirts, blouses, ties, and scarves, you can usually satisfy your need for variety with three or four suits and/or dress-jacket ensembles.

The First Ensemble

Usually the first business ensemble a person needs is a solid dark blue suit because it is appropriate for almost any interview, especially when it is teamed with a white shirt or blouse. A year-round fiber (wool or wool blend) in a year-round weave (broadcloth, hopsacking, or gabardine) is a good choice for a dark blue suit.

Additions

The next purchase for a man should be a suit from this list:

- Solid gray of any shade
- Dark blue pinstripe
- Gray pinstripe

- Blue and gray plaid

The next purchases for a woman are either dresses or suits in:

- Solid gray of any shade
- Blue in medium shades
- Maroon, beige, camel, rust, or dark brown

or dresses (not suits) in blue or gray pinstripes or plaids. If the dresses have no matching jackets, they should be teamed with a blazer of either navy, camel, or possibly black.

Some clothes and colors are not commonly worn in very conservative businesses but may be acceptable in your particular business. Avoid depending on these choices when you are unfamiliar with the peculiar dictates of your situation. Choose from this list only when you know firsthand that these clothes are acceptable.

For men, suits in

- Camel
- Beige
- Black

For men, blazers in

- Navy
- Camel

For women, dresses and suits in

- Black
- Dark Green

Shirts and Shoes

Although many colors may be attractively coordinated with the suits you select, not all combinations are suitable for business. Because shirts and blouses should be freshly laundered each time you wear them, you may want several, even duplicates, in the most commonly worn solid colors — pastel blue, pastel yellow, and white. Narrow stripes of dark blue and dark maroon on white backgrounds are also good choices. Illustration 6-14 shows shirts

and shoes commonly worn with business suits and dresses.

Most men in business get along well with two pairs of black shoes and several pairs of black socks. Women in business usually keep black, brown, and perhaps navy shoes. They may seasonally also wear beige and camel colors. Several pairs of hose in beige and light taupe are needed.

Shopping

One of the most important things you do for your wardrobe is to plan your shopping for it. Carefully note which stores sell the brands you like and when their sales are. Check on store policies, and time your purchases carefully.

Brand Names

After you have purchased clothing of the style you need for a while, you will become familiar with the brand names that seem to meet your needs best. If you already know some that you like, you can place a few phone calls to the local stores to find out whether or not they carry the lines. If they do, ask about how complete their stock is or when they expect it to be replenished. If you are not familiar with the brands that suit your needs, take note of those that you try on that you especially like if they fit and are within your price range. If you are alert when you shop, you will soon find certain stores and certain clerks that simplify your shopping by having and knowing what you need and like. After you have shopped with them a few times and they know what you want, some clerks will call you when they receive items in which they think you will be interested.

Sales

Beware of sale merchandise. Stores usually have two kinds of "sales." One sale is usually a

SUITS	Dark Blue	Gray	°Blue Pinstripe	°Gray Pinstripe	Blue Plaid	Gray Plaid	*Medium Blue	*Maroon	Beige	Camel	*Rust	*Dark Brown	Black	*Dark Green
SHIRTS AND BLOUSES –Solids–														
White	P	P	P	P	P	P	P	P	X	S	P	P	S	P
Blue	P	P	P	P	P	P	P	P	P	P	P	P	X	P
Yellow	P	P	P	P	P	P	P	P	X	X	P	P	X	P
Tan	P	X	P	X	P	X	S	P	P	S	P	P	P	P
Beige	P	S	P	S	S	S	P	P	S	S	S	P	S	P
Rust	P	S	P	S	P	P	S	P	X	X	S	X	P	S
Gray	P	P	P	P	P	S	P	P	X	X	X	X	P	X
*Navy	X	S	X	X	X	S	X	S	P	S	X	X	X	X
*Black	X	S	X	X	X	S	X	S	S	S	X	X	S	S
*Pink	X	P	X	X	X	P	X	P	S	S	X	X	X	X
*Maroon	X	S	X	X	X	S	X	X	X	X	X	S	X	X
*Orange	S	S	X	X	S	S	X	X	X	X	S	S	X	X
*Red	X	S	X	X	X	S	X	X	P	X	X	X	X	X
Stripes on –White–														
Blue	P	P	S	S	S	S	S	P	S	P	S	X	X	S
Maroon	P	P	S	S	S	S	S	P	S	S	X	X	S	X
Brown	X	X	X	X	X	X	X	S	S	S	S	P	X	S
SHOES														
Black	P	P	P	P	P	P	P	P	X	S	S	X	P	P
Brown	X	X	X	X	X	X	X	X	P	P	P	P	X	P
Cordovan	S	S	S	S	S	S	S	P	P	P	P	X	X	S
*Gray	X	P	S	P	P	P	X	S	X	X	X	X	X	S
*Beige	S	S	S	S	S	S	S	S	P	S	S	S	S	S
*Camel	S	S	S	S	S	S	S	S	P	S	S	S	S	S
*Navy	P	P	P	P	P	P	P	P	P	P	S	X	X	S

°Men's suits and women's dresses *only.*
*Women's clothes *only.* All others apply to *both* men and women.

P=Preferred
S=Sometimes
X=Not Recommended

Illus. 6-14.   Color Combinations for Shirts/Blouses with Suits and Shoes with Suits bargain and one is not. The sale which offers regular merchandise for a lower than regular price is the only one that will interest you for your wardrobe. The other kind is one in which the store buys "sale" merchandise to market during its "sale." This sale merchandise is rarely of the quality that the store usually handles and frequently is a very poor investment as a permanent item in your wardrobe. Learn which sales are the ones that offer the kind of merchandise you need.

One of these sales may be the end-of-season sale when all seasonal merchandise that has not been sold is marked down before the new season's goods are put out. Avoid, however, buying anything of an extreme fashion during these end-of-season sales, because next season you may find it passé and therefore a waste of your money. Also, avoid tying up your money in next year's clothing when you really need it for next season's clothes. In March, it would not be wise to spend the money you planned for spring clothes on next winter's coat if you don't have appropriate spring clothes for April, May, and June of this year. Taking advantage of end-of-season sales can provide quality merchandise at lower-than-normal prices, but it also ties up this year's money in next year's clothes. Be sure you can afford to do that before you indulge in the end-of-season sale.

Sale items themselves can be traps. It is important that you be objective when considering a sale item. Be sure that it is something you would buy at the regular price, if money were no object, before you consider buying it at the sale price. No matter how inexpensive an item may be, if you don't use it, it is a waste of your money. Sometimes items are on sale that have buttons missing or a belt missing. Before you decide to purchase the items and replace the buttons or belt, check the cost of that kind of replacement. If it brings the total cost of the item up to or above the price of one with all the buttons and belt in place, you will be wasting your time in repairing a sale item.

There are sales that offer the kind of merchandise you will need. Be vigilant in learning the patterns of sales of the stores in your community and in learning which ones usually offer the kind of merchandise you want on sale. A sales clerk who helps you regularly can be your best friend in helping you to know the difference between the two kinds of sales.

Timing

Try to plan to do your shopping when you are not tired or hurried. If it is possible, plan to shop when the stores are not crowded, or at least at times other than the peak crowded periods. Be considerate when you shop. Explain what you want to a clerk and consider the clerk's suggestions. If the store's stock does not meet your needs, say so, thank the clerk, and leave. Sometimes, because the clerk does not fully understand your needs or does not thoroughly know the stock, items may be shown to you other than what you have described. Be firm in sticking to your shopping plan, and resist trying on items that do not fit your plan. You will save yourself time, and wear and tear on your nerves and energy.

Store Policies

Some stores are more cooperative than others about letting you purchase items "on approval." This means purchasing something, keeping your receipt, taking the item home, trying it with whatever you plan to wear with it, and returning it (without wearing it, of course) for a refund if it doesn't work with your ensemble. Check the store policy if you wish to use this procedure. It is, of course, better to take the item you want to coordinate with you because you save yourself the trouble of taking something back that doesn't work. Too, you have a better chance of coordinating if you use the item itself, rather than your memory, to match or contrast a color, line, or texture.

Prices

Getting the most value for your clothing money involves many factors. When you compare prices of garments, consider some of the hidden costs:

- *Alterations.* Alterations on men's suits are usually free. Women very often have to pay for them. Ask before you buy.
- *Cleaning.* Light colors look soiled sooner than dark colors, and they usually need to be cleaned more often to look fresh.
- *Pressing.* Wool and synthetic fibers need infrequent pressing. Clothes that have been treated for wrinkle resistance may often be washed and worn without pressing.
- *Quality.* Narrow seams and long stitches cost less to produce than wide seams and small stitches, but they also wear out faster and rip more easily. Good workmanship may cost more initially, but it usually is a good investment.

——————— *Fitting* ———————

Getting a good fit is perhaps the most important part of purchasing your wardrobe. Clothes that are too big or too small, too short or too long, or that simply do not fit your body are not good buys. Good fit is one area you cannot ignore and be well dressed. When you fit your clothes:

- Wear the undergarments you plan to wear with the garment.
- Allow for ease in your clothes.
- Be sure you can walk, bend, reach, and sit comfortably in the garment.

Jacket and Blazer Fit

The fit of your business suit is exact. The jacket should cover, not accentuate, the contours of your body. The lapels lie flat and the collar closely follows the contour of your neck. On the underside, the collar should be reinforced and stitches should be even and small. The shoulders fit snugly but allow for free movement of your arms. Most importantly, the jacket should feel comfortable.

The chest of the jacket should fit smoothly all the way around, with no wrinkles or bulges. Horizontal wrinkles in the back usually mean that the jacket is too tight; vertical ones mean that the jacket is too big.

The sleeve length should be approximately five inches above your thumb tip. The sleeve of the jacket leaves one-half to one-fourth inch of the shirt or blouse cuff showing. The shirt and blouse collar at the neck and the cuff at the wrist protect the suit jacket from undue wear and soil, and they minimize the frequency of cleaning needed.

Jacket lengths can vary. A longer jacket tends to shorten the silhouette and a shorter jacket gives a leggier look. The length of your jacket should be approximately the point where your fingers join your hand when your arms and hands hang flat against your sides.

The lining of the jacket should blend with the fabric color, not contrast with it. It should allow for ease in wearing but should not droop into view at the jacket hem or the sleeve hem.

A vest is optional for the business suit. If one is worn, it should fit close to the body, with no wrinkling or creasing. On men the last button of the vest is left unbuttoned.

Pants Fit

Suit pants should fit at the waist with space to comfortably slip your hand in and out of the waistband, but they should not bulge under

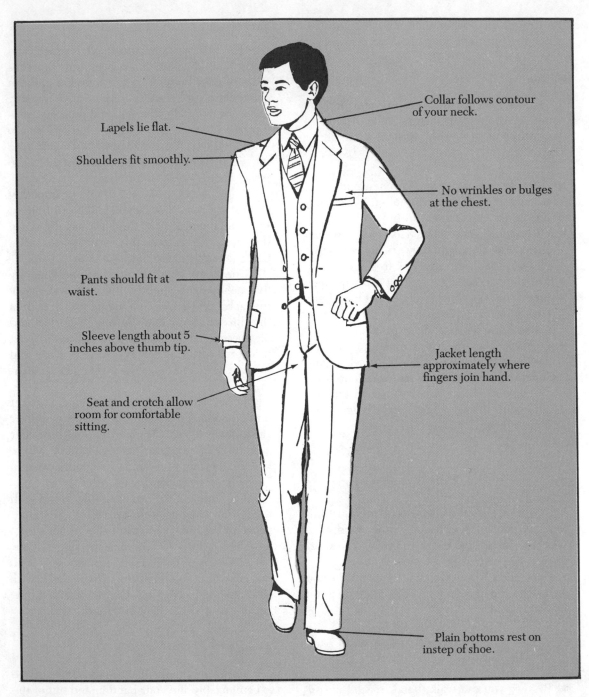

Collar follows contour of your neck.

Lapels lie flat.

Shoulders fit smoothly.

No wrinkles or bulges at the chest.

Pants should fit at waist.

Sleeve length about 5 inches above thumb tip.

Jacket length approximately where fingers join hand.

Seat and crotch allow room for comfortable sitting.

Plain bottoms rest on instep of shoe.

Illus. 6-15. Points to Check for a Good Fit in a Man's Suit

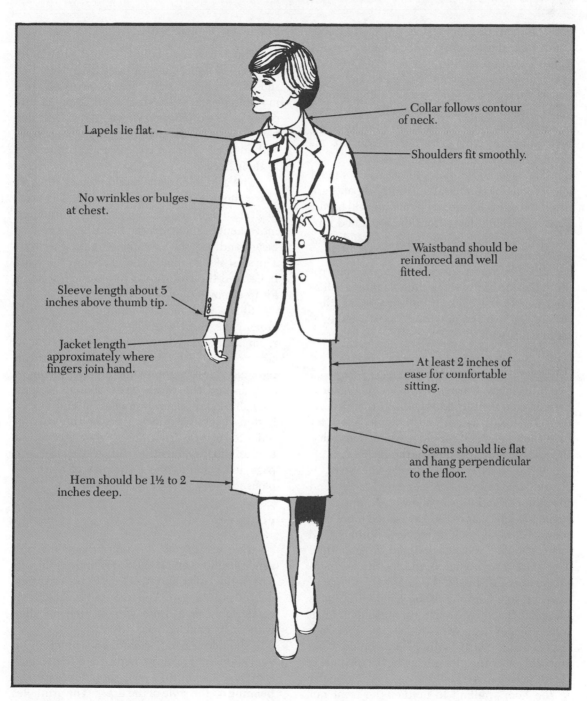

Collar follows contour of neck.

Shoulders fit smoothly.

Lapels lie flat.

No wrinkles or bulges at chest.

Waistband should be reinforced and well fitted.

Sleeve length about 5 inches above thumb tip.

Jacket length approximately where fingers join hand.

At least 2 inches of ease for comfortable sitting.

Seams should lie flat and hang perpendicular to the floor.

Hem should be 1½ to 2 inches deep.

Illus. 6-16. Points to Check for a Good Fit in a Woman's Suit your belt. Men usually wear suit pants waistbands near the navel. Women wear suit pants at the natural waistline.

The jacket chest measurement and waist measurement of a suit typically differ four to eight inches. A person with a waist size larger or smaller than those within the four-to-eight-inch range may have to have the intricate trouser recut alteration to get a good fit.

The seat and crotch area of pants should allow room for comfortable sitting. If pants are fitted too tight, horizontal wrinkling will occur. Pant legs should hang from the waist and hips without wrinkling or binding and should allow for comfortable sitting.

Plain-bottom pants should break and rest on the instep of the shoe, then slant one-half to one inch to the back. If cuffs are worn, they usually are two and one-fourth to two and one-half inches wide.

Skirt Fit

Suit skirts worn by women in business hang from a well-fitted waistband that is reinforced. The fit at the waist should allow for breathing space but should not be so loose that the waistband hangs low in the back.

If the skirt is of a straight-line style, it should have at least two inches of ease around the stomach and hips to allow room for ease in sitting. A-line shapes can have much more ease room. Closures such as zippers, buttons, and snaps should be concealed and lie smoothly. The skirt length that is most often worn in business is just below the knee.

The suit skirt should be lined with seams lying flat. The hem should be one and one-half to two inches deep with stitches invisible from the outside. Skirts with pleats should hang smoothly with the pleats hanging flat. Seams on skirts and pants should hang perpendicular to the floor, pulling to neither the front nor the back.

Shirt and Blouse Fit

The tailored collar on a shirt should fit closely when buttoned around the neck but should not be so tight that it wrinkles. Removable plastic collar stays aid in keeping this collar in place. (Button-down collars will not have stays.) Collars vary in height so that people with long necks can have collars in proportion to their necks.

The armhole seam should stop at the end of the shoulder bone or just beyond. The armhole should be large enough for comfortable movement but not so large that the sleeves are baggy and the shirt wrinkles under the arm. The shirt sleeve should fall just below the wrist bone, and the cuff should fit closely but allow for free movement.

Shirts and blouses should fit smoothly around the chest and waist with enough ease room for free movement but not so much as to cause a bulky look. They should taper gently at the waist, leaving approximately four inches of ease around the waist. They should be long enough to stay securely tucked in and have a button at least two inches below the waist in order to keep the front closed when the shirt or blouse slips out a little. Illustration 6-17 on page 103 contains the principles of shirt and blouse fit.

Dress Fit

Dresses vary in style more than suits, and generalizations about the fit are more difficult. Check the collar and neckline to be sure they do not pull or gap. You should be able to sit comfortably in a dress with a high neckline without its choking you.

Shoulder seams should end precisely at your shoulder bone or possibly one-fourth inch shorter or longer than your shoulder bone, depending on the style of the dress. The armholes should fit smoothly around your arm, not bind-

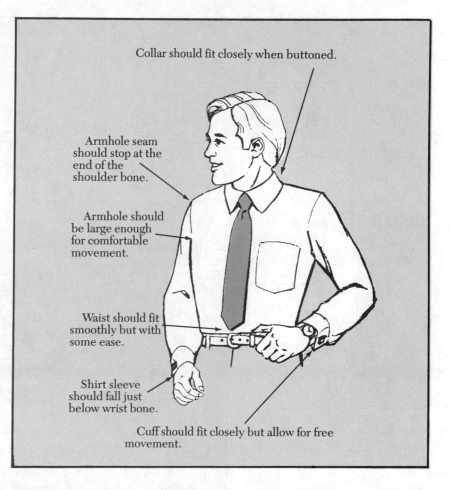

Collar should fit closely when buttoned.

Armhole seam should stop at the end of the shoulder bone.

Armhole should be large enough for comfortable movement.

Waist should fit smoothly but with some ease.

Shirt sleeve should fall just below wrist bone.

Cuff should fit closely but allow for free movement.

ing or gaping. Sleeve armholes must be comfortable — not tight, not sagging.

Bodice darts, if there are any, should end at the fullest part of your bust. If they end before that point or if the darts themselves are placed too high or too low, the dress will not fit smoothly. Side seams should be perpendicular to the floor. If they hang awry or are stretched to the back or front, the garment either does not fit or is constructed improperly.

The length should be somewhere near your knee. When you try the dress on, wear the same height shoe you plan to wear with the ensem-

ble. A higher heel usually takes a longer skirt to be in good proportion; a shorter heel, a somewhat shorter skirt.

If the dress has a natural waist, be sure it hits you at your natural waistline. It is possible to wear the waist one-fourth to one-half inch above your natural waist; but if the bodice is too long, the dress will appear wrinkled and too large for you.

Long sleeves should be long enough to cover your wristbone but not to cover part of your hand. Illustration 6-18 on page 104 contains the principles of dress fit.

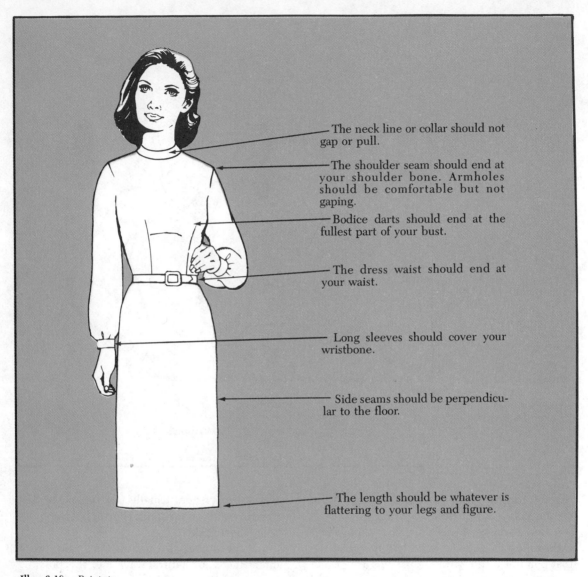

The neck line or collar should not gap or pull.

The shoulder seam should end at your shoulder bone. Armholes should be comfortable but not gaping.

Bodice darts should end at the fullest part of your bust.

The dress waist should end at your waist.

Long sleeves should cover your wristbone.

Side seams should be perpendicular to the floor.

The length should be whatever is flattering to your legs and figure.

Illus. 6-18. Points to Check for a Good Fit in a Dress

Fabric Care

When you select your clothes, read the fiber content and care labels carefully. These bits of information can make a big difference in your decision to buy or not to buy. The fiber content of the garment and whether it is washable or dry-cleanable only will appear on the label. Beyond that information, there are some other facts about fabrics that will help you in caring for them. Regardless of fiber content, garments that are lined, padded, or intricately assembled rarely should be washed.

Cotton

Cotton, one of the four natural textile fabrics (the others are wool, silk, and linen), is frequently used in clothing for warm weather and for clothes worn next to your skin because it absorbs perspiration and facilitates your body's cooling system efficiency. Cotton is usually washable but wrinkles easily unless it has been treated. The wrinkle-resistant finish may deteriorate with repeated washings. A hot iron is used on the wrong side of the dampened fabric to remove the wrinkles. Check to see whether or not any cotton garment you buy has been preshrunk or Sanforized. If not, expect it to shrink when you wash it.

Wool

Wool is often used for cold-weather clothing because its "breathing" action holds the warmth of your body. Wool, too, is absorbent and can be effectively used for warm-weather clothes. Unless wool garments specifically call for washing (which automatically means cold-water washing), have them dry-cleaned. The heat of a clothes dryer and the heat of an iron can shrink and destroy wool. To press wool, always use a press cloth, steam, and the wrong side of the fabric if possible. Wool rarely wrinkles much, and the wrinkles that do occur usually "hang out" without pressing.

Linen

Linen washes easily but wrinkles very easily, too, unless treated. A hot iron on the wrong side of the dampened fabric is necessary to remove the wrinkles. Linen is used often for warm-weather clothing because it is absorbent.

Linen is washable but is usually most satisfactory when it is dry-cleaned since moisture makes it wrinkle readily.

Silk

Silk is a fragile textile fiber usually used for soft and special-occasion clothes. It can be gently hand washed in cold water and pressed with a cool iron. Usually silk should be dry-cleaned. Silk often is blended with wool for suits.

Synthetic Fibers

There are three synthetic fibers that have similar characteristics and are important in your wardrobe: polyester (Dacron, Trevira); acrylic (Acrilan, Orlon, Zefran); and nylon (Qiana, Antron). All resist wrinkles and all wash easily and well. If pressing is needed, a warm iron on the wrong side is used very lightly. Clothes that are made from these fibers usually wear extremely well year-round and probably will be blended with one of the four natural fibers in your clothes.

Acetate is a synthetic fiber that is fragile and that does not launder well. Plan to have it dry-cleaned and to handle it carefully. It wrinkles easily and should be pressed with a warm iron on the wrong side.

Arnel is washable, but it has a tendency to wrinkle easily. A hot iron is needed to press it. Rayon, used extensively in clothing, has a tendency to stretch out of shape when wet; therefore, it usually should be dry-cleaned rather than washed. It wrinkles and should be pressed with a warm iron. Rayon is sometimes blended with wool in suits and dresses.

Frequently you will find that two or more fabrics have been blended in a garment. Be sure that you treat the garment (washing, cleaning, pressing) according to the more fragile of the blended fabrics, not the more durable. Blends of polyester and wool, polyester and acrylic, and silk and wool are common and make excellent clothing fabrics.

────────── *Upkeep* ──────────

A business wardrobe is a costly investment. Even though four or five outfits are all you really need, they can represent a large part of your clothes budget. Taking good care of them makes good sense because it adds to their lifetime.

- Your closet should provide space for air to circulate around those clothes that are not cleaned every time you wear them.
- The hangers should support the neck and shoulders of your tailored coats, jackets, and dresses. A shaped wooden or plastic hanger is best.
- Pants look better if they hang from the cuffs or hems rather than from a fold in the leg.
- Skirts hang well from the waistband.
- Shirts and blouses on the hanger keep a smooth collar when one or two buttons at the top are fastened.
- Buttons and other fasteners should be repaired as soon as they are noticed as being loose. Small rips and hems that are loose should be repaired before they become big problems. Usually a good dry cleaner will provide these services. If not, locate a tailor or alterations shop that will.

Questions for Chapter 6

1. What difference does being "in uniform" make in business?
2. What makes a "business uniform" uniform?
3. What are the characteristics of a business suit?
4. What are the best fabrics and patterns for a business suit?
5. What blouses and shirts do women wear with a business suit?
6. What are shirt colors worn by men? by women?
7. How do you decide what kind of knot a tie should have?
8. What dresses are usually worn in business?
9. How is a blazer different from a suit coat?
10. What are the coats usually worn in business?
11. What coat style does a man usually wear? a woman?
12. What shoes are appropriate for men? for women?
13. What leather accessories are appropriate for business wear?
14. What jewelry is good for men? for women?
15. Why do you need more shirts, blouses, socks, hosiery, and underwear than outerwear?
16. Are all colors that are attractively combined, good combinations for business?
17. How many pairs of shoes do you need for business wear?
18. What factors affect the price of clothes?
19. What points should you check for good fit in a jacket?
20. What points should you check for good fit in pants and skirts?
21. What points should you check for good fit in shirts and blouses?
22. What natural textile fibers are good for business wear?

Chapter 7

Dressing Yourself

Chapter Objectives

After studying this chapter, you should be able to:

1. *Select colors that give your body structure a tall, thin look.*
2. *Recognize tints, tones, and shades of primary, secondary, and inter-mediate colors.*
3. *Select colors that complement your complexion.*
4. *Use monochromatic, analogous, and complementary harmony effectively in assembling your wardrobe.*
5. *Use lines in your clothes to give yourself a tall, thin appearance.*
6. *Choose fabrics and textures to balance irregular body size.*
7. *Select undergarments to meet your specific needs.*

Wearing the right clothes for business is vital; looking good in those clothes is important, too. Even the perfectly proportioned body needs clothes with colors and lines that complement that structure. The less-than-perfect body can minimize imperfections with informed choices.

Studies done about the relationship of appearance to success in business show that people who are tall and thin have an edge over those who are short and fat. Judicious use of colors and lines can make a person *appear* taller and thinner than the person actually is and help that person reap the benefits of the tall, thin body structure.

Color Structure

To understand the effect of color, you need to understand how colors are structured. Besides the pigment, color has hues, intensities, and values that influence how colors react or harmonize with one another.

Color

Color is the term used for a phenomenon of light or visual perception that enables you to differentiate otherwise identical objects. Colors are thought of as primary, secondary, and intermediate and as pure pigment, tints, tones, and shades. An example of these relationships is shown in a hue chart (Illustration 7-1). The primary colors are blue, yellow, and red. The secondary colors, which are formed by mixing two primary colors, are violet, green, and orange. The intermediates, formed by mixing a secondary with a primary, are blue-violet, blue-green, yellow-green, yellow-orange, red-orange, and red-violet. Some of the tints of each of these colors are shown in Rows 1 through 4 of the chart. The tones and shades are Rows 6-9. The pure pigment color is Row 5. Each square on the hue chart is a different color.

The pigments of any of the primary colors (blue, red, and yellow) plus black and white, can be combined in varying proportions, yielding an infinite variety of secondary and intermediate colors. All colors, however, can be broken down finally to primary pigments (of red, blue, or yellow), black, and white.

Hue

Hue is a term used to classify gradations of a color. On the hue chart, the first square in the violet column is a tint of violet. Although manufacturers of dye or paint may give it various names, it is a gradation of violet, therefore, a

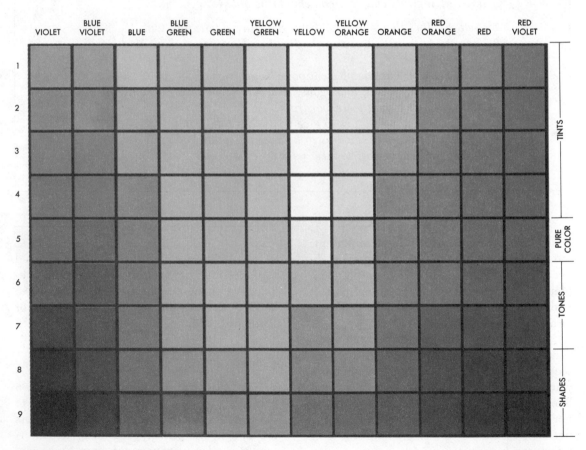

Illus. 7-1. Hue Chart

M. Grumbacher, Inc.

hue of violet. In fact, each square in the violet column is a hue of violet. Number 9, which is recognizable as purple, is obviously a hue of violet. However, Number 9s under yellow, yellow-orange, and orange (the browns) are not so obvious as hues of those colors

The hues of the primary, secondary, and intermediate colors are formed by adding white, gray, or black to the pure pigment. When white is added, the resulting hue is a *tint*. Gray added makes a *tone*. Black added makes a *shade*.

Tints, Tones and Shades

Tinting, toning, and shading may occur in many degrees. All such modifications, however, are not pleasing to the eye. An orange, for example, with a very small amount of black added looks dirty; with more black, it becomes a more appealing brown. A small amount of white added to red may make it faded and weak; but more white will make it pink and very pleasing to the eye.

The amount of pure pigment visible in a color is referred to as its intensity or saturation. Row 5 shows the most intense or most saturated of each of the colors. Tints, tones, and shades each dilute the intensity of the pure pigment that is visible.

Value describes the amount of light that is reflected by a color. The lightest of all colors is yellow. In any row across the chart, the yellow column will show the color reflecting the most light (highest value). As you move away from yellow in both directions, the lightness decreases. Violet is regarded as the color of lowest value.

The Neutrals

The presence of all three primary pigments (red, yellow, and blue) in equal amounts is black. Varying the proportions of the three and using the result for shading or toning gives another range of colors discernible to your eye. If you see a brown with a greenish cast, you will know that the black used to shade the orange is not pure; it has more yellow and blue than red. These unexpected "casts" that sometimes show in shades will be important to you in selecting colors compatible with your complexion. White is the absence of any color, and gray is the combination of white and black.

The Color Wheel

A color wheel can be used to show how colors are related so that you can use them in harmony. The three primary colors of pigment that are used as the basis of all other colors appear equal distances apart on the color wheel (Illustration 7-2 on page 110), usually with the yellow at the 12 o'clock position, blue at the 4, and red at the 8. Between the primaries are green at 2, violet at 6, and orange at 10 .

The colors formed by mixing the primaries and secondaries — the intermediate colors — appear yellow-green at 1, blue-green at 3, blue-violet at 5, red-violet at 7, red-orange at 9, yellow-orange at 11. The nearer a color is to a primary or secondary, the more of that color it takes on. However, some of the less dominant color is still visible. There are an infinite number of combinations that could be shown on such a wheel. The ones that this color wheel shows supply a frame of reference into which you can fit any color you encounter.

The relationship of one color to another is classified according to its placement on the wheel. Colors directly across the wheel (12 and 6; 1 and 7; 2 and 8; 3 and 9; 4 and 10; 5 and 11) are called complementary colors. Any five adjacent numbers are called analogous colors. These terms will be used later in discussing harmonizing combinations for your wardrobe.

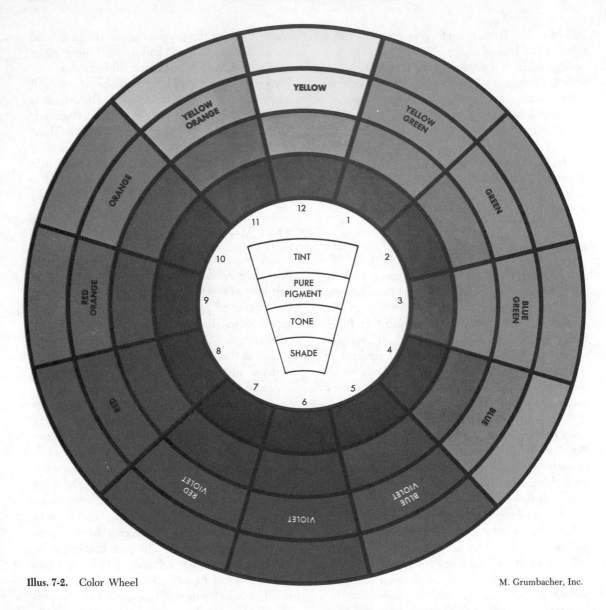

Illus. 7-2. Color Wheel

M. Grumbacher, Inc.

—— *Use of Color Structure* ——

Three principles of color structure are important to guiding you in its use for your clothes.

1. Color pigments react to one another, giving distortions.

2. Black absorbs light lowering the intensity and value of surroundings.

3. White reflects light increasing the value but lowering the intensity of surroundings.

Distortions narrow the range of pleasing combinations for complexion compatibility and harmony. Black and white, however, dilute the distortions and provide for a wide range of compatible and harmonious combinations.

Compatibility

Colors suited to your complexion, eye, and hair color should brighten and warm your face. Colors not suited to your complexion probably will seem to drain your face of its glow or distort your complexion color unattractively. They may cast dark shadows around your mouth and eyes, emphasizing lines in your face.

Distortions

Complexions may have any of the primary and secondary color undertones. Few, though, show well-defined color because of the tinting, shading, and toning pigments that are present in the skin. A person, for example, may have red, orange, yellow, green, blue, or violet undertones that are not recognizable until various other colors are placed near the face. Even then, the true undertone may be distorted because of the ways adjacent placement of colors is perceived by the eye. Also, the amount of undertone pigment varies from person to person and varies in your complexion according to your age because complexion undertones tend to fade as you age. Exposure to the sun also alters undertone pigment.

Colors appearing adjacently on the color wheel, when worn together, cause each color to "move" farther away from the adjacent color and assume some of the properties of the next color on the wheel. Red, for example, worn by a person with yellow undertones, makes the yellow undertones appear greenish. Red, worn by a person with orange undertones, makes the orange look yellowish.

Notice in Illustration 7-3 that because of its relationship to other colors, blue makes complexions of all undertones take on a warmer, brighter color. That enhancement may account for the popularity of blue in business wardrobes.

Colors appearing across the color wheel (complementary colors) brighten the undertone present. Violet, for example, worn by a person of yellow undertone, brightens the complexion. Distortions occur also when fabrics of the two colors are combined. In fabrics, though, you can select a hue that compensates for the distortion.

Illus. 7-3.
Distortions Resulting from Color Combinations

Color Causing Distortion	Color Showing Distortion*					
	Red	**Orange**	**Yellow**	**Green**	**Blue**	**Violet**
Red	Intensify	Yellow	Green	Brighter	Green	Blue
Orange	Violet	Intensify	Green	Blue	Brighter	Blue
Yellow	Violet	Red	Intensify	Blue	Violet	Brighter
Green	Brighter	Red	Orange	Intensify	Violet	Red
Blue	Orange	Brighter	Orange	Yellow	Intensify	Red
Violet	Orange	Yellow	Brighter	Yellow	Green	Intensify

*Use this chart to determine slight distortions of color that may be expected when certain colors are combined. For example, when red is combined with orange, the orange will take on more of a yellow cast; when red is combined with yellow, the yellow will take on more of a green cast.

Tinting, Toning, and Shading

The distortions of natural undertones will play a major role in the selection of colors for your wardrobe. If, for example, you have yellow undertones in your complexion, red close to your face may make you turn greenish. However, if the yellow is not too strong, shading may help. You may find that red shades (black added) may be used moderately and that blue-reds may be attractive with your complexion. Red in all its tints, shades, and tones will not necessarily be excluded from your wardrobe — just the clear, bright ones near your face that turn you "green."

Often the colors that complement your complexion will also complement your eyes and hair. You can brighten your eyes and hair with careful selection of colors. Using the same color of your eyes or hair, for example, presents a dramatic effect. Generally, however, a contrasting color near the face will be needed to provide a single point of interest and relief from the drama.

Avoid combining colors that are tinted, shaded, or toned to only a slightly different intensity. Gray eyes with a suit of only slightly grayer color will be unappealing, whereas, a suit with a considerable amount of additional gray toning may be very harmonious. If you wish to emphasize your hair with wardrobe color, use light colors to make dark hair look richer and dark colors to make light hair look brighter. Complementary colors may be used to increase the vividness of the eye color. Orange and orange hues, for example, worn by a person with blue eyes, intensify the blue.

Harmony

Appealing combinations of color are referred to as color harmony. Several kinds of harmony are available for your wardrobe. There are strengths and weaknesses for you to consider with each one.

Monochromatic Harmony

Monochromatic harmony is achieved by using one color of various values (amount of light reflected) and intensities (amount of pigment visible). Too much of one hue of a color, however, can be monotonous and should be carefully avoided. Combinations of hues of only slightly differing intensity are not appealing. The monochromatic schemes that are most successful are those that combine varying hues and fabric textures and those that are relieved by a stripe or plaid blend of the hues of the color.

Analogous Harmony

Analogous harmony is achieved by combining colors that are close to each other on the color wheel (any five adjacent numbers), blues with greens, beiges with reds, browns with yellows, greens with yellows, etc. The analogous combinations that are most pleasing are those that lie between two primary colors rather than those between two secondary colors.

There is great flexibility in analogous harmony, and the success of the harmony depends upon good choices in tints, tones, and shades. These combinations are probably the most familiar to you and the easiest of the harmonies to assemble and wear comfortably. The key in assembling analogous harmony is to skip a color on the wheel. If you have a blue, for example, do not go to a green for the accent. Skip green and use yellow.

Complementary Harmony

Complementary harmony is achieved by combining the colors that are directly across the wheel from each other — blue with orange, red with green, yellow with violet. These combinations are usually most pleasing if one color is a tint, tone, or shade, and the other is pure. Complementary colors used together intensify each other. For example, in a red and green combination, red will seem redder and green will seem greener. Complementary harmony works best with a large amount of one subdued color and an accent with the other. Shading the color used in the larger amount frequently improves complementary harmony.

Other Contrasting Harmonies

Double complementary harmony is achieved by combining two complementary combinations. Split complementary harmony is achieved when colors on each side of the complement are used instead of the complement — red with blue-green and yellow-green instead of with green. A triad is achieved when three colors touched by the points of a triangle are combined. Until you have developed a very refined sense of color, these combinations may not be easy for you to assemble or wear comfortably.

Unappealing Combinations

By definition of the harmonies, there are no colors that cannot be combined. However, you are aware that some combinations, be they monochromatic, analogous, or complementary, are unappealing. The usual reasons these are unappealing are:

1. In monochromatic color schemes, a slight amount of shading, toning, or tinting combined with pure pigment is not appealing. Beware of combining fabrics with only slight gradations of hue.
2. In analogous combinations of color, use of

colors side by side on the color wheel usually is not appealing. Better combinations are colors separated by intermediate and secondary colors.
3. In complementary harmony, intensity is usually the problem. Shades, tones, and tints are preferred over pure pigment for this harmony because the combination of complementary colors automatically increases the intensity of both colors. Equal amounts of the two colors are usually overpowering and uninteresting.

All harmony can be improved if one primary color is combined with two secondary colors rather than one secondary color with two primary colors.

Tall and Thin Appearance

You can enhance the appearance of your body and improve the balance of your proportions to some degree with color. Thoughtful placement of low and high value colors will draw the eyes to points of emphasis and away from areas you want to obscure.

Value

One of the most important considerations in altering the illusion of your size is the value of the color utilized. The colors high in value (yellow, green, orange) will appear to enlarge the areas they cover. Those low in value (blue, violet, red) will appear to diminish except for red, which because of its warmth, appears closer to the viewer and, therefore, larger. You can, of course, use shades of any of the colors to achieve a lower value and modify the illusion. You achieve the thinner look by wearing either colors of low light value or dark shades of colors of high light value.

Placement

Various placements of color can give balance to an ensemble and create illusions as well as complement your natural coloring. Black used close to the face often absorbs the face colors, whereas white close to the face will reflect the colors of the face. A black suit needs relief near the face to prevent the face from appearing drained of its glow.

Because light colors that are carefully placed attract the eye and draw it away from undesirable figure flaws, they are often used for blouses and shirts with dark suits. These light-colored shirts and blouses attract the eye to the face and hands when they are worn with dark suits. This light reflecting color appearing at the top of the suit and the end of arms tends to "lengthen" the figure and arms and emphasize the face. The dark suit tends to obscure the width of the figure making it appear thinner than it is.

Lines

The horizontal, vertical, straight, angular, and curved lines used in the design, fit, and fabrics of your clothes will create an illusion about your size and the proportion of your body parts helping you to appear thinner and taller.

A line can create an optical illusion by leading the eye in a certain direction, contrasting one area with another, dividing areas into equal or unequal spaces, yielding illusions of size, emphasis, and balance.

Straight Lines

Straight lines lead the eye and make figures seem taller if the lines are vertical and wider if the lines are horizontal. The placement of lines is vital to achieving good proportion to your figure.

- The nearer a horizontal line is to the center of your body, the more it shortens you.
- The nearer to the center a vertical line is, the more it lengthens your figure.

Adding accents to the ends of straight lines changes the illusion:

- A V at the end of a line seems to extend the figure.
- An inverted V or a – (bar) seems to diminish the figure.
- Multiple straight lines in any direction tend to widen a figure because the eye travels from side to side.
- Any line that leads the eye to the perimeter of the figure tends to widen.

Illus. 7-4. A dark suit makes the figure appear thinner than it is, but a horizontal line widens the figure.

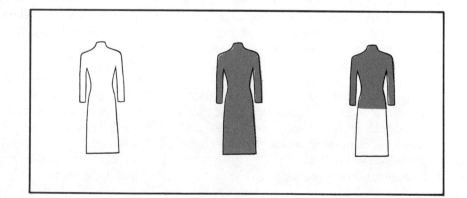

Illus. 7-5. Multiple straight lines in any direction tend to widen the figure.

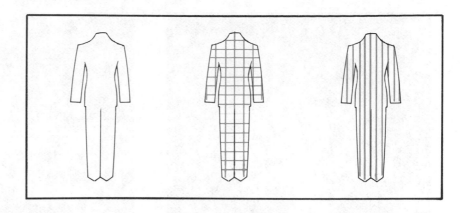

- A line that keeps the eye attracted to the center of a figure tends to narrow the figure.
- In V-lines the point of the V narrows the figure wherever it appears, and the stems that lead the eye to the perimeter of the figure widen it wherever they appear.

A suit with pants draws the eye in a straight line down the front making the figure appear taller than it is. By drawing the eye to the center, away from the perimeter of the figure, width is diminished. If a suit skirt has detailing down the front, such as a seam, it has the same effect of lengthening and slimming as the suit with pants.

A dark suit with a light shirt or blouse has a vertical line with a V at the top which further lengthens the figure. When the coat is removed, however, dark pants or skirts with a light-colored shirt make a horizontal line at the waist near the center of the figure, shortening and widening it.

Plaids, which are a combination of horizontal and vertical lines, add bulk to the figure and shorten it slightly. Most people should choose very subtle plaids if they wear them at all in order to minimize the bulky effect.

The hemline of a jacket in a contrasting color makes a horizontal line that widens the figure wherever it falls. The placement of that horizontal line also will shorten the figure and should be placed very carefully on a short per-

Illus. 7-6. The point of a V-line narrows the figure, and the stems that lead the eye to the perimeter of the figure widen.

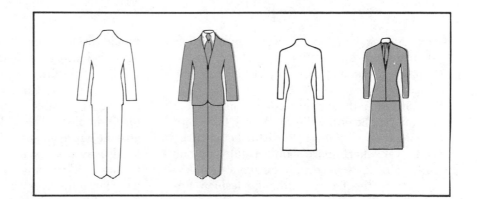

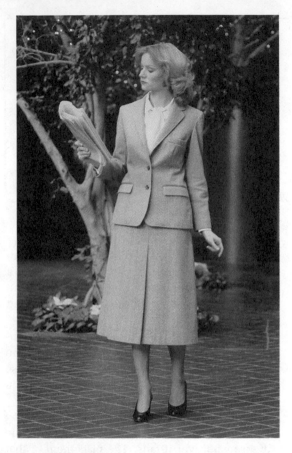

Illus. 7-7. A suit skirt with a pleat draws the eye to the center and makes the figure appear taller than it is.

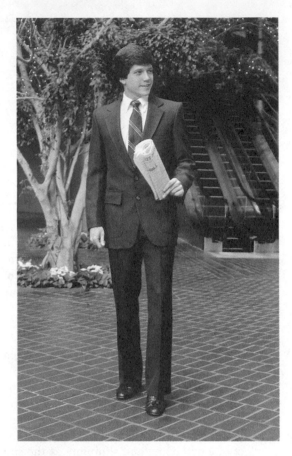

Illus. 7-8. A dark suit with a light shirt has a vertical V at the top which lengthens the figure.

son. A long jacket on a short figure further shortens the figure. Shorter jackets allow a longer leg line and tend to add height to the short figure.

Skirt lengths should be determined by the overall height of the figure. A very tall figure should avoid very short (above the knee) skirts, and a very short figure should avoid very long (mid-calf) skirts since they exaggerate the extremes of the figure. Although fashion frequently changes hem lengths, each person

should carefully consider her own figure needs before adopting a new fashion length.

Pant lengths, too, are often dictated by fashion. The short figure needs to wear slacks as long as possible without allowing them to touch the floor. The added length will tend to give the figure height. A tall figure, on the other hand, may wear pants that end at the bend of the foot, with or without a cuff. The shape of the pant leg influences the look of height of the figure. A flared leg shortens the figure, whereas

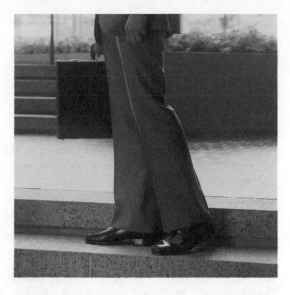

Illus. 7-9. The length and shape of the pant leg influence the look of height of the figure.

a straight, stove-pipe one heightens the figure. Cuffs on pant legs tend to shorten the figure because of the horizontal bands they create.

Angled and Curved Lines

The shape of a line, if it isn't straight, makes a definite difference in the way a figure is perceived. An angular line defines sharply the area it surrounds, whereas a curved one tends to soften the shape of the area it surrounds. Angular lines give feelings of stateliness, sophistication, dignity, and calmness. Full, curved lines are graceful and luxurious. Controlled curves are spritely and somewhat nervous in feeling. Curved lines are not usually worn for business. The angular pattern of plaids is worn, but the softly curved lines of floral prints are reserved for leisure wear.

The structure of the tailored jacket or dress presents straight and angular lines obscuring the natural curves of the body and presenting an image appropriate for business. Clothes that follow the body curves such as T-shirts and sweaters are good for leisure time activities when curves are "in."

Borders

Fabric texture and construction of clothes form a border around the perimeter of your silhouette. Clothes that are too small and those that are too big will distort your image in an unbecoming way because of the nature of borders:

- A very close border makes a figure appear larger.
- A slightly larger border tends to maintain the true proportion of the figure but tends to give it a slightly smaller appearance.
- A very large border draws more attention to itself and its bulk than to the figure.

Fabric Texture

Although your body itself forms the basic lines in your clothes, the texture of the fabric contributes to the effect. Fabric textures range from soft to stiff. The softer the fabric, the more revealing of the form it will be; the stiffer the fabric, the less revealing. Soft fabrics that cling to the lines of the body tend to give the illusion of increased size, just as a small border on a figure makes it look larger. Stiff fabrics tend to obscure the shape of the figure and reflect more of the shape of the garment than of the figure.

Fabric weights range from light to heavy. Lightweight fabrics are revealing, and heavy ones, though they add bulk, obscure the lines of the figure. A dull-surfaced, medium-weight texture will be suitable for many figures, especially stout figures, since the dull surface diminishes the size and the medium weight is not too revealing. Heavy-weight fabrics may be worn by tall, thin figures since they add bulk to the figure.

Construction

Although your figure itself forms the basic lines in your clothes and the fabric texture contributes to the effect, most lines in clothes are formed by the overall shape and interior seaming of the garment. The shape of a garment is determined by whether the cut and construction have been bloused, eased, tapered, tunneled, or flared. Bloused and eased construction generally adds bulk to the figure. Tapered and tunneled construction generally diminishes the bulk of the figure. Flared construction diminishes the small part of the flare and widens the wide part of the flare.

Proportion is important in line selection. A small figure should avoid large hats, prints, plaids, and trims (such as very large buttons), since they will draw attention to themselves and away from the person. A large figure, including the tall and heavy, should avoid small hats, very small patterns, and trims because the contrast makes a large person look disproportionately larger. Heavy, bulky items should be confined to the tall, thin figure. Only small items can be suited to the small figure.

Women's Undergarments

Undergarments for women include the bra, girdle (or support panty), and lingerie. You can make your clothes fit better and make your figure appear to be in better proportion than it really is by selecting undergarments carefully.

Foundations

The bra and girdle are the foundation garments and the foundation of the lines in women's clothes. Most figures require both under some fashions and some figures require both under all fashions. If you are considering omitting either a bra or girdle, be sure the muscles are firm and smooth and that you have not one ounce of excess fat. Carefully check your image front, back, and profile in the garment you are considering wearing without foundation garments. If your lines are not smooth and the tone of the muscles that support your breasts and hips is not firm, wear foundation garments. If your undergarments are obviously missing, you are not well dressed.

Selecting a Bra. The purpose of the bra is to support the breasts and shape the bodice so that hips that are too wide or too narrow are better balanced. The fashion looks that fade in and out of popularity are a soft, natural look, a flattened look, and a voluptuous look. Rather than trying to copy the latest dictate of fashion, decide whether you need (1) to increase the size of your bust with a padded bra, (2) simply to support a well-formed bust, or (3) to de-emphasize a too-well-endowed figure. Your purpose will dictate which kind of bra you need.

Whatever your needs, carefully measure your bust line to determine the size you need. Two measurements must be made; one is of your rib cage just under your breasts, the other over the fullest part of your breasts. Be sure that your tape measure makes an even, horizontal line around your body. Take the measurement of your rib cage and add five or six inches to arrive at the closest even number, i.e., to a measurement of 28, add 6; the size is 34. To a measurement of 29, add 5; the size is 34. Take the measurement of your fullest part to determine the cup size. If the reading is the same as you arrived at for your bra size, you wear an A cup; if it is one inch more, a B cup; two inches more, a C cup; three inches more, a D cup. (If your rib cage measures more than 38 inches, add only 3 or 4 inches, since you are harboring some excess fat that may or may not be reflected in your cup size.)

Always try on a bra before you buy it. Observe the shape of the cup and the naturalness of the curve. Be sure that the neckline is what you need for the clothes you intend to wear. Check the straps to see if they are placed for comfort over your neck bones and that you can swing your arms unrestrictedly.

Selecting a Girdle or Support Panty. Girdles and support panties are designed to provide a smooth line under skirts and pants and to control bounce in the hips as you walk. To determine your size, measure the fullest part of your buttocks. Sometimes girdles and support panties are sized simply petite, small, medium, and large. Sometimes they are sized like lingerie panties, 4, and 5, 6, etc. The measurements in inches for those designations are:

- Petite, Size 4, 34 inches and under
- Small, Size 5, 34 to 37 inches
- Medium, Size 6, 37 to 40 inches
- Large, Size 7, 40 to 44 inches

Try on your girdle or support panty before you buy it. Walk, sit, and bend in it. Be sure that the legs fit comfortably as well as the crotch and the waist. Be sure that the waist and legs do not roll.

If you are exercising regularly and keeping your muscles firm, you may be able to wear control-top hose instead of a girdle or support panty. When you try such control, observe whether or not you have bulges that show under your clothes.

Bras, support panties, and girdles come in various lengths and styles. A bandeau bra has a one- to two-inch band around the rib cage and can be worn by most figures. A long-line bra will have wider bands, ranging from three to six inches, to control midriff bulges. Girdles may have a wide waist band, ranging down to no waist band, and the length of the legs is varied so that you can get whatever meets your re-

quirements smoothing any bulges in the thigh area.

Bras are available with underwiring that provides for additional support for heavy breasts, mainly C and D cup sizes. Try on an underwired bra before you purchase it. Be sure that you are comfortable where the wires rest against your rib cage underneath your breasts and under your arms.

Lingerie

Panties and slips are not considered foundation garments but are important in the lines of your clothes. Your main concern is to select lingerie that is comfortable next to your skin and promotes a smooth line under your clothes. Bikini style panties stretched over a less-than-firm stomach may make unsightly bulges that show up under your clothes. A slip that is too full for the dress you are wearing may look bulky under it. Cotton is the most comfortable fabric for panties and bras but nylon is widely used because it is lightweight. Fabrics that resist static electricity are available in slips to keep them from clinging to your legs as you walk.

Men's Underwear

Men's underwear consists of undershirts and undershorts. The choice of an undershirt includes choosing from the "tank" style with no sleeves and a low, rounded neck or from a T-shirt style with sleeves and either a V-neck or a high, rounded neck. The lower neck style in both the tank and T is the most versatile because the undershirt remains invisible under an open-neck shirt you may wear for leisure time.

Undershorts of either the brief style, which give support, or the boxer style, which are lighter weight, are available. Choose shorts which meet your needs for support or freedom.

Important consideration for underwear is that it be absorbent. Cotton is the best fiber.

Questions for Chapter 7

1. What are the primary colors; the secondary ones; the intermediate ones?
2. What color is a shade of orange?
3. What color is a tint of red?
4. How can the undertone of a person's face be distorted?
5. What may account for the popularity of blue for business wear?
6. What is monochromatic harmony? analogous harmony? complementary harmony?
7. What are the causes of unappealing combinations of colors?
8. What are the "value" and "placement" considerations for looking tall and thin?
9. What line does a suit reflect to make you look taller than you are?
10. What part does a light-colored shirt or blouse with a dark suit play in making you look taller and thinner?
11. What effect does a hemline of a contrasting color jacket have on your height?
12. How do you decide how long to wear your pants and/or skirts?
13. What effect do clothes that are very tight have on your appearance?

Chapter 8

The Business Face

Chapter Objectives

After studying this chapter, you should be able to:

1. *Care for your skin according to its particular needs.*
2. *Develop health practices that contribute to more attractive skin.*
3. *Develop cleaning procedures for healthy skin.*
4. *Control the oil on your face.*
5. *Develop appropriate grooming procedures for your face.*
6. *Select grooming aids and cosmetics according to your particular face grooming needs.*
7. *Care for your mouth and teeth.*
8. *Maintain fresh breath.*

Like clothes, faces have a certain look in business. Very simply, they are healthy, clean, and well-groomed. They look as though they are cared for. In terms of health, they look refreshed from rest, stimulated by exercise, and nourished with good food. The *clean* face is free of dirt, pollutants, and visible oil. The *well-groomed* face is free of excessive hair and has an even skin tone, supple surface, and expressive features.

It Starts with Skin

Your skin is composed of two layers: (1) dermis, the inner layer and (2) epidermis, the outer layer. The dermis contains hair follicles, oil glands, sweat glands, nerves, and blood vessels, all held together with connective tissue. The epidermis is a tougher layer where the openings occur for hair, oil, and sweat. The tubes running from the glands and hair follicles to the skin surface are follicles that carry oil, hair, sweat, and new skin cells to the face surface.

Properly functioning oil glands produce just enough oil to flow (1) into the follicle, (2) up, and (3) out onto the surface of the face to lubricate it. More importantly the new skin cells that are manufactured deep in the dermis are pushed by newer cells, oil, and a growing hair up the follicle wall to the surface. Although they are round and plump with water when they start, by the time the new cells reach the

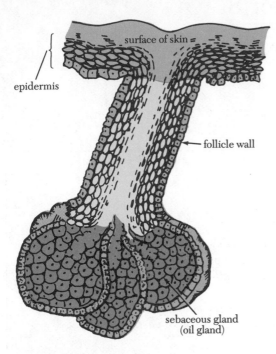

Illus. 8-1. Sebaceous glands produce oil to lubricate the skin.

surface of skin

epidermis

follicle wall

sebaceous gland (oil gland)

surface, they are flat and dead. Such cells form the surface of your skin. Eventually, they will fall off, completely replacing themselves approximately every 27 days.

──────── Health Factors ────────

The health factors that affect skin include diet, exercise, and rest. You know the reasons to observe good health practices, but do you know what the practices are?

Diet

Good nutrition for your skin means including meat, milk products, and green and yellow leafy vegetables in your diet every day. It means eliminating foods that contribute to problems to which you may be vulnerable, such as flushing.

Good Food

The vitamin generally believed to contribute to fresh-looking skin and sparkling eyes is vitamin A. It occurs mainly in green and yellow leafy vegetables and milk, not in potato chips and candy bars! The nutrient that facilitates the replacement of dying cells in your skin is protein. Protein occurs mainly in lean meat, not carbonated colas or cake! Every day some skin cells die and are sloughed off. Because the dying, shedding, and replacing process is a continuing one, your food intake daily should provide the nutrients required for such replacement.

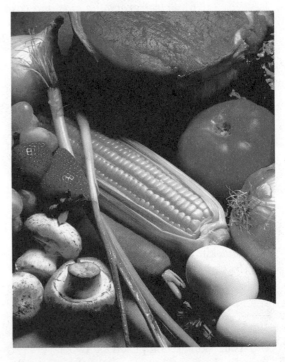

Illus. 8-2. The health factors that affect skin include diet.

Another important element in your diet is water. Your skin consists of large amounts of water evaporating and being replaced continuously. One of the most important purposes of water in your body is to flush impurities and waste from your system. You can make your entire body, skin, digestion, and elimination systems function better by consuming six to eight glasses of water a day. If it is difficult to get the amount of water you need because you drink mainly from fountains, make an effort to provide a glass for drinking water either at the fountain or at mealtime.

Not-so-Good Food

Some foods and liquids seem to harm your skin. Liquor and coffee cause skin problems, especially flushing, in some people. Over a period of time, the effect of flushing is permanent redness in the skin. You can avoid flushing by diluting liquor in mixers and water, and by drinking decaffeinated coffee of a reduced temperature.

Exercise

Skin needs stimulation, too — not the vigorous rubbing and pounding that goes with a body massage (although that is better than no stimulation at all). The skin needs stimulation from an atomsphere that relaxes you in an activity that promotes vigorous blood flow, adequate oxygen intake, and elimination of waste. As you participate regularly in activity that stimulates blood flow and oxygen intake, you care for your skin.

A brisk walk or game of tennis that causes your circulatory system to speed up its flow of blood to your cells promotes good skin. When your skin tingles and glows temporarily from increased activity, it means that additional nourishment has been brought by your blood to the skin surface. Relaxation is necessary to

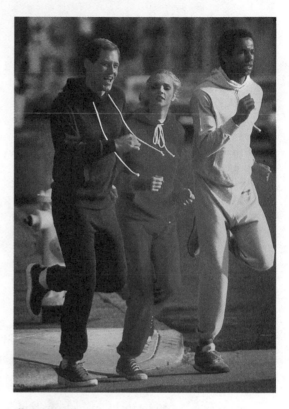

Illus. 8-3.   As you participate regularly in activity that stimulates blood flow and oxygen intake, you care for your skin.

this kind of activity. A tense or nervous body constricts blood vessels, causing the skin to be cut off from this stimulating nourishment.

Rest

If you are nervous and tense for long periods of time, your skin will reflect your discomfort. There will be no well-nourished skin simply because the nutrient-carrying blood cannot properly feed and regenerate the surface of your body. A heart that is not working at peak efficiency or blood vessels that are constricted near the surface of your body can rob your skin of the nourishment it needs.

Take a good look at your skin, especially your face, when you get up in the morning. Take another look when you begin to prepare for bed at night. Most skins look very different before and after rest. The older you get, the more obvious the difference. Rest for your body includes rest for your skin. Relaxing and sleeping allow muscles to rest and blood to flow freely into the tiniest capillaries, bringing oxygen and nutrients to nourish your skin. Without such rest, your skin competes with other organs of your body, such as your muscles and digestive organs, for those important nutrients. Without adequate rest, the skin may get only whatever is not burned as energy. If you are eating only marginally, other parts of your body may exhaust your supply of nutrients before your skin gets a chance at them.

Cleaning Supplies

Your face is constantly excreting body wastes and oils through its pores and collecting atmospheric pollution. Although your face is constantly on display and being judged by others, cleaning is more than cosmetic — only clean skin is healthy. Dirty skin has many potential problems. Because faces have soil consisting of oil, dead cells, sweat, and pollutants from the air, they require cleansers that will loosen, dissolve, and remove all this debris.

Haphazard cleaning can lead to a buildup of decomposed cells, sweat, bacteria, and pollutants which block and enlarge the pores and cause the skin to look thick, coarse, and greasy. The job of a cleanser is (1) to remove as much dirt and oil from the face as possible without harming the skin, and (2) to be completely removable from the skin itself.

The cleanser most often used is soap. Soap is not always what it appears to be; it can have

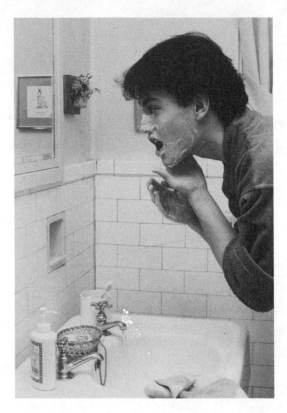

Illus. 8-4. Only clean skin is healthy.

many additives for many purposes. Basically it is a combination of fatty acids and oils which react with soil. It may be superfatted with extra oil to leave an oily residue. It may be enriched with glycerine for the same purpose. It may not be soap at all but a detergent which is easier to rinse off than soap; it may have a deodorant added to check body odor; it may have olive oil (castile), or cocoa butter instead of fat, or cold cream added for a gentler cleaning. One is perfect for you.

Other cleansers are cold cream and liquid cleansers. These are usually mixtures of water, oil, beeswax, and fragrance. The oil dissolves the debris, which can be wiped away with tissue or cloth and followed with an alcohol-based astringent. Such cleansers usually leave a greasy residue that is not left with soap and water cleansing.

Some cleansers have granules imbedded in them and may be either soaps, creams, or lotions. They are used as scrubs to loosen imbedded grime and dead cells and thereby thin the skin by hastening the sloughing off of dead cells. These abrasive cleansers are rough on skin but effective in removing dead cells. Usually scrubs are used only once or twice a week. Because such thinned skin is sensitive, it should be protected from shaving and sun for a few hours after cleaning.

Some secondary cleansers are fresheners, toners, and astringents. They are usually alcohol and water mixtures that cut through oil and freshen the skin after cleaning. After-shave often has this alcohol-water mixture and serves as an astringent (an expensive one!). Simple, diluted rubbing alcohol is probably the least expensive freshener/astringent.

Although not specifically a cleanser, the last part of a cleansing program will probably be a moisturizing agent. It seems strange to remove all the oil possible from the skin with soap and cleansing cream and then to put more oil on. Remember though that skin cells start out fat and plump with water deep in the dermis and that by the time they become part of the surface of your face they are flat and dead because most of the water has evaporated.

In addition to removing the debris, thorough washing, cleansing, and rinsing take all the oil that is imbedded in these cells, leaving them dryer than ever. If you wait long enough after washing, oil from the dermis will flow from the glands up through your pores and moisten them again, making the surface flexible and supple but dirty again from the accompanying collection of sweat and pollutants.

Most people prefer to apply a coating of oil after cleansing so that the skin will be comfortably soft and supple in the meantime. These moisturizers have a cosmetic benefit if used correctly. If the clean skin is still wet when the moisturizer is applied, the oil will trap the water in the cells, stopping it from evaporating and giving a lifelike look to otherwise dead skin cells.

One more agent is very important — water. Water is actually the only ingredient that can be absorbed by the skin cells. It is effective for mobilizing the debris and grime that is loosened by the cleanser. Using several rinses (literally splashing the face several times) is vital to a good face cleaning. All the cleansing agent, soil, and dead cells can be removed if the face is rinsed, rinsed, and rinsed. What will be left are cells not yet ready to fall off that are plumped with water, looking fresh and healthy.

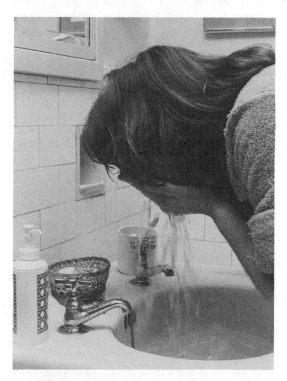

Illus. 8-5. Using several rinses is vital to a good face cleaning.

Cleaning Procedures

Because oil can be a problem by occurring in either too great or too little an amount, cleaning procedures that take that problem into account are necessary. Normal skin is described as that which has just the right amount of oil produced to both look and feel good most of the time. Oily skin is skin that looks greasy most of the time if steps are not taken to prevent the greasy look. Dry skin is actually skin that doesn't have enough water, but too little oil is the reason. Because so little oil is produced to coat the face, too much water evaporates from the cells, leaving the skin so dry that it is taut, uncomfortable, and often superficially wrinkled. You may even be unlucky enough to have a combination of these problems — dry skin on one part of your face and oily skin on another. If so, you have two sets of cleaning procedures to follow.

Actually, throughout your lifetime you probably will experience the whole range of oily-dry skin problems because age itself affects the production of oil on your face. As a teenager you probably produce more oil than at any other time, usually too much oil, especially on your forehead, nose, and chin. As an adult, you probably will have dryness around your eyes, where oil glands are most scarce. As it works out, just about the time the glands in your forehead, nose, and chin calm down to normal oil production, those around your eyes get too lazy to meet your needs. Caring for your needs, however, is not that much trouble, no matter where you are in the oil cycle.

Ideal Skin

Characteristics of a skin with just the right amount of oil are a firm texture; buoyant tone; fresh appearance; good color; a supple look; no visibly enlarged pores; and no flakiness. Other complexions usually strive for this balance because the skin looks and feels better than it does with too much or too little oil. With care and attention, anyone can achieve the appearance of this kind of skin. The amount of care and attention needed is related to how much your skin varies in either direction from just the ideal amount of oil.

Because you care for your face according to how much oil occurs naturally on it, the frequency of cleansing, type of cleanser, choice of astringent or after-shave, and moisturizers vary according to the degree of oiliness in your face skin. A skin with neither too much nor too little oil usually can take either soap and water or a cream or lotion cleanser. If soap and water are used, you may want to use a moisturizer immediately after cleansing to keep your skin from feeling taut. If either cream or lotion is used, you may want to use an after-shave or astringent to clean and close the pores and to give a refreshed feeling similar to that obtained with soap and water. Depending upon its exposure to dirt and grime, this face should be cleansed once before bedtime and possibly again in the morning. Sometimes astringent on a cotton ball will substitute for morning cleansing of this ideal skin.

This ideal skin may need a scrub once in a while to remove dead skin. If so, use the scrub before bedtime so that the skin has a rest before shaving or makeup is considered. Particular occasions that may call for a scrub are when the summer's tan is fading or when you have had exposure to grime in the air for a long period of time.

During the day, this skin may benefit from the use of a prepackaged astringent pad for the nose, forehead, and chin to take off the shine of accumulated oil. The packages are easily carried in a pocket or briefcase. They can be used easily and quickly, and discarded. They leave your face feeling very refreshed as well as very clean.

Normal skin usually needs moisturizing after every cleansing. Men will clean their faces, shave, perhaps apply after-shave, rinse, and then apply the moisturizer. After-shave balm is a moisturizer but an expensive one. If a fellow's masculinity is not offended, he can get off much more cheaply by using less expensive moisturizing lotions packaged for women. Skin cells have no gender; they respond the same way to moisturizers, regardless of which sex the container was designed for. Women will clean their faces, apply the astringent, rinse, and apply the moisturizer. Men and women with normal skin who use soap and water to clean their skin can skip the astringent/after-shave step and apply the moisturizer after the last rinse while the cells are plump with water.

Too Much Oil

Normally at puberty the oil glands in the skin become very active. You probably will have more oil from approximately age 12 to age 25 than at any other time in your life. Frequently, the oiliest part of your skin is from your forehead down the center of your face to your chin. This area is known as the T Zone. The easiest way to check for oiliness is to wash your face carefully with soap and water, dry it, apply nothing to it, and check it approximately four to eight hours later. If it is moist with oil, it is oily. If it has a dry, tight feeling, it is not oily. The problem is to achieve some oil but not too much. Too much oil contributes to blemishes, large pores, and flakiness. Too little oil contributes to dry, rough skin.

Oily skin should be washed a minimum of twice a day, once in the morning and once at night. You may want to wash it more often. If you do, keep in mind that the excessive oil is produced deep in the dermis and only shows up on the surface. You may be robbing your surface cells of water by washing too often while doing nothing about the real problem deep within the skin.

Soap and water are considered the most efficient cleansers for oily skins. Superfatted, cream, and cocoa butter soaps should be avoided. Rinsing is vital to cleansing oily skin because the pores are usually larger and more easily clogged than the pores of dryer skin. The thorough rinsing is helpful in flushing the surface debris from those pores.

Scrubs, too, because of the grains, help to dislodge the accumulation of oil and soil in the large pores of the oily skin. A complexion brush will do a better job than your fingertips can. Cellular buildup which may flake off is reduced by these scrubs, but be sure the buildup is due to oil rather than to dryness before you give yourself a vigorous scrub. The flakiness, characteristic to both conditions, one because of too much oil and one because of too little, is treated differently. Scrubbing should be done at bedtime and never just before shaving. You probably will want to avoid astringents and after-shaves after scrubbing because skin becomes somewhat tender after it is so thinned.

Even an oily skin can benefit from a moisturizer at bedtime if it is applied properly. Wash the face as usual but don't dry it. Leave as much water on it as your skin will hold and put a very light moisturizing lotion (maybe as light as baby oil) over the water to keep it from evaporating. Remember, your problem is excess oil production, not excess water.

To cut down on the excess oil, you can apply drying agents to your face periodically. Such chemicals as benzoyl peroxide, salicylic acid, resorcinol, and sulfur put on a clean face and left for a few hours (overnight) dry oil in the follicles that soap and water cleansing cannot. The frequency of such applications depends on the degree of oiliness you suffer. If you have acne in addition to oily skin, you will find these chemicals helpful in controlling acne because they also peel surface cells of your skin. All the chemicals are available in over-the-counter preparations in the drug department. Most are advertised as acne treatments.

Astringents and alcohol-based after-shaves are especially useful to people with oily skin. Astringent after every cleansing helps remove remaining oil, and packaged astringent-soaked tissues are valuable to use throughout the day when oil accumulates on your skin. Blotters such as tissue and those prepared especially for oily skin can be used periodically. Even a good rinsing when a soap and water cleansing is not needed is good. The important point to remember is that your skin needs water even though it is oily. "Watering" it now and then while removing the oil will give it a fresh, clean look.

Extremely hot weather seems to stimulate the production of oil in oily skin. Take care to cleanse it more often and to blot the oil more frequently in hot weather if you are treating oily skin. Clay-type face masks and drying masks are good to use on oily parts of your complexion. They serve to remove the flakiness that occurs from excess oil as well as that which occurs from the natural deterioration of skin cells.

Too Little Oil

You may have dry skin when you are young if your oil glands are not very active; you are almost sure to have it when you are older because oil production slows down with age. Care of dry skin means cleaning it without drying it out further. The lack of oil leaves what moisture you do have exposed to air so that it can evaporate. Oil on the surface protects the water so that it does not evaporate.

Dry-skinned people are the only ones who can use superfatted soaps and cleansing creams without worrying about having too much oil on the skin. Your degree of dryness will determine how often you use such special cleansers. Regular soap and water can be used if you replace oil immediately after washing. The best prac-

tice is to leave as much water on the face as possible while you apply the oily moisturizer. You attempt to seal the moisture in the skin cells with the oil. Neither men nor women want a greasy look, so be careful to blot off excess oil and creams. Remember, it is water you want in the cells, not any more oil than that which protects the water from evaporation.

Fortunately, dry skin attracts less debris than oily skin and may need fewer daily cleansings. Once-a-day cleaning is not unusual for dry skin. If you need only one cleaning a day, do it at night. Rinse again in the morning to replace water and refresh your skin. Because cleansers left on the skin can be very drying, dry-skinned people need to rinse more than others. Splash, splash, splash with warm water after you have cleansed. A toner or balm with very little alcohol should be used generously after a cleansing done with cream or lotion. Water is best for rinsing after a soap cleansing.

Scrubs for dry skin are questionable. As cells flake off, they may look rough and you may be tempted to scrub with a granular cleanser to smooth your skin. This procedure can irritate very dry skin, which tends to be somewhat thinner than other skins. As an alternative, a mask that replaces oil while peeling dry skin cells probably will be more satisfactory.

Other Skins

You may have areas that are too dry *and* areas that are too oily. Those that typically are too oily are the forehead, nose, and chin. They need the soap and water cleansing twice a day. The areas that are often very dry are around the eyes and mouth. They often need tender cleansing, perhaps only with a cream once a day. Such combination skin is more trouble to care for than others but with a little effort and attention, it can present the face that is well-groomed.

Grooming

The finishing touches for faces vary for men and women. Men usually shave the hair off their faces, and perhaps apply a bronzer to even the skin tone. Women skip the shaving, use a foundation to even the skin tone, and accent facial features that may need it. Because men's faces usually have stronger features (larger cheek bones, darker eyes, distinctive mouths), men often have expressive faces without cosmetics. Women, however, use a cosmetic touch here and there to accent features such as pale eyelashes and skin.

Men's Shaving

Anyone with a razor can shave his face. Right? Maybe. The goal, of course, is to remove the growth of hair. Such removal, however, should not irritate the skin in the process. Getting a mild shave is the key to shaving successfully day after day. The process of shaving varies according to whether an electric shaver or a razor blade is used.

Razor Blade Shaving

Although both kinds of shaving begin with a thorough cleansing to remove oil from the beard, there the similarity of the two processes ends. Blade shaving requires the wettest beard possible. The thorough removal of oil with a good cleansing begins the process of wetting the beard. It is followed with the application of an appropriate shaving preparation designed to wet the beard and to lubricate the skin under the beard. These preparations swell the hairs of the beard, making them stand upright and thus be better targets.

Because water is the best moisturizer, splash water on the beard repeatedly before applying the shaving preparation. Your choice of preparation is usually between foam and gel.

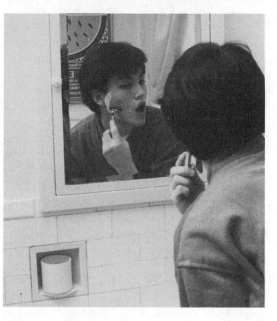

Illus. 8-6.   Getting a mild shave is the key to shaving successfully day after day.

The foams are wetter because they have more water. The gels usually lubricate the skin under the beard better because they have more oil.

Whatever preparation you choose should be allowed to do its work a couple of minutes before you start shaving.

Electric Blade Shaving

Electric shavers operate best on dry beards, whose hairs don't bend. Because oil softens hair, a thorough cleansing is necessary. Such cleaning softens the beard and must be followed by a preparation that will dry it but leave the skin underneath smooth. Pre-electric shaving preparations are just such drying agents. They usually have enough astringency to stiffen the beard and to evaporate quickly. They also coat the skin so that the shaver can glide across it.

Cutting the Beard

All the preparation in the world is lost if the blade used is not sharp. Whether manual or electric, be sure the blade is clean and sharp. Then apply it methodically going *with* the grain of growth. Save the heaviest growth, usually the upper lip and chin, until last so that the preparation has longer to work. Gentle is the word with both blades. Remember, skin is just beneath the beard, and it may be irritated and cut easily.

After dewhiskering, you should rinse, rinse, rinse to remove the remaining preparation. What follows the rinsing depends on the condition of the skin and how much oil it produces. If the skin is not tender and produces plenty of oil, an alcohol-based astringent or after-shave is good. If the skin is irritated or tends to be dry, an after-shave balm is better. Such a balm also serves as a moisturizer to seal in the moisture left from the rinse. If a balm is not used, some other moisturizer is appropriate to finish your shaving routine.

Skin Tones

If the face skin is blotched, or has uneven colorations, both men and women look better when they apply a light color that evens the skin tone. Men's products are called bronzers. Although women can use the bronzers, they usually use foundations.

Bronzers

Strictly speaking, bronzers are translucent gels that contain harmless dyes to color the skin more or less permanently (remember, skin replaces its topmost layer as often as every 27 days). The best ones produce what looks like a summer's tan without subjecting the skin to the harmful rays of the sun. These bronzers do not cover blemishes, and they are less effective than foundations for evening radically uneven skin tones.

Bronzers are applied with clean hands, on a clean, moisturized face. If you use a well-lighted mirror and start with a little of the gel on your fingertips, you can apply it lightly, beginning with the forehead, being careful not to leave a line of demarcation at your hairline. Work down your nose, cheeks, and chin carefully blending it under your chin to your neckline leaving again no line of demarcation. Bronzers dry quickly and usually won't run if you are caught in a rain shower. Perspiration, however, can discolor them, so be sure to blot perspiration carefully to keep it from running on your face. The lightest coat you can use to get even color is best. Let it dry completely. Nothing is used over it — you have already cleaned and moisturized.

Like anything foreign on your face, you should clean bronzers off your face at night. Some dye may have colored the cells, and a harmless residue of color may remain after cleaning. Your regular cleansing routine should remove the gel easily before you go to bed.

Foundation

After applying under-makeup moisturizer, women who need it (men if they dare!) are ready for foundation. The purpose of a foundation (sometimes called base) is to give your skin uniform color and texture. Slight imperfections in your complexion will be covered giving you a smooth, even skin tone.

Selection. Selecting a foundation includes decisions about form, color, formula, coverage, and finish. Consider your complexion coloring and problems when making each decision.

Foundation comes in liquid, cream, gel, and pancake forms. Apply liquid and cream formulas with your fingertips, but remember not to put your fingers into the bottle or jar.

Pour the liquid onto your fingertips. Use a wooden or plastic spoon to get cream and gel foundation out of the container. Pancake foundation, especially good for oily skin, is applied with a wet cosmetic sponge.

The color of your foundation should be selected to match the color of your skin as nearly as possible. Experimentation is the surest way to select the right color. Most cosmeticians at department stores and drug stores have testers available that you can sample on your skin. With their help, apply several shades to your face. (You can test on the back of your hand, but your face is better.) Check them in direct daylight with a mirror to select just the right one for your own complexion. Make a note whether the shade you choose is a rose, beige, pink, cream, or brown tone, and be guided in the future when you change brands or kinds of foundation. You may need to change the color of your foundation seasonally as your complexion color changes.

Foundations come in nonallergenic, medicated, and astringent formulas. If you are experiencing frequent blemish problems, try one of these formulas. In general, the medicated and astringent foundations have a more drying effect on your skin than the normal formula. The nonallergenic formula does not contain the substances to which people are commonly allergic.

Foundations are available in varying degrees of coverage. If you have near-perfect skin, a translucent foundation to provide protection and a glow will be best for you. Gels and water-based liquids frequently are the most translucent of foundations. Oil-based liquids and creams provide the coverage needed by many people. Pancake provides the best coverage for blemished skin.

A matte or shiny finish foundation formula is available. Matte finish foundation usually does not require powder because it is considered to be an all-in-one (foundation and powder) formula. Most foundations, however, give some sheen, which may be worn as is or changed to a matte finish with the application of face powder.

Application. Foundation may be applied to your entire face and on your neck and ears if they are exposed. Do not try to cover your face all at once. With your fingertips or a wet makeup sponge, begin with your forehead, and then cover your cheeks, nose, chin, ears, and neck. Place dots of foundation at strategic places and blend them over your face.

Apply foundation sparingly to the hairy parts of your face, such as your upper lip and near your hairline. Very carefully blend the color into these areas, removing with a tissue any foundation that appears matted by the hair. There must be no line of demarcation between the foundation and natural skin. There should be an illusion of a smooth, even, unblemished complexion. If you have difficulty achieving this illusion, you may have chosen the wrong color. Too light a color of foundation gives a chalky appearance. Too dark a color is impossible to blend without lines of demarcation.

Cleaning foundation off your face at night is as important as putting it on. Follow your cleansing routine scrupulously, especially at night, if you decide to wear foundation during the day.

Highlighting Your Features

Because women's features are smaller and usually less defined than men's, women often choose to use cosmetics to emphasize them. Cheekbones can be emphasized with color, eyes with mascara, and lips, of course, with lipstick. Most businesswomen wear mascara and lipstick. Men, of course, do not. Other cosmetics, if worn at all, are very subtle. People should not notice your makeup; they should notice the expression of your face. Use of eye-

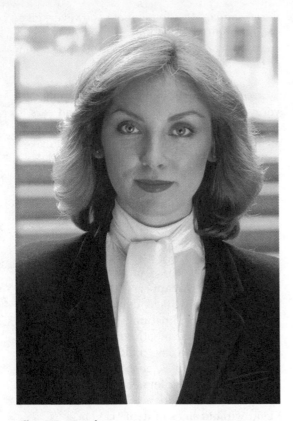

Illus. 8-7. People should notice your expression, not your makeup.

shadow is often criticized by business people. If you choose to wear it at all, choose brown or gray and be aware that you risk losing "face" with your colleagues. Eyeliner is also under attack and probably should not be worn in business.

Cheek Color

The purpose of rouge and blush is to contour your face and give you a healthy glow.

Selection. Rouge and blush are available in a large array of colors from light pink, to peach,

to dark brown. Your color choice depends on the color of your complexion. Choose a pink tint if you are fair, a pink-orange ("peach") or blue-pink ("plum") if you have a medium or dark complexion. Darker tones are for darker complexions and provide more of a contouring effect than a brightening one.

Cheek color comes in liquids, creams, and gels that are applied before your face powder. Powder blush is applied after the powder.

Liquids can be poured or squeezed onto your fingertip and gently applied to your cheekbone. Creams and gels should be scooped from the container with a cotton-tipped stick or a wooden or plastic spoon and placed on your fingertip. Powder blush that is brushed on with its own applicator is easiest to apply but has less staying power.

Application. To apply, you begin at the high point of your cheekbone, approximately aligned with the center of your eye, and move out toward your ear to the hairline. Cheek color should not be near your nose or eyes. It is applied no lower on your face than even with the bottom of your nose. A triangle with softened corners is the usual shape of the cheek color. Blend the edges of the color carefully so that no lines of demarcation are visible. The color should be more intense in the center of the area to which it is applied than it is near the edges. If cheek color is noticeable, it hurts rather than helps you.

Mascara

Mascara is used to color the lashes uniformly, making them appear thicker and longer. It is available in cake, cream, and liquid form. Some liquid mascara has tiny fibers that make the lashes appear longer and thicker than they really are. Apply mascara with either a brush or a stick applicator that comes with the liquid. An alternative to using mascara is to have your lashes dyed in a beauty salon. Men whose lashes are light may want to consider dyeing them.

Selection. The color of mascara you wear depends upon your eye and hair color. Usually black mascara is good only for people with very dark hair and eyes. Most brownettes, redheads, and blondes fare better with a lighter color mascara. It is wise to start with a dark brown for daytime and save the colors to dramatize your leisure-time wear.

Application. To apply mascara, brush the lashes upward and outward. Don't forget to color the top of the upper lashes. For more color, allow the first application to dry and apply another coat. Mascara should be applied sparingly, if at all, to lower lashes. Mascara applied on lower lashes tends to smear on the skin just below your eye; so be careful to keep this area clean throughout the day if you wear mascara on your lower lashes. Before your mascara dries, use a clean lash brush to separate the lashes for a full, natural look. After your mascara dries, place a tissue under your lower lash and brush your upper and lower lashes again to remove loose makeup and prevent it from falling on your face or in your eyes during the day.

Eyelash Curling

After your mascara is dry and you have brushed away any debris, you may want to use an eyelash curling appliance for a flattering, wide-eyed look. Gently squeeze the lashes with the curler and hold for ten to thirty seconds. Practice with this appliance will make you expert in curling your lashes.

Lip Color

The purpose of lip color is to shape and emphasize your lips. Your mood is usually expressed by the way your lips look. It is im-

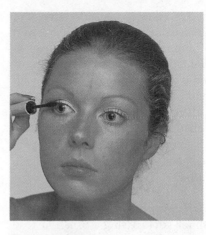

Illus. 8-8 (above). Mascara is used to make lashes appear thicker and longer.

Illus. 8-9 (below). You may want to use an eyelash curling appliance for a flattering wide-eyed look.

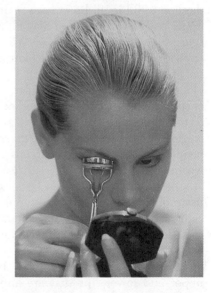

portant that lip color be applied correctly and kept fresh throughout the day. If you have good natural coloring, a moisturizer may be all you need.

Selection. Lip color is available in gel and cream form. The color you wear may be keyed to the color of your costume or of your complexion. Experimentation with a tester at your cosmetic counter is the best way to select a lip color. Dark and bright colors fade in and out of fashion. For daytime wear you probably will find lighter shades most flattering. Men, of course, do not wear lip color. They usually do, however, need good moisturizers, especially in extreme weather.

Application. Apply lip color with a lip brush or lip liner stick. Using a brush instead of the gel stick itself reduces the bleeding of color and improves wearability. Put plenty of cream or gel on the brush bristles to make an even line. Keep your lips closed but relaxed and draw a firm outline on half of the upper lip from center to outer corners. Next, open your mouth, stretching your lips taut, and retrace the line to fill in all lip creases. Complete the upper and lower lips. You may fill in with the brush or with the stick. DO NOT BLOT. Today's formulas do not require blotting; indeed, the texture and gloss are distorted when you do blot them. Along with the lip color, a clear gloss or conditioner may be applied either beneath or on top of the color. The use of such a conditioner or gloss gives a sheen that is flattering to most people, and it protects your lips from harsh weather.

Before you reapply your lip color, carefully tissue off the remains of the last application. Lip color is most attractive and remains true in color longer when it is applied to clean lips.

Shaping. The most desirable lip shape is upper and lower lips that are approximately equal in size. If yours are not, you can create some illusion by outlining the fullest lip just inside the natural line and outlining the thinner one exactly on the natural line. Do not try to compensate for unequal lips by putting lip color

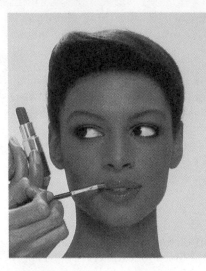

Illus. 8-10. A lip brush reduces the bleeding of color and improves wearability.

outside the lip area. The skin around your lips is somewhat different in texture from your lips, and the color will not look the same as it does on your lips. You will merely look as if you made a mistake in applying your lip color.

Eyeshadow

The purpose of eyeshadow is to make your eyes distinctive. It is worn between the brow and the lashes of the upper lid.

Selection. Eyeshadow is available in stick, cream, powder, gel, and cake form and in matte and frosted finish. The most suitable business shades of shadow are brown and gray.

Application. Different colors and various placements can give you a variety of looks. If you select an eyeshadow cream or gel, stroke on a band of color from the inner to the outer corner of the eye. With your fingertip, blend the color upward and outward, making certain that the deepest color tone is near the crease, blending and shading off as the brow line and outer portion of the eye area are reached. Cake and powder shadow are applied with a brush or a sponge. Apply from the inner to the outer portions of the eye, blending and shading to the brow line. Remember to make the color very subtle. A hint of color is usually much more flattering than strong, harsh colors. If your eyeshadow is noticeable, you have used either the wrong color or too much.

Face Powder

Face powder is applied to set your foundation. It can provide a sheen, matte, or luminescent finish and can be obtained in loose or pressed form. Loose powder is most efficient for use at your makeup table. You may want to carry pressed powder for quick touch-ups during the day. Don't confuse pressed powder with pancake foundation. They serve different purposes.

Selection. Face powder is available in colors and in a transparent form. Transparent powder adds no color. If you select a colored powder, which gives a slightly heavier look, it should match your foundation. When cream or liquid cheek color has been used, transparent powder is especially recommended because it cannot distort the color. Face powder is sometimes omitted entirely to achieve a sheen, which fades in and out of popularity.

Application. Apply the powder carefully with a clean puff, brush, or cotton ball over your entire face, or just in the oily sections, such as your forehead, nose, and chin. Pat the powder on; do not rub or stroke. Carefully blot with a tissue near your hairline, on your chin, and especially around your neck to avoid soiling your collar. Blotting is a pressing motion, not a

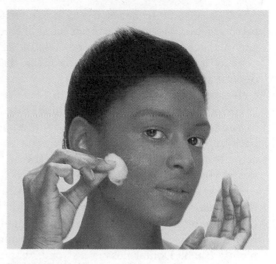

Illus. 8-11.   Apply powder with a clean puff, brush, or cotton ball.

rubbing one. Powder may be omitted in the drier areas of your face and where you have facial hair. Brush the powder away from your eyebrows and lashes.

Inside the Mouth

The business face does not end with grooming only the outside. Clean teeth are essential to the well-cared-for look. Your mouth is a special area of your body in terms of care. It should reflect a refreshing smile, clean, white teeth, healthy gums, and a fresh breath.

Teeth and Gums

Usually a dentist can help you with any problems you have with your teeth or gums. Many people, however, need a checkup only once or twice a year and have their teeth professionally cleaned of built-up plaque and stains at that time. The rest is easy to do daily at home.

It is absolutely necessary to brush your teeth at least twice a day to clean them of food and plaque. More often may be helpful, especially if you eat sweet or gooey foods that deposit sugar or food on your teeth. Tobacco, coffee, and tea may stain your teeth. Don't try to correct stains with vigorous brushing. Brush in a circular motion, being careful not to scrape back and forth over the same area. You can actually dig grooves in your teeth with the bristles of your brush by brushing improperly.

Food and plaque that collect between your teeth cannot be removed completely with a brush; therefore, you must floss your teeth either before or after brushing to get them completely clean. Dental floss is a strong, white, waxed string that you draw between your teeth to remove debris. It is available wherever you buy your toothpaste and toothbrush. Use it at least once a day. Toothpicks are dangerous to your gums and should not be used. They are never acceptable for use in public. It is better to carry a small container of floss to use privately if you get food between your teeth.

Only your dentist can treat gum problems. If you notice soreness or your gums pulling away from your teeth, consult your dentist. Early treatment of gum problems may mean avoiding much pain and eventually saving your teeth.

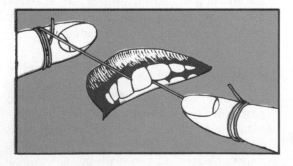

Illus. 8-12. You must floss your teeth to get them completely clean.

Fresh Breath

Your breath may be affected by many things: what you eat, your sinuses, tongue, teeth, gums, and the condition of your digestive system. It is not normal to have offensive breath. If you have it regularly, you should consider it the sign of a problem and start immediately to determine the cause and eliminate it. Bad breath is one of the most offensive of the body odors and definitely detracts from your grooming.

Foods with strong odors frequently leave an odor in your mouth and may contribute to bad breath long after you have cleaned the odor from your mouth. Brushing your teeth, rinsing your mouth thoroughly, and gently brushing your tongue will eliminate from your mouth any odor left from offensive foods. If the food odor still is apparent in your breath, an antacid tablet may aid in diluting the odor in your digestive tract.

Bad breath may result from sinus drainage. Frequently, an infection in your nose that accompanies a cold causes bad breath. Antihistamines are available to dry up the drainage of your sinuses and your nose and therefore are somewhat helpful in controlling the breath odor caused by this drainage. Breath mints actually do more to alleviate the bad taste such drainage leaves in your mouth than they do for your breath. They are better, however, than nothing at all for temporary relief.

Certain normal bacteria grow on your tongue. These in their normal balance do not cause bad breath. If you are under treatment with certain antibiotics, some of these bacteria may be killed. The result will be an imbalance that may cause bad breath. The doctor who prescribed the antibiotic can correct the condition.

Unclean teeth and unhealthy gums, of course, will cause unpleasant mouth odors. You know already how to clean teeth and care for gums. If you still suspect your teeth and gums as causes for unpleasant breath, consult with your dentist.

The condition of your digestive system affects your breath. An acid stomach can cause bad breath, and people with diabetes or other internal disorders frequently suffer from bad breath. Ulcers in the stomach and improper elimination can also cause bad breath. Frequent acid stomach and the other problems described, of course, should be treated by a physician.

If bad breath is caused by something you can correct, there is no reason to tolerate it. If it is a symptom of a more serious problem, consult a doctor without delay; and use temporary breath fresheners and mints until it is corrected permanently. Remember, though, that breath mints, fresheners, and gargles are temporary. You want permanent control of your mouth scent. There are few more offensive odors than bad breath. Freshen yours by correcting the problem that is causing it. You can do yourself no greater favor in terms of human relations.

Questions for Chapter 8

1. What are the characteristics of a well-groomed face for business?
2. Describe the cells that form your skin. How often do they replace themselves?
3. What are the health factors that affect skin?
4. What is the job of a cleanser for your face?
5. What are some of the cleansers you can use?
6. What is the job of a moisturizer?
7. What is the cleaning procedure for ideal skin? oily skin? dry skin?
8. What are the differences in procedure for razor blade and electric shaving?
9. What is a bronzer, and who should use it?
10. What is a foundation, and who should use it?
11. Why do women usually highlight facial features when men don't?
12. What products can you use to highlight eyes? lips? cheekbones?
13. What can you do to keep your breath fresh?

Chapter 9

Business Hair

Chapter Objectives

After studying this chapter, you should be able to:

1. *Adapt your hair according to its texture, thickness, oiliness, and curl to a well-groomed business look.*
2. *Develop a hairstyle that balances irregularities in your facial features and your body size.*
3. *Select a hairstyle that fits your personal life-style.*
4. *Design a care program for healthy hair.*
5. *Select grooming aids that enable you to keep your hair well-groomed.*

Like the business face, business hair doesn't call attention to itself with either extreme styling or unusual color. Neatness is the main criterion for business hair. The styles for both men and women are simple and well-suited to the person. A well-groomed appearance is expected for success in today's competitive world.

Business Styling

The main business requirement is that hair be neat. Unruly styles on either men or women will hamper them in business.

No specific criteria for length are available for hairstyles as are available for clothing. Most successful businessmen wear their hair shorter than a rock star (rarely letting it reach their shirt collars) and longer than Telly Savalas; all of them wear it neatly arranged. Successful businesswomen wear their hair many lengths, from slightly longer than that of businessmen to almost shoulder length, again neatly arranged.

Gently waved and somewhat full hairstyles are preferred to very curly or "glued-to-the-head" styles for both men and women Selecting the style for yourself that helps you in business involves accommodating your hair type and your physical features.

Adapting Your Hair

If you have some special problems with hair, you need to consider these problems when you are selecting a style. Hair that varies far from medium texture, average bulk, oiliness,

Illus. 9-1. Well-groomed hair is expected in today's competitive world.

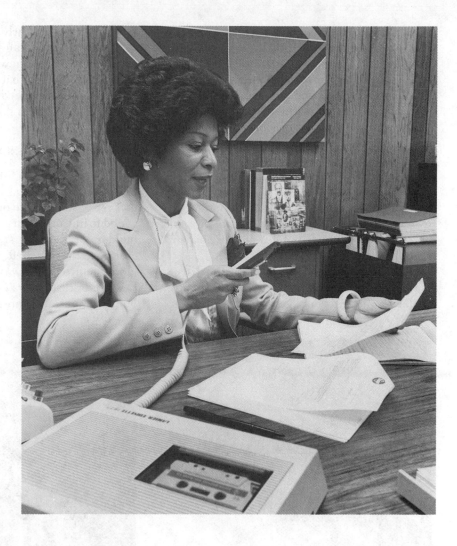

and curliness, or hair that is in poor condition needs special care in styling.

Hair Texture

Just the right texture probably doesn't exist. Most hair is too fine for some styles and too coarse for others. You can either (1) choose a hairstyle to meet the needs of your hair texture, or (2) alter the texture of your hair to meet the needs of the hairstyle you choose. Doing a little

of each will probably be of little trouble and allow for some freedom in selection.

Choosing the Hairstyle

Very fine hair will not hold a style very long without help. If your hair is fine, a good idea is to choose a style that (1) does not require much arranging and (2) looks good after a few hours at work. It is true that you can force fine hair into many styles with permanents, spray, and constant grooming; however, you may end up with fine but brittle, dry, unattractive hair, suffering from too much handling. You will be better off with a style that requires a minimum of processing if you can find one.

A blunt cut that is well shaped rather than a layered one, usually is easier to handle with fine hair that is dry. Fine, oily hair usually does best with a short, layered cut that has a body wave that doesn't allow it to cling to the scalp.

People with coarse hair need very careful haircuts that keep this hair-with-a-mind-of-its-own under control. Coarse hair has to be kept clean or it looks matted (if it is oily) or spiky (if it is dry).

For women a good idea for very coarse hair is a well-shaped blunt haircut that turns slightly under on the ends or slightly up on the ends.

Don't try for a very curly style if you have coarse hair; you will spend all your time setting it or needing to set it. Men with coarse straight hair need to avoid cuts that are too short on top. Coarse, curly hair needs more frequent trimming to keep it from growing "twigs."

Altering the Texture

Too much or too little texture can be controlled with products designed especially for that purpose. Texture or manageability can be added to fine hair with products labeled as body builders or texturizers. These products add a coating to the hair shaft, making it seem to have more bounce of its own. You can accumulate a buildup of texturizers on your hair, making it dull, if you use them regularly and if your hair

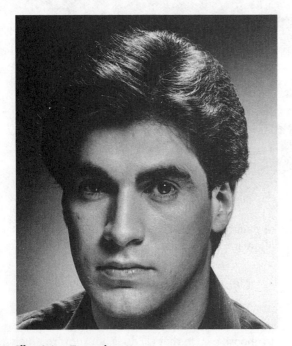

Illus. 9-2. Fine, oily hair usually does best with a short, layered cut that doesn't cling to the scalp.

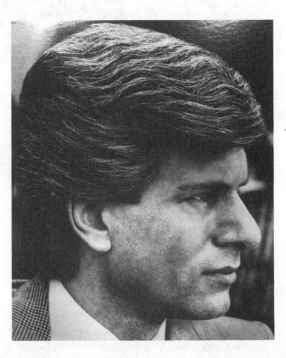

Illus. 9-3. Men with coarse hair should avoid cuts that are too short on top.

is very porous. When this seems to be happening, refrain from using the texturizer for a couple of shampoos to see whether or not the shine returns to your hair.

Too much texture or coarseness can be tamed with a cream rinse, which makes coarse hair much softer. The cream rinse is rinsed into your hair after you shampoo it. Try to keep the texturizers and cream rinses away from your scalp. They were intended for your hair, not your skin.

When you are arranging or setting fine hair, try drying it before you spray setting lotion on it. The setting lotion holds better because it is not diluted by the water on the hair. Lotions with body builders or texturizers are good for fine hair.

Hair Thickness

Few people are satisfied with the amount of hair they seem to have growing on their heads. There are some products to help give the illusion of more hair, but few to give the illusion of less hair. Body builders coat the hair, causing it to appear fuller. Also, you can color your hair, which tends to make the hair shaft swell, seeming to give it more bulk. Hair cuts and styling are important in reflecting more or less bulk in your hair. Hair setting lotions frequently add bulk to your hair by coating it, especially near the scalp. It is important to keep hair setting lotions off the scalp itself, though, because they tend to flake off your scalp when they are dry, making it look as if you have dandruff.

Thin hair should receive your utmost attention. If it is thin naturally, that is one thing; if it is thinning because of some problem, that is quite another. All of us lose up to 50 hairs a day. Don't worry about that. If you are losing more than your share, review your handling techniques and consult a doctor if it seems necessary. Some heads of hair are so thin naturally that the scalp shows through unattractively.

Coloring the hair blonde makes the scalp less obvious because the hair becomes approximately the same color as the scalp. However, not every complexion looks good with blonde hair. Very thin hair usually should be short because length tends to pull it very close to your head and makes it look even thinner. Thin hair can be gently curled or straight.

Hair that is very thick usually is a blessing. Thick hair generally needs some layering, though, especially if you wear a short style. It usually looks good either gently curled or straight with a slight curve under or up at the ends for women. Men with thick hair can get good layered cuts that give a full but controlled look.

Oiliness and Dryness

Hair is frequently either too oily or not oily enough. If it is too oily, frequent shampooing is

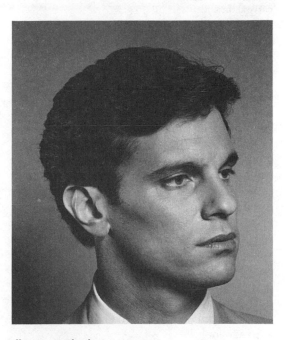

Illus. 9-4. Thin hair usually should be short.

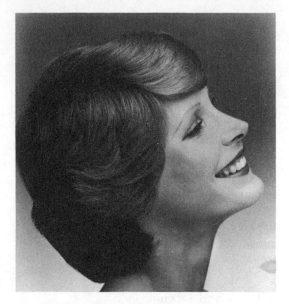

Illus. 9-5. Thick hair usually looks good either gently curled or straight with a slight curve at the ends.

a must. Use shampoos and aids designed especially for oily hair. Avoiding cream-based rinses, shampoos, and grooming aids will help control oil, too.

Very oily hair should be styled so that you can wash your hair every day if it needs it. A simple style will be best. Avoid styles that require hot hair dryers because these seem to stimulate oil production in your scalp. Although a conditioner may be needed occasionally, don't use one routinely since it tends to make your hair oilier. Use a vinegar or lemon rinse and warm-to-cool water when you wash your hair as well as a specially formulated shampoo for oily hair. Because it needs frequent washing, oily hair needs to be short. A permanent wave lifts the hair away from the scalp and helps keep this oily hair from packing close to the scalp, giving a greasy look.

Dry hair, too, should never be subjected to hot hair dryers. While it is stimulating the scalp, the hot air is drying — really drying — your hair. A quick conditioning treatment each time you shampoo your hair is a good idea. A thirty-minute conditioning treatment approximately every third or fourth shampooing will help. Try to space your shampooings a week apart since dry hair does not attract dirt like oily hair does. Try to protect your hair from dirt in the air and the drying rays of the sun with a head covering when you are outside. Specially formulated cream shampoos are good for dry hair. Avoid hairstyles that require frequent color or chemical treatments since these tend to dry your hair even more. A style for dry hair should be one that requires infrequent blow-drying, setting under the dryer, or curling with hot rollers.

With regular conditioning, dry hair can be styled in a variety of lengths and cuts. Only dry, fine hair tends to be fly-away and usually should have fewer layers than other dry hair.

Curl

The permanent curl in your hair can be increased or decreased at your pleasure — almost. There are, of course, permanent wave solutions that alter the structure of your hair shaft to make it straighter or curlier. These, applied to your hair when it is rolled on a permanent wave rod, will permanently curl your hair. Applied to your hair while it is pulled straight, these solutions will permanently straighten your hair. The permanence of either process depends upon the strength of the solution.

The main consideration is not how long your hair remains either curled or straightened but how much of the chemical it can take without damaging the hair. Very curly hair must take much abuse if it is to be permanently straightened. Very straight, lank hair likewise suffers strong assaults from powerful solutions if it is to be very tightly curled. The point is,

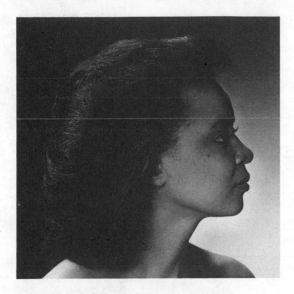

Illus. 9-6. The permanent curl in your hair can be increased or decreased.

spiky. Keep it in good condition to keep it under control and neatly arranged.

Physical Features

When you have learned to care for your hair and to accommodate any peculiarities it may have, you have the opportunity to style your hair so that it suits your physical and personal characteristics exactly. Consider your face and head shape and the relative size of your body in height and width. Be careful to examine any style you may be considering in light of how you will look in a full-length mirror, front, side, and back. The front should frame your face according to its best features, and camouflage your weaker ones. The side view should balance a high forehead, protruding nose, and any irregularities in your chin line. The back should reflect a hairstyle that is in proportion to the size

don't try to permanently change your hair too much in either direction.

Select a style that uses at least a degree of curl or straightness that is native to your hair shaft so that you won't be tempted to damage the shaft with strong solutions in an attempt to permanently curl or uncurl it. Once hair has been permanently curled or straightened, it should not be redone until new hair grows out and all the hair already exposed to the solution has been cut off.

In business, very curly hair often looks too casual. To relax the curl you can have a permanent on large rollers that relaxes tight curls into soft body waves, which are better suited to a professional look.

Curly hair should not be cut in many layers if it is to be kept under control. It does need expert shaping to avoid curlicue ends from sprouting like twigs. Curly hair that is very dry often looks bushy; very oily hair often looks

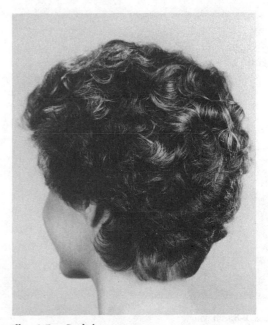

Illus. 9-7. Curly hair needs expert shaping to avoid curlicue ends.

of the remainder of your body, balancing an irregular width or height of your frame.

Facial Features

The idea in selecting a hairstyle to complement your facial features is to balance any irregularity in breadth or width in your forehead by not repeating a bad line in your face. The style should also provide a clear view of your strongest features, such as high cheekbones or expressive eyes. If, for example, your chin line is wider than your forehead, select a style that is wide at your forehead and temples and narrow at your chin. If you have a broad forehead and a pointed chin, select a hairstyle that covers part of your forehead on each side. If your forehead is very wide in proportion to the length of the rest of your face, select a hairstyle that conceals at least part of your forehead, giving your face better overall

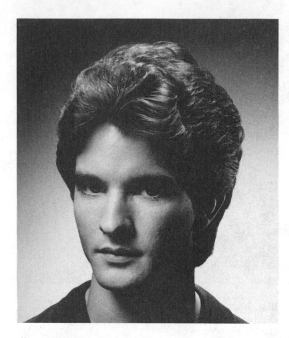

Illus. 9-9. If you have a broad forehead, select a style that covers part of your forehead on each side.

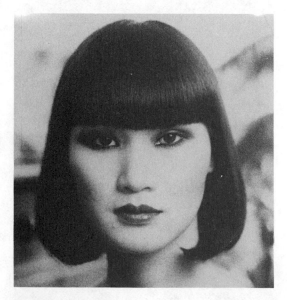

Illus. 9-8. If your chin is wider than your forehead, select a style that is wide at your forehead and temples.

proportion. If your eyes are close-set, choose a hairstyle that is full and widened at the temples. This will draw the eye in a horizontal line, widening the illusion of your eyes. If you have high cheekbones, select a hairstyle that shows the profile of your distinctive bone structure — never one that covers it.

Profile

Your profile may be the least important consideration in your hairstyle. If you must fudge on any point, do it on this one. The idea in selecting the right style for your profile is to consider the size and shape of your nose and chin. If either has an extreme shape, you should be especially careful that your hair does not contribute to the irregularity. A long nose under hair that is rather flat on top, slanting

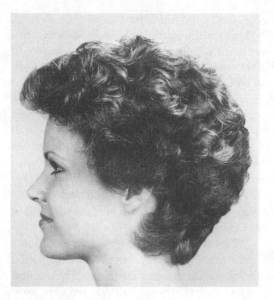

Illus. 9-10. In selecting the right style for your profile, consider the size and shape of your nose and chin.

upward to the crown will emphasize the length of the nose. A little height and softness on the top with a rounded profile will de-emphasize the length of the nose. A receding chin requires hair curling and slanting to the front on the ends to "bring the chin out." Never comb the hair back at the chin line if the chin is receding. To do so emphasizes the receding line by re-peating it.

Body Size

The relative size of your body should be balanced by your hairstyle. If your body is small, choose a small hairstyle, not too long, not too full. If your body is wide, choose a style that is "tall" and of medium width so that your head will contribute to the illusion of height but will balance your width. The width in your hair-style, however, should be above your earlobes.

Width in your hairstyle near your shoulders tends to widen your body. If you are unusually tall, don't wear your hair too short or too "tall." A longer style that is more nearly flat on top will balance your frame size better.

Personal Characteristics

How willing are you to learn the techniques needed to keep the style you select? How much time are you willing to spend daily on it to keep it attractive? How appropriate is the style for your life-style? Remember that the reason you are developing these dimensions of yourself is

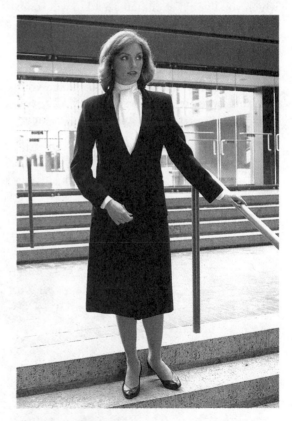

Illus. 9-11. If you are unusually tall, don't wear your hair too short or too "tall."

that you want to attain certain goals. Well-groomed persons always are preferred in business and public life over those who are not. Learning to care for your hairstyle is not difficult, and it becomes habit after a little practice. A few minutes at night and each morning spent in caring for your hair can make a tremendous difference in your all-day confidence in your appearance.

Select a hairstyle that fits your activities. Too casual a style that swings free and has loose, fly-away strands is inappropriate for the tailored appearance needed in business.

Take into consideration the climate in which you live. Wet climates tend to wilt some hairstyles and to make curly styles unruly. Dry climates tend to aggravate thin, fly-away hair that is short, and windy ones tend to destroy free-swinging styles of little body. Consider also your personality. Do you need to change your hair somewhat to be happy with it? Can you wear the same style for long periods without becoming bored with it?

Make a thoughtful inventory of ways you have worn your hair in the past, ways you would like to wear it, and what your hair actually will and will not do without excessive use of chemicals and handling. For example, if you have very fine, curly hair, it will never be coarse and straight without chemically altering it. Be realistic about your inventory items. Cross out styles that you have worn in the past that were too difficult to maintain or that you felt uneasy with. Disregard the styles that did not look good on you or that were faddish and are now out of date.

When thinking of the ways you would like to wear your hair, consider its texture, bulk, oiliness, condition, and curliness. Then eliminate styles that are not suitable because your hair is too fine or coarse or too thin or thick. Forget about styles that would not allow you to wash frequently or that would require too frequent washings. You should not consider a style

Illus. 9-12. Select a hairstyle that fits your activities.

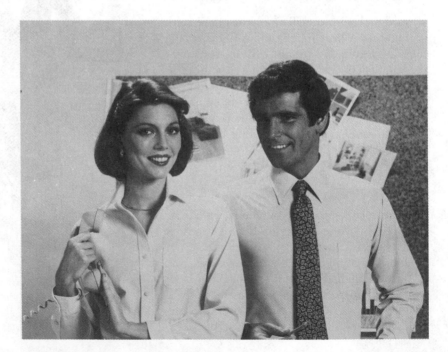

that would require straightening or permanent waving hair that is in poor condition or a style that would not suit the natural curliness or lack of it in your hair.

Hair Care

To have the best-looking hair you can have, you must have clean, healthy hair. If your hair is currently in poor condition, it probably got that way from abuse. Check the procedures you have used on your hair: Too much shampooing? Too much sun? Too much chlorine water? Too much permanenting? Too much coloring? Whatever the cause of your damaged hair, re-evaluate your practices and techniques. No hair looks truly good when it has been damaged. It does not heal. You simply must wait for new hair to grow (at the rate of one-half inch per month on the average).

In the meantime, damaged hair can look better if you use conditioners, texturizers, and body-building solutions that are fillers and that add some shine and body. A short hairstyle that allows you to cut most of the damaged hair off probably will be the most attractive way to wear your hair until new, healthy hair grows in. Avoid styles that require chemical curling or coloring of hair that is in poor condition.

Dandruff

Dandruff is a problem that is shared by many people. There is no known cure for dandruff. It is believed to be excessive flaking of the skin cells of the scalp, and there is no way to prevent it. You should shampoo when your scalp begins to flake. Massaging your scalp gently with your fingertips before shampooing may loosen scale that is ready to fall so that you can shampoo it out. Use of dandruff-control shampoos will help control your dandruff, but they will not cure it. With continued use, your scalp may build up a tolerance for the active ingredients in your dandruff-control shampoo, making it lose its effectiveness. Switch brands if your shampoo seems to quit working. Be very careful about allowing the "fallout" to rest on your clothes. A bit of flaking scalp on your collar or shoulders is unattractive.

Shampooing

Basic to well-groomed hair is regular shampooing. Shampooing is more than wetting, pouring on a little soap, and rinsing. You can give yourself a really good shampoo with very little effort.

Before you wet your hair, brush out all the loose spray, dirt, and dust you may have in it. If you are washing your hair in the shower, brush your hair back so that it will require a minimum of rearranging once it is wet. If you are bending over the sink to wash it, brush your hair forward.

A wide-tooth comb is handy to have beside you when you are shampooing your hair. You can comb conditioners down through your hair, making sure that each hair is coated and that the ends are saturated.

When you wet your hair use warm — not hot — water. Hot water seems to have a drying effect on dry hair and to stimulate oil gland production in oily hair. Warm-water-saturated hair is ready for shampoo. Start with your scalp, sudsing it and rubbing it with your fingertips — not your nails — to remove any scale and dirt. Add more shampoo if you need it, and clean your hair next, working from your scalp to the ends. Try to work quickly because leaving shampoo on too long seems to dry your hair out. If your hair is not exceptionally dirty or oily, one soaping is sufficient.

The rinse should be warm-to-cool water, if you can stand it. The rinse cannot be too well done. Rinse and rinse and then rinse some more. This is where most people shortchange their hair — soap left in dulls the hair and makes it tacky so that it attracts dirt and grime. What a mess! Try a cold water rinse at the end of your shampoo to give your hair shine.

Gently squeeze the water out of your hair, being careful not to pull or twist any of it. Wet hair is very fragile. Wrap a towel around your hair and let it soak up the excess water. Gently blot it with the towel, trying not to tangle it. Avoid rubbing the hair strands together when they are wet. After your hair is towel-dried you can use conditioners, cream rinses, and setting lotions if you wish.

The shampoo you use should suit the needs of your hair. There are shampoos designed to combat excessive oil, dryness, and dandruff; and you can get shampoo designed for use on hair that is colored. There are even some made for use without water. They are rarely satisfactory for regular use, though, and are used mainly when you cannot possibly wet your hair.

Conditioning

Conditioning does not heal or permanently change abused hair. It does add strength, though, and helps prevent further damage or breaking. Hair that has been subjected to harsh weather or to chemicals, such as those used to permanently curl or color it, needs to be conditioned frequently. The chemicals used for coloring and curling penetrate the hair shaft, causing tiny breaks in it. Conditioning temporarily fills these tiny breaks, giving some strength to the hair, making it smoother looking and usually more manageable. The longer and more often hair is subjected to chemicals or weather, the more often it needs conditioning. The ends of the strands need more conditioning care than that part which has newly grown from the scalp. Concentrating the conditioner where your hair is in poorest condition corrects damage without softening the hair too much near the scalp, where you may want more body.

Conditioners are applied to your hair after you shampoo, rinse, and towel-dry it. They may be left on for twenty to thirty minutes with or without heat, or they may be required for only two or three minutes. The hair is then flushed with cool-to-warm water, blot-dried again, and ready for hairsetting lotion.

Conditioners work by coating the hair shaft to make it much smoother. If they are designed to stay on for twenty to thirty minutes, they penetrate the hair shaft, adding strength. If they are designed for two to three minutes or less, they merely are coating the shaft. It is possible to get a buildup of the quickie conditioners if you use them after every shampoo. If you notice a dulling near the ends, or if they seem sticky when they are dry, you may need either to refrain from using conditioners for a while to allow the buildup to be stripped from the ends or begin using a vinegar or lemon rinse to strip the buildup. The occurrence of buildup depends upon how porous your hair is and the chemical makeup of the particular conditioner you are using.

Coloring

In business, you may have an advantage if you have brown hair, probably because most people do. On men, gray, especially salt and pepper, gives a distinguished appearance. Gray and white hair on women, however, are not popular in business.

At some time in their lives, both men and women will probably want to alter the color of their hair. There are some basic principles of hair coloring that will help you make and execute these decisions.

You can have attractive highlights and colors with little trouble if you stay with your own basic color. Coloring can be a great deal of trouble, however, if you have dark brown hair and decide to change it to flaming red or blonde. The new growth of hair (approximately one-half inch per month) must be colored as soon as it begins to show. However, if you have dark brown hair and add red or auburn highlights, or frost parts of the hair blonde, you may not need to retouch the hair for several months. Because coloring is a chemical treatment that can damage your hair, it is better to select a color not very different from your own so that the treatment will not have to be repeated frequently.

Personal Coloring

If you wish to change your hair color, be sure first of all that the color will look good with your complexion. If you have a dark complexion, do not try to change your hair to a very light red or blonde. If you are in doubt about how a color will look with your complexion, try on a wig of that color, and check your face in daylight and artificial light. Frequently it is necessary for women to change their makeup colors to a shade darker or lighter when they change the color of their hair. Sometimes it is helpful to darken or lighten eyebrows. While your wardrobe colors may remain basically the same, you may find that brighter or darker hues of your basic colors will enhance your new hair color.

There are several disadvantages to changing the color of your hair. Frequent coloring without regard to regular conditioning can permanently damage your hair. You will need to use a shampoo that is formulated for colored hair so that it will not strip the color each time you shampoo. Conditioning must be done at least once a month, perhaps more often. Most people need to condition when they touch up the new growth of hair which occurs approximately every four weeks.

The advantages to coloring your hair depend upon how it improves your appearance and the manageability of your hair. As you age, lighter hair tends to look better with your complexion and may be well worth the effort it takes to maintain it. If your hair is fine and thin, coloring it will give it more body because the chemicals in the coloring process swell the hair shaft. It can also make your hair dry and coarse, though, and you must be alert to these problems.

When you decide to change the color of your hair, decide whether you wish to go lighter or darker. If you are going lighter or highlighting, you will be involved in a two-step process unless your hair is very light already. This will involve stripping your hair of its color (the first step) and adding the color you want in the form of a toner (the second step). If you are already very light and want only to go a bit lighter, or if you want to darken your hair, you will probably be involved only in a one-step process. In a one-step process the chemical agent that causes the color to penetrate the hair shaft is mixed with the color itself and both are applied at the same time.

It is wise to let a professional hair colorist permanently color your hair for the first time. The hair colorist will want to give you a patch test for allergic reactions to the chemicals, and you will want a strand test before you actually submit to the color change. The patch test can save you much physical discomfort if you are allergic to the chemicals used. The strand test, in which a small amount of your hair is colored as a test to see how the color turns out before you do all of your hair, can save you much emotional discomfort if you do not like the resulting color. Hair that is permanently colored cannot be changed at will; it must have a resting period between color changes. You will have to live with whatever you get, at least for a while.

Temporary Color

There are coloring products designed for temporary changes. Instead of penetrating the hair shaft, stripping and replacing your natural color, they simply coat your hair, covering your natural color. Only slight changes can be achieved if you are trying to lighten because your natural color shows through the coating.

Temporary hair coloring products are designed mainly for covering gray and restoring faded color. They may last only until you shampoo again or through four or five shampoos, depending upon which kind you select.

Handling Hair

The less you have to handle your hair to keep it well-groomed, the better it is for your hair. The key to well-groomed hair every day, without excessive damage from handling, is to get an expert cut of a good style for your particular hair and become an expert in setting and/or arranging it so that it stays put without frequent handling.

Haircuts

The basic cuts available are variations of four styles. The first three are blunt cuts and the fourth one is a layered one. The blunt cuts (for women) can range from your chin line on down in length. The differences are: (1) the length is even all around, the sides being the same length as the back; (2) the sides are longer than the back; (3) the back is longer than the sides. Each of these blunt cuts can be with or without bangs, with a side or center part. The fourth cut is a layered one (for men or women). The layered cut seems to have more body if the layers are blunt cut with scissors rather than a razor.

Setting

Setting can be accomplished by blow-dry setting, with flat curls clipped or pinned in, and with rollers. Hair can also be wrapped around your head and dried for a very straight look. Most setting works better with a setting lotion.

If you use a blow-dry set, you will need a brush or a wide-tooth comb. The hair is usually towel-dried — blotted, not rubbed — and setting lotion is combed through. The hand-held hair dryer should be held approximately ten inches away from the head and moved from the scalp to the end of the hair while you comb or brush it in the direction opposite to what it will be when you are through. Move the dryer quickly enough so that not too much hot air is applied for too long a period to the hair. You can burn your hair very quickly. With short hair you can start at the crown or at the front hairline. With long hair you will probably find it easy to start at the hairline, combing forward as you dry it. Dry thin sections of hair at a time. When you use thick sections, the outer hair dries but the hair underneath remains damp.

Blow-dry styles can be shaped with a curling iron; or you can use a few hot rollers at the crown or near the ends to give them shape. If your hand-held dryer has a styling comb or brush attachment, use it just before your hair is completely dry.

When you need just a curve around the edges of short hair, use a styling brush attachment on damp hair. You can also create a curve with hairsetting tape or a curling iron. Usually, you get a longer lasting set if you pin or tape the hair while it is damp with setting lotion.

Plastic curlers are usually used in hair that is wet with setting lotion and dried under a hair dryer. The longest lasting set is achieved with this procedure. There are some basic hair setting procedures that you can use to achieve several hair styles. To set your hair on rollers, start at the front top and make a row down the center of your head to your neckline. Starting at the top, roll two rows down each side. This basic pattern will comb into many styles. You can angle the top and side rows to achieve different effects. The same pattern can be used with hot rollers on dry hair.

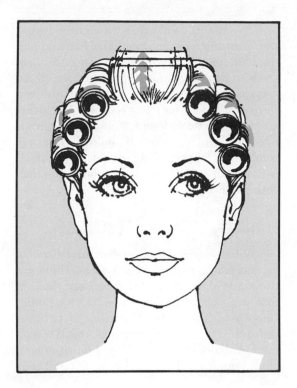

Illus. 9-13. A basic setting pattern will comb into many styles.

In-between setting can be done with a curling iron. Hot rollers and curling irons with mist give a longer lasting set than those without mist. Be sure to protect your ears and neck from the heat of the rollers with cotton or tissue. Allow hot curlers to cool completely before removing them. The curling iron usually is left in the hair for ten to thirty seconds and gently removed, disturbing the curl as little as possible until it cools. The hot curl can be pinned or clipped in until it is cool, if you like.

Arranging

Keep in mind when you brush and comb your hair that the less wear and tear on your hair, the better its condition will be. Very gentle combing and brushing is recommended. However, the frequency of the handling is important, too. It is better, for example, to do whatever is necessary at one time, even if it requires back-combing gently and use of hairspray. The style should not need rearranging again for several hours. This is far better than giving your hair a few quick "run throughs" with a comb several times a day to keep it well-groomed.

Very few people need to brush one hundred strokes a day. The only known benefits are that brushing spreads the scalp oil throughout the hair and it stimulates the scalp. The damage resulting from brushing is worse for most people than the benefit gained.

When you are combing your hair into place, do so gently. Some back-combing, especially near the crown and near your temples if you need fullness, may be done without harm to your hair if you do so gently. Back-combing, because you are combing the hair against its natural grain, can increase damage to hair that is split by splitting it more. However, back-combing it gently near the scalp where the hair is the healthiest and strongest should not damage your hair, and it can add much to the shape of your hairstyle.

Hairspray can be used to hold your hair in place with no damage to the hair. It can prevent tangles by holding your hair in place against onslaughts of wind and other tangling agents. The can should be held away from the hair approximately ten to twelve inches while you are spraying so that the mist will settle evenly on your hair.

The Appliances

A professional hairdresser can do things for your hair that you cannot do as well for yourself. You owe it to yourself, however, to learn all you can about keeping your hair as attractive as possible between visits to your hairdresser. It will take a little practice to learn to use some of the products and aids that will help in caring for your hair, but your reward will be well-groomed hair every day.

Combs and Brushes

The comb and brush you've been using all your life are your most basic tools. Be sure that the teeth of the comb and the bristles of the brush have rounded ends. That is the main criterion. They can be plastic, rubber, or some natural substance; the substance makes little difference. The teeth on your comb should be spaced far enough apart to comb through your hair easily but close enough, of course, to arrange your hair. If your hair is heavy, thick, or very curly, try a synthetic brush, which is stronger than a natural bristle one.

Force yourself to replace your comb or brush when they show signs of wear, such as bristles or teeth with jagged or sharp edges. These can damage your hair. Hair grooming aids should be washed as often as your hair is. Combs and brushes other than those with wooden handles can be immersed in warm, soapy water to be cleaned. Use a fingernail brush to clean your comb, and swish your brush back and forth in the water to clean it. Rinse them carefully and dry them on a towel.

Heated Curlers and Curling Irons

Heated curlers and curling irons are aids for curling and smoothing your hair. Heated curlers come in several sizes and may be mist, dry, or conditioner curlers. Curling irons may be with or without steam. It is a good idea to plan to use end papers to protect the ends of your hair from drying out if you use hot curlers or curling irons regularly on your hair.

To smooth your hair with a curling iron, start near the scalp on a section of hair and pull the hair smoothly through the iron. The heat tends to straighten and smooth the hair. If you want a slight curve near the end, take one or two turns and hold it for a few seconds. Curls that are set with heated rollers and curling irons need to cool completely before they are combed. A longer lasting set can be obtained with mist or a heat-activated setting lotion than with dry heat.

Rollers

Rollers for setting wet hair are made of various materials and in many sizes. There are two kinds of materials that rollers are made of that are gentle to your hair: (1) magnetic, smooth plastic and (2) wire-mesh without brushes. Your style determines the size you need. Usually rollers are clipped in with metal clips, but pins will work if they do not pull your hair.

The correct amount of hair for each roller is the amount of space the roller takes up when placed against your head. It should rest on the area where the hair that is wrapped around it grows. Be sure that when you put a roller in your hair you do not roll it tightly. The strain on the roots of your hair may damage them. Carefully enclose the ends of your hair in end papers, and smoothly wind the hair and papers around each roller so that you will not crimp the ends of your hair unattractively.

Hair Dryers

A home hair dryer is a good investment. There are several kinds. A hand-held blow-dryer is used for drying hair before it is set or while you are setting it with a comb or brush. A flexible bonnet-type hair dryer is one that is designed to be placed over hair that is set wet on rollers. Bonnet dryers will work but they do not distribute the air as evenly as the third kind of dryer, a hard-hood type similar to that in a beauty salon.

A hand-held blow-dryer usually has several heat settings for drying your hair. Usually you comb your hair with a wide-tooth comb in the direction opposite to the way you will eventually set it, while you let the warm air blow it dry. It is best to dry a small section at a time. Trying to dry thick sections at one time tends to burn the outer hair, leaving the hair underneath slightly damp. You can severely burn your hair with a hand-held dryer if you hold it too close or too long over one section of hair. Many people blow-dry their hair prior to setting it on hot rollers. Others blow-dry, combing the hair into place as it dries so that it does not require a set. Your haircut determines which method you should use.

Hand-held dryers with combs and brushes attached are best for styling while you dry. They have warm instead of hot air temperatures so that you can use them close to your hair.

Bonnet and hood-type dryers should have warm air settings because too much heat may damage your hair. The curls should be cooled before they are combed, and you can plan for this by turning the dryer to "cool" a few minutes before you are ready to comb.

Setting Lotion

Most hair styles last longer when setting lotions are used. Even if you are blow-drying your hair prior to setting it or while you set it, setting lotion combed through towel-dried hair will give you a longer lasting and more manageable set.

Some lotions are conditioners and setting lotion in one and are not designed to be rinsed out before setting as most conditioners are. These combination lotions are good for occa-

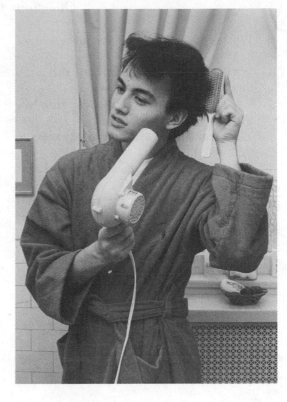

Illus. 9-14. Hand-held blow-dryers can be used for styling while you dry.

sional use but may build up and dull your hair if they are used too frequently.

Hairspray

Hairspray fell into disrepute when it was used to construct elaborate hairstyles that could not be combed. When used correctly, however, it can give you hours of well-groomed hair through wind, rain, and sleet. Don't be afraid of its ill-gotten reputation. Try it on your hair a little at a time, holding the can 10 to 12 inches from your hair so that it lands in a fine mist wherever you need control.

Questions for Chapter 9

1. What is the main business requirement for hair?
2. What hairstyles are good for hair that is too fine? too coarse?
3. What can you do to alter the texture of hair that is too fine? too coarse?
4. What can you do to make hair that is too thin look thicker?
5. What hairstyles are good for hair that is very oily?
6. What difference does the amount of curl native to your hair make when you select a hairstyle?
7. How can you balance uneven facial features with your hairstyle?
8. What personal characteristics should you consider in selecting a hairstyle?
9. Describe good shampooing procedure.
10. How do conditioners work?
11. What are the disadvantages to changing the color of your hair?
12. What appliances are helpful in setting your hair?

Chapter 10

Business Postures

Chapter Objectives

After studying this chapter, you should be able to:

1. *Develop standing posture for good physiological functioning.*
2. *Develop walking posture for good physiological functioning.*
3. *Develop sitting posture for good physiological functioning.*
4. *Perform exercises that contribute to good posture.*
5. *Adopt postures that will improve your appearance.*
6. *Recognize nonverbal language communicated by postures.*

Business posture requires you to consider three aspects: your physiology, your appearance, and your kinesic communication. Fortunately, all three aspects are enhanced by good posture: your body will function more efficiently; you will be perceived as an alert and efficient person; and you will "say" to others you are a competent person.

Positioning your body and moving to get yourself from one place to another are so automatic you may not give them a second thought. Researchers tell us, though, that there is good reason to devote attention to the positions and movements of our bodies.

Besides placing us where we want to be, the posture we exhibit does two additional things:

1. It provides for body functioning both physiologically and cosmetically.
2. It is a means of communication.

Physiological Functioning

Physiologically, muscles and bones are designed to function in a particular way. They suffer strain and sometimes permanent disfigurement when they are continually misused. Incorrect postures can result in low back pain, strained muscles, permanently deformed shoulders, and curved spines. The muscular and skeletal machinery of the body also works in such a way as to provide for unobstructed internal functioning with little strain, tension, and possibility for injury. This superb design provides for efficient physiological functioning.

Standing Posture

Standing posture is a basic one and it influences all other postures. There is a center of gravity for your body in every posture. That

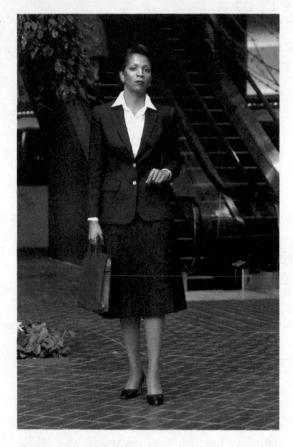

Illus. 10-1. Business posture requires you to consider three aspects: your physiology, your appearance, and your kinesic communication.

Correct Alignment

To assume the correct posture, develop a mental routine that you can perform anytime with or without a mirror. If you are strengthening your muscles with regular exercise, the correct posture will be easy to maintain once you assume it.

Unless you have skeletal malformations from genetic defect, too many years of poor posture, accident, or disease, good body alignment is not only possible; it is preferable to any other alignment.

1. With your feet slightly apart, distribute your weight equally between them.
2. Stand as "tall" as you can with comfort.
3. Check your eyes to be sure they are focused neither up nor down, so that your head is level.
4. Straighten your neck so that your chin is directly over the "u" shaped notch of the breastbone at the base of your neck.
5. Shoulders are down and slightly back although not abnormally so.
6. Straighten your backbone at the waist by tucking your buttocks slightly under and pulling your stomach up and in.
7. Give your knees a little flexion so that they are not locked.
8. Now, concentrate on how correct body alignment feels. Most of the time you must depend on how alignment feels, since a mirror usually is not available. Also, the more comfortable you become with this aligned feeling, the more often you will notice when it is lacking.

Checking Alignment

You can check that alignment by taping a string to the top center of your full-length mirror and allowing the string to fall freely, making a straight line through the center of the mirror. Align your body by positioning your earlobe

center is the point at which the entire weight of your body is concentrated so that, if supported at this point, the body will remain in equilibrium in any position. That center, when your body is properly aligned in a standing position, passes through the midpoint of your body. Specifically, from a side view, this imaginary straight line passes through the earlobe, center of the shoulder, center of the hip, slightly to the back of the kneecap, and slightly to the front of the ankle bone.

along the line. Ask someone to help you position yourself and to evaluate your body alignment. From the front view, points to check are:

1. Head and neck centered between your shoulders with shoulders relaxed and even.
2. Pelvis and hipbones even and centered squarely over your feet.
3. Feet pointed straight ahead.

From the side view, points to check are:

1. Chin parallel to the floor.
2. Shoulders neither too far back nor too far forward.
3. Abdomen flat.
4. Small of the back straight.
5. Buttocks tucked under.
6. Knees straight but relaxed.

If a single point is out of alignment, some other part of the body will disalign itself to make it easier for you to maintain your equilibrium. For example, if your buttocks are protruding abnormally, your stomach will protrude to maintain your equilibrium. If your head is held forward, some other part —probably your upper back — will be curved out abnormally to compensate. These abnormalities look unattractive, and they will strain muscles and disfigure bone structure, eventually causing you pain.

Walking Posture

The posture developed for standing applies to walking. The straight line from your earlobe through your hips remains the same. Your legs simply swing from the hip joint in the way they were particularly designed to do. The arms should swing gracefully at your sides to maintain that delicately balanced center of gravity as your legs alternately swing forward.

Alignment and Movement

The idea is to stand tall, tuck buttocks under, keep shoulders low, take steps about as long as your feet are, and swing the arm of the same side back approximately the same distance as the length of the step. The swing of the arm is very gentle — not stiff or awkward. In fact, it should hardly be noticeable. The knees are kept slightly flexed. If they are stiff, the weight of the body is bounced on the cartilage of the knee, which eventually causes pain. If they are slightly flexed, the bend cushions the weight of the body, not allowing it to destroy the structure of the knee. A stiffened knee also will give a bouncing walk that jars your head. *Smooth* is the key word. If you glide along smoothly, your walk is correct. If your head or body is bobbing, something is wrong.

Correct Walking Posture

Some of the common problems occurring in walking are:

1. Feet that point out or in. Frequently this causes a twisting motion that is not healthy for the spine.
2. A stride that is too long, causing the head and body to bob up and down at the beginning and middle of the long step.
3. Feet kept too far apart. This looks like the walker is straddling a ditch and makes for an uncomfortable bounce of the torso. The feet should pass closely together, not touching, maintaining parallel lines.
4. Too much bend in the knee, sometimes accompanied by slumped shoulders, giving an apelike appearance.
5. Heavy steps caused by striking the foot to the floor very hard, as if to make an imprint in the floor. Actually, the heel should gently strike the floor first, followed by a roll to the ball of the foot from which you push off for

the next step. The gentleness of the foot-work provides the basis for a gliding motion of the upper body.

6. Those who look like they are walking a tight-rope, placing one foot directly in front of the other instead of maintaining parallel lines.
7. Tiny steps that appear to be mincing the floor as the walker moves along.
8. Hands clutched tightly and jerked back and forth. Your hands should be relaxed with fingers slightly curved. The swing of the arm should be from the shoulder in a graceful arc.
9. Leaning the body backward or forward with each step. The chin should remain level as your body moves forward with a smooth, gliding motion.

Taking A Seat

The way to take a seat is to approach the chair from an angle and walk close enough to touch one leg to the edge of the seat of the chair. Then turn, allowing the back of your leg to touch the chair, placing one foot slightly in front of the other so that the magical center of gravity won't fail as you propel your body into the sitting position. Slowly bend only at the hip and knee joints. Keep the upper part of the body straight. Use your hands and arms if necessary only to guide yourself into the seat of the chair if the chair has arms. Otherwise, the hands and arms will not be needed during this maneuver.

If you do not turn your head to look at the seat of the chair as you sit, your balance will be easier to maintain and you will appear less awk-ward and more sure of yourself. Allow the leg that is touching the chair to be your guide. Using this procedure usually places your but-tocks on the front part of the seat of the chair. When your weight is on the chair, use your hands on the chair seat to gently lift yourself back into the chair so that the back of the chair braces your back. It is normal to lean forward

when you talk from a sitting position, but it must be done from the hip joints, not the waist. A slumped, curved spine results from leaning from the waist.

Good sitting posture maintains the same alignment from the hips to the head as good standing posture. You should be sure that you sit well back into the chair, keeping your spine straight but allowing the back of the chair to support your back. Your thighs should rest on

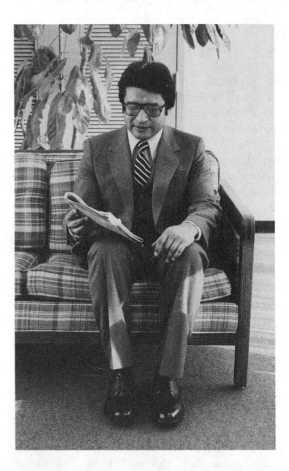

Illus. 10-2. Good sitting posture maintains the same alignment from the hips to the head as good standing posture.

the seat of the chair almost to the bend of the knee, and your feet should rest comfortably on the floor.

The structure of the chair is important. A chair that has a seat too deep to allow you to sit back and bend your knees simultaneously will be uncomfortable. When you sit in such a chair, sit forward far enough to allow your legs to bend naturally from the knee; but concentrate on keeping your hips, back, and head aligned as if you were standing. This kind of chair simply will not support your back properly.

One of the most comfortable positions is to place your feet flat on the floor, one foot slightly in front of the other, or to position your feet with the arch of one near the heel of the other, similar to the standing position. However your legs are arranged, try to maintain the alignment from your head to your hips.

Although physiologically it is better not to cross your legs while sitting, they may be crossed at the ankles and positioned slightly to the side of your body on the side of the front foot. Also, they may be crossed near the knee, preferably well above the knee. The ankles are kept close together but not wound around one another. If the chair is low enough, the crossed legs may be moved slightly to the side of the lower leg. An exaggerated side placement can throw the upper part of the body out of alignment.

Some of the common problems with sitting posture are:

1. Bending at the waist as you sit. It is infinitely better if you bend only where you have joints designed for such bending. In this case those joints are the hip joints, where the thighs of your legs are joined to your torso. Keep the waist straight so that the spine is not bent out of shape as you sit.
2. Slumping the shoulders. Shoulders should be kept level and in line with the hips. Slumping forward stretches the muscles in your back and contracts those in the chest.

3. Crossing legs too close to the knees. Legs, if they are to be crossed at all near the knees, should be crossed above the knees to allow for proper circulation in the lower leg. The back of the knee should not be pressed hard against the thigh of the other leg because to do so will restrict circulation. Crossing the legs higher puts much less strain on the cardiovascular activity in the leg.
4. Letting knees fall apart when legs are crossed at the ankles. Sitting with your knees apart makes you look sloppy. It gives your entire body the illusion of being wider than it is. If you stand or sit with knees apart, you widen the line of your body. When you cross your legs at the ankle, sweep your feet to one side so that your knees fall together naturally. Legs crossed at the ankles are easier to sweep to the side of the forward foot.

The position of your hands has nothing to do with bone and muscle support and alignment, but their placement can affect the appearance you project. Some common hand postures are:

1. Cupping your hands in your lap.
2. Crossing your arms with fingers along opposite upper arms.
3. One hand in your lap, the other hanging loosely from the arm of the chair.
4. One hand in your lap, the other resting on the chair seat, palm down.

Exercises for Good Posture

Exercises to help you attain good posture are those that strengthen the muscles in your neck, back, stomach, and legs. If you have problems with your posture or body movement, use the exercises below daily until you are able to maintain the posture you desire.

1. Neck — Upright position, place palm side of interlaced fingers behind your head. Push

head backward, resisting with a forward pull of the hands.

2. Neck — Lying, face-up position with head hanging off a bed or couch. Arms alongside body. Curl chin upward to chest, using neck muscles. Lower slowly. Vary exercise by turning head to right or left and raise head. 15 to 25 repetitions.

3. Neck and Abdomen — Lying, face-up position, hands at sides. Using tightened abdominal muscles and neck and chest muscles, curl head and shoulders off the floor. Hold this position for five to eight seconds. Return head to floor slowly. 10 to 15 repetitions.

4. Abdomen and Back — Standing. Heels 3 to 5 inches from wall, back to wall, knees bent slightly. Using gluteal and abdominal muscles, push as much as you can of your back against the wall. As strength is gained, move heels closer to wall and straighten knees. This exercise is your major posture building aid for the pelvic area.

5. Back — Lying, face-up position. Draw knees to chest, tightening abdominal muscles. Grasp legs below knees and pull them toward head.

6. Thighs — Sitting position, leaning backward, bracing with hands behind, palms down, knees bent, feet lifted from floor. Alternately straighten each leg and return to bent position. 15 to 25 repetitions each leg.

7. Calves — Standing position, hands on hips, knees half bent. Raise heels from the floor, balancing weight on toes. Lower heels to starting position. 15 to 20 repetitions.

——————— *Cosmetic Functioning* ———————

Posture and body movement have a major impact on the way we are perceived by others. We are presumed to be confident or self-conscious, nervous or relaxed, comfortable or uncomfortable according to the postures and body movements we exhibit.

Illus. 10-3. Posture and body movement have a major impact on whether or not you will be perceived as a confident leader.

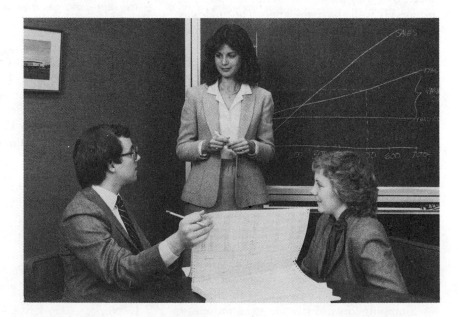

A good bit of what we believe about others and what they believe about us comes from the cosmetic arrangement visible to us. You don't need someone to tell you that downcast eyes, drooping shoulders, and a shuffling step are not signs of a confident, happy person. You make that interpretation yourself. You don't need someone to tell you that the leader of a group meeting is not the person huddled in the corner of the sofa with arms and legs tightly crossed. You don't need to be told that a person who stares into space and turns away while you are talking is not enthusiastic about what you are saying.

People generally interpret erect posture as meaning you are interested, ready, and cooperative — that the persons with whom you are communicating deserve your utmost attention. A casual posture may communicate comfort and enjoyment and that the persons with whom you are communicating may be taken for granted.

Walking

The length of your stride in walking and the pace at which you walk may communicate emotional states. Generally, the lighter the step and the quicker the pace, the happier the person is believed to be and the more ready to pursue goals. People who walk as if they have lead in their shoes may be perceived as sulky, and slow to move in making decisions. People who half-heartedly shuffle along appear dejected and may communicate a lack of goals and direction.

Sitting

One professional interviewer, when asked to name the two most important things for an applicant to do, said, "First of all, dress right; second, sit right."

When you seat yourself, you show an alert person ready for communication by placing your feet comfortably close together, flat on the floor; resting your hands on your lap; keeping your back straight, leaning slightly forward; and holding your head erect. You show less enthusiasm by either sprawling your feet and legs across the floor, by crossing them tightly, or by hanging one foot across the other leg. You may show nervousness or boredom by swinging a leg, tapping a foot, or fidgeting with your hands. You show lack of alertness by slumping in the chair.

Some of the body movements and postures people find distracting are:

1. picking at or stroking one's own hair, face, or clothing.
2. resting one's head on a hand.
3. chewing on glasses, or worse, on gum.
4. looking too much or too little at the speaker.
5. constant movement of either hands or feet while you are speaking or while others are speaking.

The cosmetic functions of posture and body movement include providing for a professional image. Well-tailored clothes fit well on a well-postured body, not on slumped shoulders or bulging stomachs.

The tall, thin look can be achieved by polishing your standing posture. The arch of one foot is placed against the heel of the other. In bringing the foot back, the body is slightly turned so that there is more of a profile view than a broader front view. The idea is to avoid a full front presentation. By rearranging your foot position and your face direction, you can present yourself from the thinner appearing profile view.

Communicating

Besides giving signals about yourself with your postures and movement, you may be communicating (to those able to understand) more specific messages. Researchers say that whether we want to or not, we identify ourselves with our postures and body movements. They say that all social animals of a common species when they encounter one another identify themselves to the other with behavior which:

1. Signifies membership in the species.
2. Signifies membership in a group.
3. Signifies a particular state of "readiness."

This encounter behavior is easily observed among cats and dogs. It is not as easily observed among people — unless you know the signs of identity.

Identity as a member of the species is automatic for people: few of us appear to be members of any species other than *homo sapiens,* the thinking species of the *homo* genus.

Our group membership and state of readiness is not an automatic identity. We exhibit behavior including posture and body movement we have learned to show that identity.

Group Posture

Posture and body movement communicate whether we intend them to or not. What they communicate depends on the body "language" we adopt in our group and the understanding of the person observing us. Some important facts about posture and body movements that define group behavior are:

1. They follow definite patterns within a social group and may vary somewhat from group to group.
2. The patterns and systems are a function of the social system of which they are a part. Those used in an office, for example, are uniquely adapted to the communication needs of that situation.
3. Body movement of one member of a group influences other members of the group. The most obvious group influence is that we

tend to imitate postures and movements of those we support and agree with, and we unconsciously shift away from those with whom we do not agree.

People who study social groups believe that body movement and postures are therefore a learned form of communication. Like language, this form of communication varies from group to group; a particular posture in one group will not necessarily mean the same thing in another culture. We learn to communicate with language by hearing and practicing it. We learn to communicate with posture by observing and practicing it. Having people nod their heads to answer our questions affirmatively teaches us to nod to signify agreement.

The head nod is an easy one because we see people using it from the time we learn to focus our eyes. Postures and body momements in situations such as interviews, meetings, and other business situations may be unknown, like a foreign language, until we have time to observe and learn them. Unlike a head nod, which everyone in our culture agrees is an affirmative sign, other postures and movements may not have universally known and agreed upon meanings. They may even have meanings varying according to the context of surrounding circumstances.

To say that a given posture or movement means a certain thing in all circumstances is risky. However, learning to observe and interpret these nonverbal communications in context in the groups of which you are a part (a) among others, (b) from someone to you, or (c) from yourself to others can vastly expand your understanding and communicating abilities within your group.

To begin understanding body movement and postures in unfamiliar contexts is to:

1. Notice the mere *presence* of body movement with or without the accompanying words.

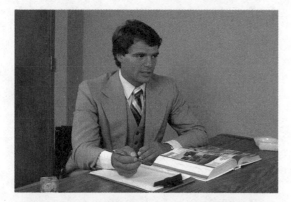
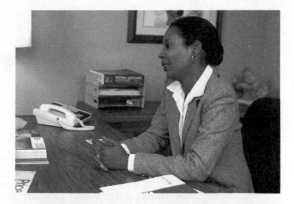
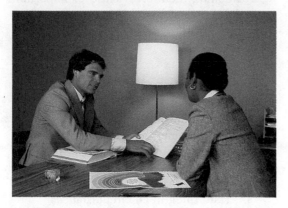
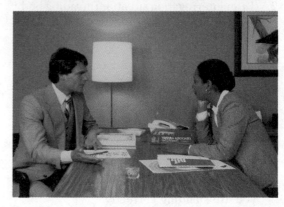

Illus. 10-4. Posture and body movement in an office are uniquely adapted to the communication needs of that situation.

2. Notice the *absence* of body movement with or without the spoken word.

Next, you can characterize the posture and movements you observe as:

1. Appropriate or inappropriate within a given scene. Ask yourself if the movements seem to occur naturally and fit the surrounding scene.
2. Reinforcing or contradicting the spoken communication. Do the movements belie

what is being said? Do the actions express the same things as the words?
3. Having placement, physiological, or cosmetic purpose. Are the movements serving some purpose other than communicative?

It will help you learn to interpret and use posture and body movements to communicate if you learn to observe the space people maintain between themselves and others. We seem to set boundaries around ourselves, defining our personal space, which varies in size according to the relationship we desire with a person during a particular encounter. We set closer boundaries for encounters which are more emotionally intimate and larger ones for those from which we maintain emotional distance.

You can get an idea of how an encounter will go by observing the positioning of the participants. You may usually assume that people will not have close give-and-take communication when one is:

1. (In an office) sitting behind a large desk while the other stands some distance away.
2. (In an interrogation situation) invading body space in a threatening way by standing close to the other who is sitting.

3. (In a lecture) standing in a solitary leadership position while others are in an audience position.

You can usually recognize the relative importance people feel in relation to others by the way they position themselves. People may show importance by:

1. Sitting comfortably while others stand.
2. Standing close to and over a sitting person.
3. Summoning people to their own offices rather than going to someone else's office.
4. Positioning themselves close to important people, such as by selecting an office close to those in recognized powerful positions.

Questions for Chapter 10

1. What three things does posture provide for us?
2. What can be the result of incorrect postures?
3. From a side view, where does an imaginary straight line pass through your body when you are standing correctly?
4. What points can you check on your standing posture from the front view?
5. What are some common problems occurring in walking?
6. What is the best way to take a seat?
7. What are some of the common problems with sitting posture?
8. What are the cosmetic effects of good posture?
9. What are some of the body movements and postures people find distracting?
10. Describe the "encounter" behavior of

members of a species.
11. What are some facts about posture and body movement that define group behavior?
12. Can you say that a body movement means a certain thing in all circumstances?
13. What can you do to begin to understand postures and body movements in unfamiliar contexts?
14. What ways can you characterize posture and movement?
15. How do we decide how large our personal boundaries will be in various situations?
16. What positions usually mean a give-and-take atmosphere will not prevail?
17. How can people show you their relative importance?

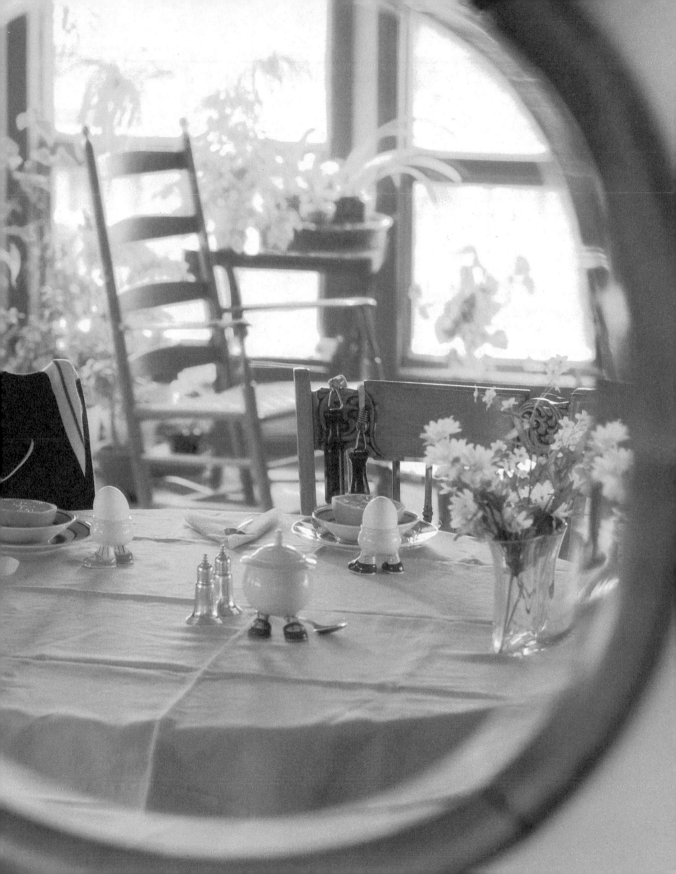

PART THREE: *Individual Matters*

Part Objectives

After studying this part, you should be able to:

1. *Understand the impact your personal appearance has on your success in dealing with people.*

2. *Keep your heart and lungs healthy with appropriate exercise.*

3. *Select and perform exercises that aid you in achieving good body proportion and good body movement.*

4. *Groom your skin, fingernails, hands, toenails, and feet.*

5. *Maintain a healthy diet and your weight at a healthy level.*

Chapter 11

Program for Success

Chapter Objectives

After studying this chapter, you should be able to:

1. *Increase your awareness about quality and the role it plays in your success.*
2. *Link personal appearance to (a) the way you perceive others, (b) the way others perceive you, and (c) the reasons people choose their associates.*
3. *Understand the implications of personal appearance for succeeding in business.*
4. *Show awareness of timeless style and simplicity as they relate to your personal grooming.*

Your program for success calls for you to learn about quality and the practical reasons for choosing to surround yourself with quality items and associate yourself with people who value your efforts. Because quality rarely comes easily and cheaply, your program for success should prepare you for selecting carefully and wisely. The aura of quality radiates to all parts of your life and brings you advantages that enrich yet simplify living.

Evaluating Quality

People entering jobs are moving toward making lasting choices. The word *quality* is one that correlates well with *lasting*. Although diffi- cult to define, most people agree that an item of quality is reliable, has long-term durability, and consistently functions as it is designed to. A sense of timeless style, simplicity, and a pres- ence that makes people comfortable are associ- ated with quality.

Although the word *quality* may not strictly apply to people, the components of quality re- late to the way we perceive people. Everyone appreciates a person who is reliable, whose personality "wears well" in the long term, and who has consistently appropriate behavior. Al- though not so well known, people appreciate a person with timeless style, simplicity, and a presence that makes people comfortable, and they associate many other positive character- istics with such a person. To enjoy such appreciation and association, you should know how to achieve an appearance that bespeaks quality.

Overcoming Resistance

To suggest that appearance affects the quality of a person's life seems undemocratic to most people. Indeed, if people are asked whether or not they judge others by the way they look, they will answer negatively and may even be insulted by the question. However, when their behavior is observed, their responses consistently show that they do, indeed, respond to attractive people positively and to unattractive ones negatively.

Psychologists explain this inconsistency by saying that because we believe our own characteristics emanate from internal workings of our minds and bodies, we consider judging others or being judged by outer appearances unfair. Overlooked in such reasoning is the fact that we can neither see the characteristics of others nor

show our own characteristics to others without long-term association. We, therefore, depend upon what we do see and have learned to associate with positive and negative characteristics to make decisions about people.

Learning to associate visible signals with characteristics starts early in our lives. When people tell their children stories, they make the beautiful princesses good and the ugly ones bad. They turn a prince into a frog to punish him and require that he be kissed by a *beautiful* princess to regain his princedom. They make Cinderella beautiful and good and her stepsisters ugly and bad.

Beyond selecting people because of their appearance, other selections are made based on appearance. Few people select unattractive surroundings in which to live if they have a choice; few select food that is not visually appealing to eat; few vacation in places they consider ugly. Such preference for attractiveness may be more than the result of early conditioning we have in children's stories.

Illus. 11-1. You should know how to achieve an appearance that bespeaks quality.

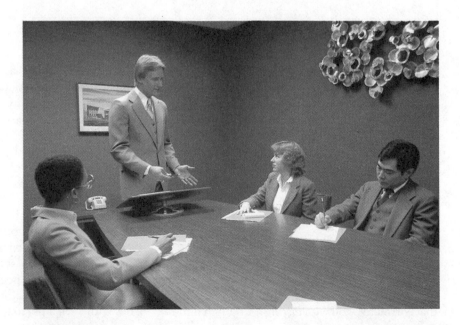

Evaluating Appearances

Because physical appearance has such a profound impact on a person's life, many studies have been done to learn what people believe about appearance. Some of these studies can guide you in evaluating responses you get to your own appearance, and perhaps in understanding some of your feelings about yourself.

About Ourselves

Social psychologists believe that a person's self-concept often develops from observing what others think about him or her. Knowing that attractive persons are treated as if they have more positive characteristics, the researchers set out to learn if the general population responds with self-concepts that reflect their treatment by others.

Although when people are asked if they believe themselves to be attractive, they often answer with modesty, those that are believed attractive by others, when asked to rate themselves, consistently rate themselves higher than unattractive persons rate themselves. For example, physically attractive individuals believe themselves (1) to be more popular, (2) to have a better personality, and (3) to be more able to get dates than unattractive persons believe themselves to be. Physically attractive women report more satisfaction with their general popularity, their leadership ability, and their degree of self-consciousness than unattractive women do.[1]

The more attractive a person is, the more attractive, personable, and considerate he or she expects his or her date to be.[2] Thus, attractive individuals expect more of their associates than unattractive people do.

About Others

Because we hold higher opinions of ourselves according to our degree of attractiveness, researchers have studied how others perceive people according to their degree of attractiveness. It is expected that members of the opposite sex are influenced by appearance. Not so well known is the fact that interpersonal attraction is influenced by physical attractiveness regardless of whether men are relating to men *or* women.[3] In general, interpersonal attraction is greater toward physically attractive strangers regardless of sex than toward unattractive ones.

People believe attractive people possess more socially desirable personality traits than unattractive persons.[4] For example, they rate attractive people as more likely to have higher occupational status, more marital competence, more parental competence, more social and professional happiness, and more total happiness than unattractive people. In general, they believe that attractive people lead better lives than unattractive ones.

People who participated in a study asking what they liked and disliked about their dates found that physical attractiveness was the most important determinant of whether or not a first-

---

[1] E. Walster, G. Walster, E. Berscheid, and K. Dion, "Physical Attractiveness and Dating Choice: A Test of the Matching Hypothesis," *Journal of Experimental Social Psychology*, Vol. 7 (1971), pp. 173-189.

[2] E. Walster, V. Aronson, D. Abrahams, and L. Rottman, "Importance of Physical Attractiveness in Dating Behavior," *Journal of Personality and Social Psychology*, Vol. 4, No. 5 (1966), pp. 508-516.

[3] D. Byrne, O. London, and K. Reeves, "The Effects of Physical Attractiveness, Sex, and Attitude Similarity on Interpersonal Attraction," *Journal of Personality*, Vol. 36 (1968), pp. 259-271.

[4] K. Dion, E. Berscheid, and E. Walster, "What Is Beautiful Is Good," *Journal of Personality and Social Psychology*, Vol. 24, No. 3 (1972), pp. 285-290.

time date was asked out again or accepted again if asked.[5]

Students aspiring to management positions should know that people try harder to please attractive people than they try to please unattractive ones.[6]

About Associates

Attractive people seem to have more friends than unattractive ones do. Researchers have discovered that people believe that the benefits they associate with attractive people will "rub off" on them if they are closely associated.

Acceptance or rejection in professional groups is influenced by your appearance and the way it is perceived to reflect on members of the group. Men participating in a study believed that associating with an attractive female would cause others to perceive them more favorably,[7] and they were right. The study paired the men with a woman made attractive and the same woman made unattractive and recorded others' responses to the man. The men created more favorable impressions for themselves when they were observed with the woman while she was made attractive than when she was made unattractive. Attractive women associating with attractive men are perceived to have more positive characteristics than those associating with unattractive men.[8]

Implications

The studies that have been done have important implications for people who want to gain advantages while they are becoming better known. Good-looking people have greater social power; they can be more persuasive, and their evaluations have more impact than those of their unattractive counterparts.[9] Therefore, you can increase your effectiveness while proving yourself if you make yourself as attractive as you can.

All other things being equal, physically attractive individuals are liked better than unattractive individuals;[10] therefore, you can gain the opportunity to increase your circle of friends and your professional opportunities by making yourself as attractive as you can. Socially, professionally, and personally, attractive people of both sexes seem to associate closely leaving unattractive people out.

——————— Achieving Success ———————

Whether you can improve your competence and poise by improving your appearance is still being studied. In the meantime, people believe you are more competent and poised if you make yourself attractive, and they react to you accordingly. Therefore, if you want to have the opppportunity to prove yourself under preconceived positive conditions rather than under preconceived negative conditions, make yourself as good-looking as you can.

[5]Walster, Aronson, Abrahams, and Rottman, loc. cit.

[6]H. Sigall and E. Aronson, "Liking for an Evaluator as a Function of Her Physical Attractiveness and Nature of Evaluations," *Journal of Experimental Psychology*, Vol. 5 (1969), pp. 93-100.

[7]H. Sigall and D. Landy, "Radiating Beauty: Effects of Having a Physically Attractive Partner on Personal Perception," *Journal of Personality and Social Psychology*, Vol. 28, No. 2 (1973), pp. 218-224.

[8]D. Bar-Tal and L. Saxe, "Perceptions of Similarly and Dissimilarly Attractive Couples and Individuals," *Journal of Personality and Social Psychology*, Vol. 33, No. 6 (1976), pp. 772-781.

[9]J. Mills and E. Aronson, "Opinion Change as a Function of the Communicator's Attractiveness and Desire to Influence," *Journal of Personality and Social Psychology*, Vol. 1 (1965), pp. 173-177; Sigall and Aronson, loc. cit.; H. Sigall, R. Page, and A. Brown, "Effort Expenditure as a Function of Evaluation and Evaluator's Attractiveness," *Representative Research in Social Psychology*, Vol. 2 (1971), pp. 19-25.

[10]Byrne, London, and Reeves, loc. cit.; Walster, Aronson, Abrahams, and Rottman, loc. cit.

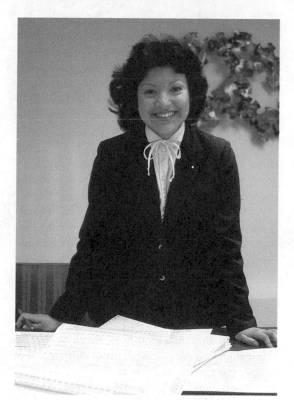

Illus. 11-2. People believe you are more competent and poised if you make yourself attractive.

It is grooming, not birth, that makes the difference. The most attractive person can be made to look unattractive with sloppy grooming habits and the most unattractive person can be made to look attractive with good grooming techniques. To say you were not born beautiful and thus give up on achieving the advantages associated with beautiful people is not justified. People have differences in what they have to work with to achieve attractiveness but they all have the ability to exert effort to achieve attractiveness. Such an effort combined with knowledge about what it takes to make yourself

attractive is sure to gain you advantages in the business environment.

Clothes

Don't settle for clothes that look unattractive on you. Being in "style" in something that does not make you look your best is not a good idea. Wearing something that doesn't fit perfectly because you got it at a good price may "cost" you a great deal in effectiveness. Wear clothes that enhance your profile. Make sure that your clothes always are pressed, clean, well tailored, and of a color that not only fits the situation but that looks good on you.

Avoid sacrificing quality for quantity in clothes. A few quality garments give you a better-groomed appearance than several shoddily made ones. Never wear anything that needs repair. Keep your shoes shined and well heeled. Keep buttons sewn securely on, rips repaired, lengths even, and waists well fitted. Among the many reasons to choose "quality" items is that they require less maintenance than shoddily made ones.

Timeless style and simplicity associated with business clothes, such as the business suit, require a standard of maintenance that is minimal compared to more exotically designed and constructed clothing and grooming concepts. The savings in never having to replace something because it is out of style but because it is worn out makes a quality purchase actually more economical than items that may have lower initial purchase prices.

Well-fitting clothes are less likely to have split seams, buttons falling off, and loose threads. Quality clothing of simple styles gives an appearance that the wearer and viewer do not tire of as quickly as more "fashionably" styled clothes; therefore, fewer of them are needed and they need to be replaced less often. The timeless appearance does not draw attention to itself as such but gives the aura of quality without specifically defining it.

Grooming

Simplicity and timeless style in grooming render the aura of quality in the person just as they do in clothing. Elaborate hairstyles, strong fragrances, or excesses in any area of grooming —even extremes in weight—detract from the overall impression a person makes.

Don't settle for a hairstyle just because it is in fashion if it doesn't allow you to look your best. Hair that is appropriately styled for business success is often styled simply. It is always clean and always of a classic style—for both men and women. Its timeless appeal is most apparent in the businessman's style, which rarely varies more than an inch in length and even less in fullness. Women will do well to recognize and employ classic simplicity in hairstyling to achieve the look of quality.

Don't allow someone to give you "the latest" just because the cut and style are "in." Experiment with lengths within those that are appropriate for business to see which ones make you most attractive. Experiment with fullness and other styling techniques that show a conservative but well-groomed appearance that make you look your best. Keep your style one that works for you not one that works for the "season" or for your hair stylist. Keep a length that gains advantages for you in business and personal endeavors, not one that is simply convenient for the swimming pool or jogging track. Learn what it takes to make your hair attractive *every day*, how often it needs cutting, washing, conditioning, curling, or straightening to give you just the well-groomed look that gains you the advantages of an attractive person.

Don't settle for skin and facial flaws and irregularities that make you unattractive. Learn to camouflage and conceal what can't be changed. Change whatever needs changing if you can. Good hairstyling makes irregularities in facial structure more appealing for both men and women. Makeup for women helps, too.

If you have poor skin, use appropriate medications to keep it as clear as possible. Keep yourself abreast of developments in the area of improving problem skin and find a physician who knows how to help you.

If your teeth detract from your smile, have them straightened, or cleaned, or capped, or whatever you need to gain the advantages of a more attractive appearance.

Don't settle for a body profile that is unattractive. Training yourself to have posture that makes you more attractive takes effort but can be achieved by almost everyone. Learn to stand and sit as tall as you can. In business, tallness often is equated with power. Even if you are only five feet tall, stand as if you are the tallest person in the room. You will develop a presence about you that makes others think of you as taller than you are. Sit with erect alertness that makes your presence distinctive.

Keep your body healthy. Being around people who look ill and feel weak makes others uncomfortable. Learn to keep your body in good health by exercising and eating appropriately. Take care to maintain good health. It will attract people to you. Stay in shape. If you currently have bulges or hollows where you shouldn't, begin exercising so that you tone up and fill out those irregularities that make your body unattractive. Design yourself a specific time and a specific set of exercises that do for you just what you need to give yourself the shape that makes you attractive.

Don't settle for fat. If you are overweight, you are incurring many disadvantages that you don't need to suffer. Most of the health disadvantages are well known. The disadvantages and prejudices against people who are overweight that result in lower incomes, less prestige, less power, fewer friends, and generally poor quality life-styles are less well known but just as real. Keep abreast of what is being learned about body weight and how to control it. Practice good eating habits that take off the excess weight you carry around needlessly.

Working

People in business, especially in the hiring of people to work in business, consistently stress the appearance of job seekers. Those working stress the need for good appearance to progress on the job. Everywhere you turn, your ability and character will be evaluated according to your personal appearance by those who see you and don't know you. Place yourself in a position to gain the support of people who don't know you and to reinforce the perception of those who do by making yourself as attractive as you can every day.

Questions for Chapter 11

1. Describe the components generally associated with the word *quality*.
2. How do the components of quality apply to people?
3. Why do people resist being judged by their personal appearance?
4. What characteristics do attractive people rate themselves higher in than unattractive people rate themselves in?
5. What characteristics do people believe attractive people are likely to have more of than unattractive people?
6. What are the implications of the studies about personal appearance?
7. What makes the difference between being attractive and unattractive?
8. How can your clothes contribute to your aura of quality and attractive appearance?
9. How can your grooming choices influence your aura of quality and attractive appearance?

Chapter 12

Exercising for Health

Chapter Objectives

After studying this chapter, you should be able to:

1. *Determine the benefit from increasing your cardiovascular endurance through exercise.*
2. *Select an exercise plan for yourself that fits your schedule, facilities, environment, personal preference, age, size, body type, and social needs.*
3. *Choose exercise that meets your cardiovascular fitness needs.*
4. *Measure your level of fitness using a target heart rate and the Kasch Pulse Recovery Test.*

To be a healthy person, you need several areas of activity in your life. Attendance at your job or school probably takes the bulk of your daylight time if you include the time you spend getting ready to go in the morning, the seven-to-eight hours you actually spend there, the time going to and from work or school, and your lunch hour. That accounts for ten or eleven hours of your time. After your household and personal care duties are fitted into your schedule, the remainder of your day is normally referred to as your leisure time. In order to have a healthy mind and body, you need to spend part of your leisure time in recreative physical exercise.

Recreation includes not only time for relaxing in a quiet place with a good book or a favorite television show, but it also includes physical activity designed to provide variety for your body from its everyday routine at work or school. If you are in a sedentary job (sitting most of the day or in activities requiring little strength), your body is suffering atrophy. Very simply, you will lose the ability to do much of anything else. It is important, then, to conscientiously plan part of your recreation time to develop power in your body to do something more than routine work. The nature of your body is such that if muscles are not used or are used only to a limited extent, they lose their capacity to be used. Unfortunately, that description applies to your heart, lungs, and vascular system also. Leisure time, then, becomes very important in terms of keeping your body physically fit.

There are two approaches to take in saving

your body from atrophy. One is to use your recreation time for active sports that condition your vascular and pulmonary systems while you are relaxing. The other way is to look for opportunities in your day to add regular physical activity to your routine. Some of the very pleasant ways to condition your body are with active sports like hiking, bicycling, tennis, racquetball, swimming, badminton, fast dancing, fencing, rowing, skating, skiing, and volleyball. However, unless you have been utilizing your heart-lung capacity beyond routine sedentary requirements, you will not be able at first to enjoy these activities regularly. You will need a plan to work up to them.

In addition to using part of your leisure time for activity that builds physical fitness for your body, it is helpful if you look for opportunities during your day to involve yourself in activity that contributes to conditioning your body. Such activity as stair climbing several times a day, a brisk walk from a bus stop to your office building every morning and night, and a quick walk in a park before eating lunch each day are good ways to work physical conditioning into your regular schedule.

Recreative Exercise Benefits

Before you decide whether or not to obligate part of your leisure time to conditioning activity, consider whether or not the benefits outweigh what they cost in terms of your leisure time.

Basic Fitness

The fitness of a human body is measured according to its development in three areas: endurance, strength, flexibility. The levels of each of these areas are the result of the activity in which a person engages. Various kinds of activity can be specifically designed to achieve in one area, but each activity contributes somewhat to the level of development of the other areas.

Endurance is achieved by exercising to condition the cardiovascular and pulmonary systems. Basically, endurance depends upon how efficiently your body uses the oxygen you breathe every day in fueling the food you eat so that it can be used as energy. Cardiovascular endurance is not easily built by short periods of exercise, calisthenics, or isometrics. It can be developed best by exercise that requires you to breathe deeply and rapidly and requires your heart to pump more rapidly than it normally would in everyday routine activity. Such endurance is built by exercise programs that include jogging, brisk walking, swimming, cycling, stair climbing, and other active sports.

The theory of developing endurance by conditioning your cardiovascular system is that if you don't use your heart muscle, it atrophies. You lose that capacity which you do not use. If you call upon your heart to supply just enough power to get you through the routine activity of your day, that is all it is able to do after a period of time. If, however, you participate in an exercise program designed to expand the efficiency of your heart so that it has power to supply you with oxygen for fueling your body beyond your daily routine requirements, you become able to live beyond your routine activities.

Some of the basic benefits you can enjoy are:

1. Your heart will operate more efficiently, beating stronger and slower but delivering more oxygen to the cells of your body to convert more of your food to energy, even during periods of routine activity.
2. Your vascular system actually will increase in the number of blood vessels available to transport blood from your heart to your cells, opening more opportunities for converting your food into energy.

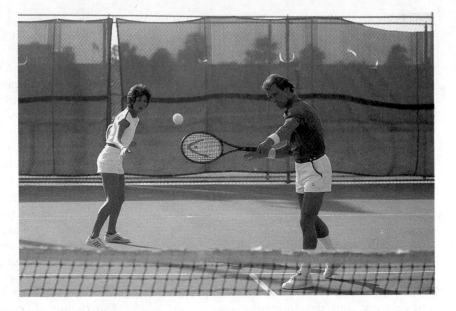

Illus. 12-1. Keeping in shape will help you to have enough energy for activities in addition to those required by your work and home responsibilities.

3. Your blood will be circulating more often because of the stronger heartbeat and additional vessels, making the supply of oxygen to your cells richer.

4. The muscles of your chest will become stronger, as will the muscles of the heart and the blood vessels themselves, in response to the increased requirement placed on them during your conditioning exercise.

Cardiovascular endurance is necessary to maintain good health. Since the basic truth is that the less a muscle is used, the less capacity it has for use, then the less you require of your heart and lungs, the less capacity they will have to perform. You should examine your daily routine. If all you do daily is ride to work, sit at work, ride home, and sit in front of television in the evening, you are not requiring much of your heart and lungs. Should you ever require more from them, for example, to swim, play tennis, go shopping, or walk a mile when you run out of gasoline, you might overtax them,

resulting in abnormal fatigue because their capacity and efficiency have been allowed to deteriorate. Should you become ill, the normal production of your heart and lungs may not be sufficient to bring your natural defenses into action efficiently if there is no reserve power. Recovery will take you longer, and your fatigue will be so great that you will not feel well as soon as you would had you been in good physical condition with reserve endurance.

To distinguish exercise that conditions your cardiovascular system from that which conditions your surface muscles, cardiovascular exercise is termed recreative exercise; the other, calisthenics and isometric exercise. Many recreative sports and activities serve to fulfill your need for recreative exercise. They may also provide some calisthenic and isometric benefit.

Illustration 12-2 shows where you can expect various sports to build endurance, strength, and flexibility. Illustration 12-3 on page 178 shows how some of the sports rate in building physical fitness.

Illus. 12-2.
Fitness
Benefits of
Selected
Sports

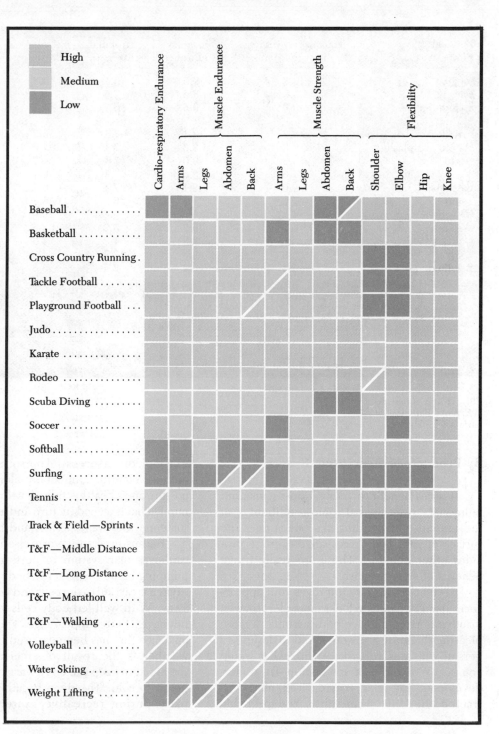

Physical Fitness	Cardio-respiratory Endurance (Stamina)	Muscular Endurance	Muscular Strength	Flexibility	Balance
Jogging	10.0	9.5	8.1	4.3	8.1
Bicycling.........	9.0	8.6	7.6	4.3	8.6
Swimming	10.0	9.5	6.7	7.1	5.7
Skating (Ice or Roller)........	8.6	8.1	7.1	6.2	9.5
Handball/Squash ..	9.0	8.6	7.1	7.6	8.1
Nordic Skiing	9.0	9.0	7.1	6.7	7.6
Alpine Skiing	7.6	8.6	7.1	6.7	10.0
Basketball........	9.0	8.1	7.1	6.2	7.6
Tennis	7.6	7.6	6.7	6.7	7.6
Calisthenics	4.8	6.2	7.6	9.0	7.1
Walking	6.2	6.7	5.2	3.3	3.8
Golf[2]	3.8	3.8	4.3	4.3	3.8
Softball	2.9	3.8	3.3	4.3	3.3
Bowling	2.4	2.4	2.4	3.3	2.9

[1]Seven experts used a scale of 0-3; thus, a rating of 21 indicated that all seven rated the sport as being of maximum benefit. The experts assumed a minimum of 4 times per week for 30 to 60 minutes per session of vigorous participation. To facilitate comparison, the ratings above have been converted to a scale of 1-10, with 10 indicating maximum benefit.
[2]The ratings for golf are based on the use of a golf cart or caddy. If you walk, the physical fitness value moves up appreciably.

Source: The figures above have been adapted from C. C. Conrad, "How Different Sports Rate in Promoting Physical Fitness," *Medical Times*, May, 1976 (Reprint), pp. 4-5.

Illus. 12-3. A Summary of Experts' Ratings of Various Sports[1]

By-Products of Recreative Exercise

Besides benefit to your cardiovascular and pulmonary systems and some conditioning to the muscles surrounding the bones near the surface of your body, recreative exercise provides other benefits. These are really fringe benefits of your exercise.

Recreative exercise improves your appearance. An active person looks more alert than an inactive person, and the body assumes a more pleasing shape. If you were asked to describe a person who was very successful, what would you say? Would the person be thin, fat, underdeveloped, muscular, rested, tired, alert, distracted, healthy, unhealthy? You probably would picture a successful person as one in good physical condition, mentally alert, with good posture and a healthy, fully developed body and mind. That is a good picture and a good goal for someone who wants to feel and be successful.

Because recreative exercise requires your cardiovascular system to perform efficiently, pumping blood through the body rapidly, vital oxygen is carried to the cells and waste is carried away. With well-fed body cells you can't help but have a better appearance. The flush of pink on a face that has been exposed briefly to cold weather is the result of efficient activity of the blood to keep the body warm when it is exposed to cold. The deep breathing that takes place during recreative exercise rids your body of carbon dioxide and feeds your body with fresh oxygen. Deep breathing also causes you to lift your diaphragm off your stomach so that you can fill your lungs with air. The result is improved posture.

Recreative exercise aids your body by utilizing muscles other than those of the heart and lungs. If you have chosen to walk or to jog, you will be exercising and toning muscles in the lower part of your body. If you have chosen tennis, you will tone muscles both in the lower and upper parts of your body. The natural use of your arms and legs in the activity you have chosen will incidentally tone the muscles in them. The more side benefits you can attain from these activities, the less isometric and calisthenic exercises you will need for body contouring. Your recreation may do that work for you if it is well chosen.

Another important by-product of recreative exercise is the feeling of success you get. The self-image of a person who practices good recreative exercise and rest habits is enhanced as much by the intense feeling of being alive as by the increased symmetry, muscle toning, and overall conditioning effect on the body. Conversely, one who does not exercise frequently suffers more than increased risk of occurrence of heart attack or high blood pressure, flabby muscles, and poor body condition. You may suffer a poor self-image simply because you are not feeling the rewards of success from developing all that you have.

Frequently, getting up out of a bed or a comfortable chair to begin a period of vigorous recreative exercise is not easy. However, with the first few deep breaths and strong heartbeats that spur the refreshing exchange of oxygen for carbon dioxide in your body, you begin to feel the reward of having made the effort. There is an exhilarating stimulation that sets this kind of exercise apart from any other. You truly develop the good "glow of health." Because you feel better when you exercise regularly in

a recreative way, you will reflect this well-being in your appearance. People who feel good — really good — look good!

Recreative exercise provides for social contacts and the development of friendships in many ways. Just the fact that you are exercising for good health makes you desirable as a friend because of the good influence you will have. Since you are doing something that all would like to do but for various reasons (usually lack of discipline) do not, people will want to know you to find out how you do it. They will be attracted to your dedication and your zest-for-living attitude.

Participating in a recreative sport for exercise provides for social contacts by bringing you around persons who are concerned with the same problems that you are. They are interested in doing more than the minimum — in living to the fullest of their capabilities in addition to benefiting their bodies. Right away you have a common bond and ground on which to start a conversation.

People who are in recreative exercise are anxious to find others who like the same kind of activity, and generally you will find them receptive to your offer of friendship. An activity that no one requires of you and that you don't have to do to earn a living is easier to stick to if you have friends who participate. The camaraderie among the participants in recreative exercise is hard to achieve in many other areas of life.

Your recreative exercise is always a good topic for conversation even with those who do not participate. There is something special about your character that is attractive because you do something for which there is no scheduled payday and for which you get no special recognition from the community. You do it because it makes you a healthy, invigorated, and more attractive person. It takes tenacity, a strong character, and real insight to work daily at a plan that requires not only time but energy, with no financial reward or recognition. Those are desirable traits for people engaging in any endeavor, especially making friends.

Recreative exercise is really so easy to take part in that the lack of difficulty may lead you to believe that anything that easy cannot be good for you. Not true! What is true is that your body is uniquely constructed to be active—your muscles, joints, and bones were designed to move—and that makes exercise easy. Walking, running, bending, swinging a racket or club, and many more activities are easy simply because your body was designed to be active. It is inactivity that destroys the body, making it stiff, achy, misshapen, and increasing its vulnerability to disease.

What conditioning and physical fitness really amount to is having more energy to enjoy life. If you have only enough energy to get by with the necessary activity required by your job, personal care, and household chores, you have none left for recreation. That can make for a life without variety. It takes energy beyond the minimum to enjoy life, and you can develop it with a good recreative exercise program.

Usually it is a good idea if you can make recreative exercise an integral part of your day, as a well-known congressman did. He jogged to work at Capitol Hill in Washington, D.C., every morning to keep himself in good condition. If you cannot jog to work, consider parking a mile away or getting off your bus or subway a mile from your place of work and getting in a brisk morning and afternoon walk. This is an excellent way to schedule exercise. It occurs regularly, it is timed, and it serves the purpose of getting to and from work. The regularity of the exercise will become habit; and with such a sensible plan, you may be able to enlist the participation of fellow workers and develop some new friends along the way.

If it is not practical to schedule your recreative exercise in such a way as to serve as a substitute for a regular part of your day, or if you choose to vary your recreative exercise, be sure that you plan for regularity, such as three to five times per week. It is always good to have an alternate indoor plan for your recreative exercise in the event of inclement weather. If you cannot jog, walk, or play tennis outdoors because of extreme weather, you may want to run in place indoors or use a stationary bicycle. These alternatives also serve to add variety to your exercise.

Often a person who has chosen well will not like to vary the routine of recreative exercise. People are protective of their time because of the vitalized way that regular exercise makes them feel. They unfailingly avoid any activity that may infringe upon their schedule for performing it. Joggers and walkers frequently are people who jealously guard their schedule of exercise because they enjoy it so much.

Regular Recreative Exercise

Since the regularity of your participation in recreative exercise is the most important part of your physical conditioning program, consider some ways to make it more appealing and easier for you to take part in regularly. Timing is of prime importance. The availability of facilities, the climate, and the environment in which you exercise are other vital considerations. On the personal side, you want to suit your exercise to your innate preferences, your age, and your size. You may want to recruit a buddy for morale purposes.

Time Schedule

Take stock of your time and how you spend it. Conditioning your body will take some of your day, approximately three to five times a week at first. Think about how much time you are willing to invest regularly in getting your body into condition. Many programs begin with as little as thirty minutes a day. After you

Illus. 12-4. Make your recreative exercise one that you will do regularly.

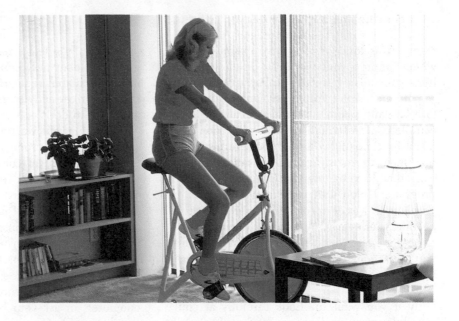

reach the level of fitness you desire, you may want to alternate long exercise periods with an exercise that does not take as much time. For example, if tennis is your sport, you can play tennis perhaps only two or three times a week and alternate with a 30-minute walk or cycling interval.

You are more likely to participate regularly if you set aside a certain time of day for your exercise. You will not plan other things during that time, and your family and friends will become accustomed to allowing you that time for yourself.

When you schedule your recreative exercise program, take advantage of your built-in body time clock. If you are an early riser who is wide awake at six a.m., plan your exercise for early in the morning. If you are a night owl, plan to run in place during the evening news. If you have an hour for lunch, take advantage of your lunch schedule by planning to use the first 30 minutes for your recreative exercise and the last 30 minutes for eating your lunch.

Some people find it beneficial to get up a little earlier in the morning to get in the recreative exercise before other events of the day begin. The advantages of this time of day are that few things are going on to distract or interfere with your exercise and that once you do it, you do not have to plan around it later. Also, you get the benefit of that increased blood flow and oxygen intake all day long. A person who participates during this time of day rarely has a day of the "blahs." The body is too vital and alive to be "blah." Morning exercise, though, should be taken before breakfast, since you should not have vigorous exertion within two hours after a meal.

Often, part of the noon hour can be utilized for exercise. A nutritious lunch can be brought from home and eaten in the park after you walk or jog. It really gives you a break from your work, and this is time that usually is wasted. An additional benefit is that such a plan keeps you from shopping during lunchtime—probably saving you money.

Stair climbing can be done as you arrive at work, if you work on an upper floor. An advantage of this kind of recreative exercise plan, which fits into your work schedule, is that it frees your leisure time for other activities.

If you haven't gotten your exercise in before late afternoon, set aside a certain time to complete it. Although the late afternoon is a beautiful time of day for outdoor exercise, you may have to guard against the fatigue of the work day discouraging you from your exercise program. If you wait until after dinner, or if you live in a section of the country where it becomes dark early, outdoor activity may have to be done after dark. Be sure that it is safe for you to participate at that time outdoors so that you won't be discouraged.

The time is there for you to condition your body if you want to. Look carefully at your schedule, your preferences, and at what will work for you. Then make a plan that is easy to keep, so that you can be physically fit with energy to spare.

Facilities

Carefully select a recreative exercise program that does not require facilities that may not be available regularly. The easier it is to take part in the activity, the more regularly you will want to do it.

Running and walking require only good, supportive shoes; rope skipping, only a rope. Some programs, of course, require a swimming pool, a bicycle, or other facilities. Be sure that you can afford the costs of whatever program you select. If facilities or equipment are required, they must be available to you three to five times per week.

If you are using part of your workday for walking or jogging, keep your extra shoes at work. Arrange to measure your route with a car odometer, or ask your bus driver to measure the distance between the two points on your planned route. You can, of course, use an odometer that straps to your body or one attached to a bicycle to measure your distances.

Illus. 12-5. Be sure you have regular access to the facilities needed for your exercise program.

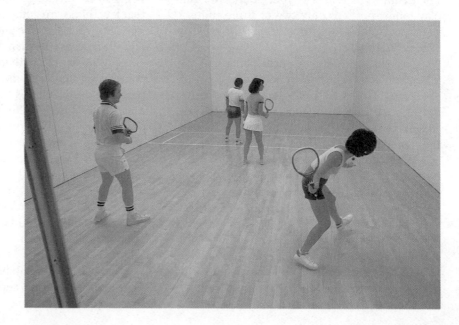

Climate and Environment

Your climate makes a difference in whether you should choose an indoor or outdoor exercise activity. Cold weather, unless it is below freezing for long periods of time, generally does not deter an outdoor program because you can dress for it. Hot weather, though, above 95 degrees, may deter you somewhat. If you live in an area that is subject occasionally to such extreme conditions, be sure that you have an alternate indoor exercise to substitute during such weather so that your conditioning goes on. Running in place indoors is a good alternate to jogging outdoors on a regular schedule. Stationary cycling is a good alternate to walking and cycling outdoors.

The environment of your exercise area is important. If you live in a wet climate, where it rains five out of ten days either seasonally or throughout the year, select an outdoor activity only if you are willing to go out in the rain regularly. If your environment is near a freeway or factory where the air is polluted heavily, you may want to select an indoor recreative exercise for your conditioning program. If you live where bicycling is hazardous because of heavy traffic, choose another activity. It may be pleasant, however, if you go to a park or area of clean air and serenity on a weekend occasionally, to ride on a bicycle trail or to take a walk through a wooded area.

Personal Preferences

Your goal is to get your body in good condition so that you have reserve power when you need it. You also want to enjoy your recreative exercise. If you are operating only marginally now, with little energy beyond that which you need for routine daily activity, the idea of beginning a recreative exercise program may appear to be beyond your endurance, making all exercise unappealing. You must select an activity and start just where you are if you are ever to improve. If you don't start an exercise program, you will forever live marginally with no physical resources to enjoy the extras of life.

At first you will be borrowing against endurance that you will develop in the future, and you may get discouraged. The human body responds quickly though, and sooner than you think you will be easily accomplishing your daily and weekly exercise goals with little effort. Once you reach increased levels of energy and endurance, you will never again want to live marginally with only enough stamina to get through the workday.

Make your recreative exercise something you enjoy so that you will want to participate regularly the rest of your life. Start by investigating the fringe benefits of the various recreative exercises available to you.

In walking and jogging, for example, you may vary the route and learn a great deal about the neighborhood in which you exercise. You probably will meet people in the neighborhood. If you like outdoor air, new acquaintances, and the excitement of what may be just around the corner, you may like jogging or walking. Bicycling is another recreative exercise that exposes you to new scenes. You are less likely to meet people than when you are walking or jogging, though, unless you join a bicycling club or others in your neighborhood are cyclists. However, if you like the wind in your face and the thrill of maneuvering under your own power, you will like bicycling.

After you've reached your desired level of fitness, add activities such as tennis, volleyball, and dancing, which are active recreative exercises that aid you in meeting people. The skill required in these activities frequently is attractive to those who like to work toward mastery while exercising. If the challenge of skill mastery appeals to you, you may enjoy these recreative exercises.

Illus. 12-6. After you've reached your desired level of fitness, add activities such as dancing which are active recreative exercises that aid you in meeting people.

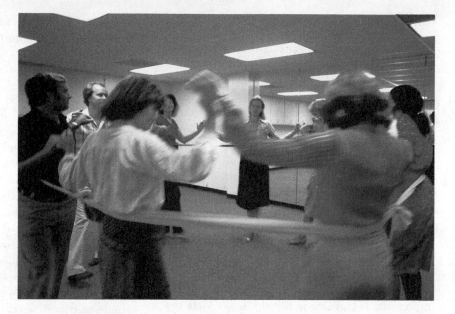

Swimming, rope skipping, stair climbing, skiing, skating, and rowing all have benefits to offer to make them attractive to you while you build the fitness of your body. You may even try several that you think you will like before you settle on one. When you are evaluating your choices, notice all the benefits of each activity, the facilities, the environment, the equipment, and anything else that may make it more attractive and enjoyable. Make your choices those that truly suit your personality preferences.

Age and Size

Age and size can make a difference in the rate at which you progress in your recreative exercise program. The usual plan of one-week steps may be changed so that the same level is maintained for two weeks before the next level is undertaken. This allows the heart and lungs a more gradual adjustment when it seems wise because of age or size.

It is important not to suddenly ask your heart and lungs to support an activity that is vigorous if for thirty or more years you have not made such a request. Most people under thirty, who have participated in school activities and other youthful endeavors within the past ten years, can select almost any recreative exercise they wish at the rate suggested. Those over thirty should consider the present condition of their bodies and what they can and cannot do without undue strain from the beginning.

If you are a large person, either overweight or exceptionally tall, it takes more endurance from your heart to supply your body during exercise than it does for a person of normal or small size. A large person may need to progress at a slower rate than usual, taking two weeks at each level instead of one until the heart is built up to the endurance needed for the extra size.

If you are small or of normal size, the usual rate of progress probably will feel only slightly tiring to you. Constantly try to increase your weekly rate, though, so that the conditioning effect works to your advantage in increasing the efficiency of your heart and lungs.

Body Type

You should also take into account your body type. The classifications of body types are based on five characteristics: strength, endurance, power, agility, and body support. If you select wisely as shown in Illustration 12-7, you can succeed in activities regardless of whether or not you possess these physical characteristics.

Buddies

Because your exercise program needs to go on, whether you have company or not, it is a good idea to be able to function at your exercise program without a buddy so that you won't be dependent in case your buddy leaves or discontinues exercising for some reason. However, it's always nice to have someone to do things with, and recreative exercise is no exception. If you have someone who is as conscientious as you are about your program, you can be of great benefit to each other for encouragement, especially when one of you is a little out of sorts and wants to shirk the exercise program for the day.

	Physical Qualities That Are Typical of Certain Body Types					Activities in Which You Can Expect to Experience Most Success													
	Strength	Endurance	Power	Agility	Body Support	Archery	Badminton	Basketball	Bowling	Cycling	Golf	Handball	Hiking	Jogging	Skiing	Swimming	Tennis	Running	Wt. Training
Endomorphy						X			X	X						X			
Meso-Endomorphy	X		X	X		X			X	X	X	X	X	X	X	X			X
Mesomorphy	X	X	X	X	X	X	X	X	X	X	X	X	X	X	X	X	X	X	X
Meso-Ectomorphy	X	X	X	X	X		X	X	X	X	X	X	X	X	X		X	X	X
Ectomorphy		X		X	X		X	X	X	X	X		X	X			X	X	

Reprinted from: C. T. Kuntzlemen (ed.), "Body Type," *The Physical Fitness Encyclopedia* (Emmaus, PA: Rodale Books, 1970). p. 58.

Illus. 12-7. Body Type and Activity Participation

Illus. 12-8. A buddy can offer encouragement when you want to shirk your exercise program for the day.

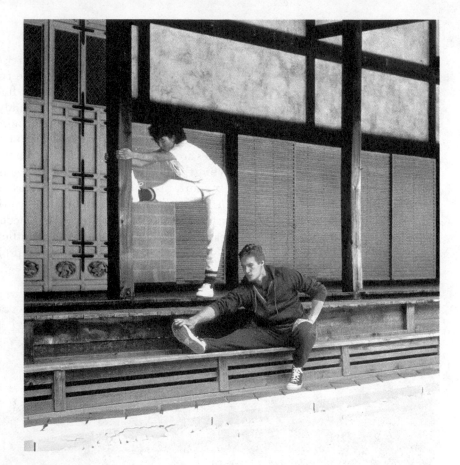

There are several ways to recruit a buddy. If you have a friend who rides the same bus to work with you, suggest that the two of you get off a mile away from work and walk briskly on to your building each day. You will be doing him or her a favor in terms of health and the quality of life. If you regularly eat lunch with someone at work, suggest as an alternative that you exercise part of your lunch period, and picnic in the park during the remaining time. If you ride home on the bus with a friend, suggest that you get off a mile before your regular stop so that you can get in a brisk walk. Suggest to a friend who works in the same building that you climb stairs for exercise.

— *Recreative Exercise Programs* —

There are various levels of conditioning that can be attained. A program can be designed to provide for whatever level you wish to attain. Any level above atrophy that you choose is better than what you will achieve without a program. Some fitness programs that are good for cardiovascular fitness are described in the following books:

Jogging by Bowerman and Harris
Canada's Fit Kit
Aerobics for Women by Cooper
The Aerobics Way by Cooper

Physical Fitness and Dynamic Health by Cureton
Vigor Regained by deVries
The Complete Book of Running by Fixx
Prescription for Life by Graham
Keep Your Heart Running by Kiell and Frelinghuysen
YMCA Physical Fitness Program by Myers
Complete Conditioning by Shepro and Knuttgen
Beyond Diet by Zohman

Target Heart Rate

What makes these fitness programs good for you is that they expand your fitness by causing you to exercise enough to achieve a target heart rate that steadily increases your heart's efficiency. You need to be sure that the exercise plan increases your heart rate to the appropriate number of beats per minute for your age group for 15 to 30 minutes a day for three or four days per week. Use Illustration 12-9 to make your comparison by taking your pulse count immediately after exercising, before you have time to rest.

Kasch Pulse Recovery Test

Stress tests are often given by physicians. If you wish, you can test yourself after you consult your doctor by taking the Kasch Pulse Recovery Test. You will need:

1. A bench or step 12 inches high,
2. A clock or watch with a sweep second hand, and
3. A friend to help you with the counting.

To take the test:

1. Don't smoke or engage in physical activity for two hours before starting.
2. Step up onto the bench or step.
3. Stand fully erect.
4. Step back down from the bench.
5. Repeat items 2, 3, and 4 for three minutes at the rate of 24 steps per minute (one step up and down every 2.5 seconds), being sure that both feet step onto the bench and return to the floor each time. Don't jump or hop.
6. If you find the procedure too vigorous, stop. Rate your fitness level as poor.
7. When you have completed the three minutes, sit down and relax for 5 seconds.

Illus. 12-9. Target Heart Rates

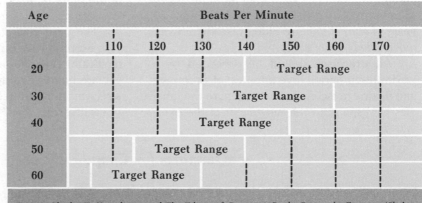

Age	Beats Per Minute						
	110	120	130	140	150	160	170
20				Target Range			
30				Target Range			
40			Target Range				
50		Target Range					
60	Target Range						

Source: Charles T. Kuntzleman and The Editors of *Consumer Guide, Rating the Exercises* (Skokie, IN: Publications International Limited, 1978), p. 55.

Illus. 12-10. Circulo-Respiratory Endurance Ratings, Measured by Pulse Recovery Rate (In Beats/Minute)

Age (In Years)	Fitness Level				
	Excellent	Good	Average	Fair	Poor
For Men...					
18-26	69-75	76-83	84-92	93-99	100-106
33-57	63-76	77-90	91-106	107-120	121-134
For Women..					
18-26	76-84	85-94	95-105	106-116	117-127
33-57	73-86	87-100	101-117	118-130	131-144

8. Take your pulse rate for 60 seconds.
9. Use the chart in Illustration 12-10 to gauge your fitness level.

Common-Sense Considerations

There are some common-sense cautions and precautions to consider. It is a good idea to have a check-up by your doctor before starting any exercise routine. The doctor will tell you if there should be any restriction on your planned activities.

It is wise not to try to build up faster than the beginning programs suggest. A sedentary heart, although grateful, will suffer shock enough with the suggested speed of progress. Many programs given are for people under 30 years of age. If you are older, take them even more slowly than suggested.

All exercises should be preceded by a warming-up period (five minutes) of stretching and flexing muscles slowly to prepare the muscles to respond to the movement of the exer-cise. Equally important is the cooling-down period that consists of mild exercise, such as walking slowly and swinging your arms so that your heart will not be overtaxed. Because the movement of your arms and legs during exercise aids your heart in pumping blood to your body, if you stop your movement suddenly, your heart bears the entire burden in pumping extra blood until your body cools and your breathing rate slows. Since your digestive system needs the services of your cardiovascular system for digestion after you eat, don't plan to exercise within two hours after a meal. Your digestion will suffer if you direct the blood and oxygen to other parts of the body by exercising vigorously too soon after a meal.

The most vital common-sense rule is that your exercise must be regular. To exercise spasmodically is dangerous for your heart. While you are building to the level of fitness you desire, you must exercise three to five days out of each seven.

Questions for Chapter 12

1. What happens to your body if you don't exercise?
2. What are the two ways to save your body from atrophy?

3. In what three areas is fitness measured?
4. How is endurance achieved?
5. According to Illustration 12-3, which two activities will help you most with

(a) cardiovascular endurance?

(b) muscular endurance?

(c) muscle strength?

(d) flexibility?

(e) balance?

6. What are the by-products of recreative exercise?

7. What considerations will help you get *regular* exercise?

8. What is a "target" heart rate?

Chapter 13

Exercising for Shape

Chapter Objectives

After studying this chapter, you should be able to:

1. *Analyze your body proportions.*
2. *Analyze your grace and flexibility.*
3. *Restructure your proportions, strengthen your muscles, and increase your endurance in specific parts of your body by isometric, isotonic, and weight training programs.*

Basically, endurance exercise or recreative exercise conditions muscles and tissue inside your body, such as your heart and lung muscles. Isometrics, calisthenic exercise, and weight training condition muscles surrounding your bones. Conditioning is necessary to a well-developed, healthy body. Isometrics, calisthenic conditioning, and weight training, by contributing to the strength and flexibility of your body, aid you in keeping your balance, giving your body symmetry and grace. Muscles on the surface of your body, like the muscles of your cardiovascular system, become incapable of functioning if they do not function for long periods of time. The tissue around them turns mainly to fat, which is rarely shaped to suit your aesthetic tastes. Using muscles on the surface of your body by isometric and calisthenic exer-cising and weight training increases the blood flow and oxygen input to those muscles, and stored fat tissue is replaced with muscle tissue.

The increased strength of well-developed muscles gives you better control of your body movement. You have the strength in your legs to walk and raise and lower yourself from a chair with more control. You are able to carry a grocery sack without strain on your arms when the muscles are as strong as they should be.

Not only is strength increased with calisthenics, but flexibility and suppleness are increased. When muscles are not used, they may simply stretch or shrink. They become inflexible. Exercising them by flexing and contracting the muscles gives you more suppleness. You are able to move not only with more control but also with more grace.

Exercise Benefits

The shape of the body that is desirable is one without excess fat but with some degree of fatty and muscle tissue to form round curves over the bones underneath. Most of the padding should be muscle because control and flexibility depend upon well-developed muscles. Only a thin layer of fat near the skin is considered desirable. Muscles characteristically assume a shape that is desirable; fat rarely does.

Movement and flexibility depend upon the development of muscles used in movement. Graceful movements will not be possible without well-developed muscles that both stretch and contract with ease. Stretching exercises combined with bending ones make the muscles in your form smooth and flowing and enable your body to move lithely and with flexibility rather than with rigid, board-like jerks.

A body without exercise becomes lumpy with fatty deposits in inappropriate places. Muscle tissue is so shaped that when it is developed in place of fatty tissue, it provides a gentle curve where it is becoming and a firm, smooth look where it is desired. Fat has no orderly shaping; it generally just bulges if it occurs in large quantities.

Proportion Analysis

One of the best ways to determine whether or not you need exercise for reshaping your body is made visually by simply standing nude in front of your full-length mirror, observing bulges and hollows where there should be smooth curves. With a hand mirror check the side views and back view. After all, you are seen from those directions as much as or more than you are from the front.

Another check is to compare your relative measurements with those of the "average" body that is appropriately developed. Only your scale will tell you if you are too fat or too thin. However, your tape measure can reveal whether what you have distributed on your bones is distributed in an aesthetically pleasing proportion. See Illustrations 13-1 and 13-3 on pages 192 and 193.

Movement Analysis

A well-proportioned body that moves without grace, flexibility, efficiency, and internal order is a shameful waste of beauty. Exercise aids the development of each of these areas.

Grace

Gracefulness is a balance between flexibility and strength. To check the gracefulness of your body, perform your everyday movements in slow motion to see if you can move with ease and grace.

Stand with your back to a chair, place one leg so that the back of your knee touches the chair, and without the use of your hands (since you may be holding something) very slowly lower yourself into the chair by bending only your knees and hip joints. Do not curve your back as you sit. The more slowly and smoothly you can perform this slow motion sitting, the better your flexibility and strength, and of course, the more graceful you are.

Now, without the use of your hands and with one foot slightly in front of the other, rise from the chair with the same slow motion. Remember to let the leg and thigh muscles perform the work. Do not curve your spine.

Climb stairs in slow motion speed without the use of your body movement to swing you up or down the stairs. Steady yourself with the use of the bannister, but do not allow your head and trunk to bob back and forth for balance or momentum. Let the muscles that were designed for climbing and lowering your body do the work. Keep your spine straight. Good control gives a gliding feeling and graceful appearance.

Illus. 13-1. "Ideal" Proportions for Women and Men

	On Women	On Men
The largest part of the		
CHEST AND HIPS should measure	the same.	the same.
THIGHS should measure..........	6-7 inches less than the waist.	8-10 inches less than the waist.
CALVES should measure..........	6-7 inches less than the thighs.	7-8 inches less than the thighs.
The smallest part of the		
WAIST should measure	10 inches less than the chest.	5-7 inches less than the chest.
ANKLE should measure..........	5-6 inches less than the calves.	6-7 inches less than the calves.
The **UPPER ARM** midway between the elbow and shoulder joint, arm extended, palm up, should measure.......................	twice the circumference of the wrists.	twice the circumference of the wrists.

If you have trouble with any part of these activities, you need to build strength and flexibility in the muscle masses that are weak.

Flexibility

You need flexibility in your body, especially in your spine and neck. If you are flexible in the trunk of your body, your walk will be smoother. Flexibility makes all movement more graceful and easier for you to perform. Check your flexibility with some bending, twisting, and stretching motions. Stand with your heels against a wall; twist the trunk of your body with your arm extended so that it touches the wall on the opposite side of your body (Illustration 13-2). Now with your toes to the

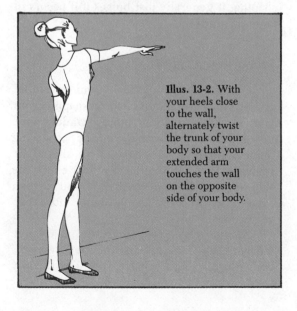

Illus. 13-2. With your heels close to the wall, alternately twist the trunk of your body so that your extended arm touches the wall on the opposite side of your body.

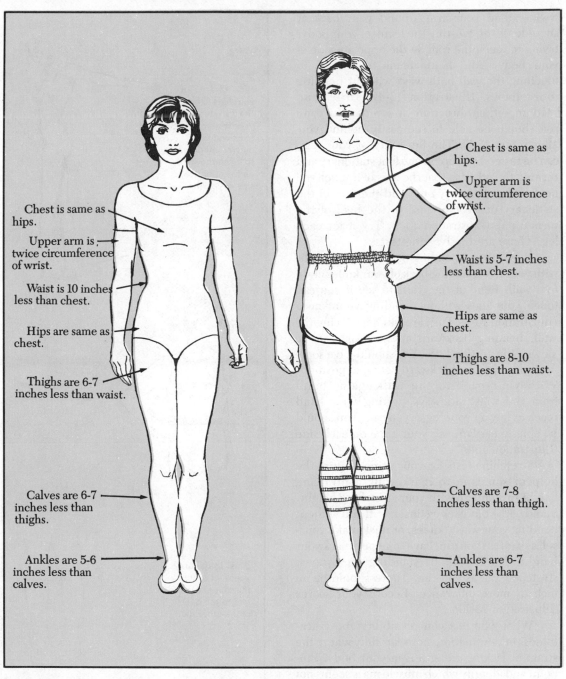

Chest is same as hips.

Upper arm is twice circumference of wrist.

Waist is 10 inches less than chest.

Hips are same as chest.

Thighs are 6-7 inches less than waist.

Calves are 6-7 inches less than thighs.

Ankles are 5-6 inches less than calves.

Chest is same as hips.

Upper arm is twice circumference of wrist.

Waist is 5-7 inches less than chest.

Hips are same as chest.

Thighs are 8-10 inches less than waist.

Calves are 7-8 inches less than thigh.

Ankles are 6-7 inches less than calves.

Illus. 13-3.
Proportion Analysis

wall, extend your arm around your back at shoulder level, twisting the trunk of your body, trying to touch the wall on the opposite side of your body. You should come very close to touching the wall both ways without bending your elbows (Illustration 13-4). Turn your head in either direction as far as you can. You should be able to see easily behind you (Illustration 13-5). The flexibility of your legs can be tested by keeping one foot stationary and turning the other so that the toes of it touch the heel of the stationary one, and the toes of the stationary one come close to the heel of the turned one (Illustration 13-6). Try it for each leg. Those are the twisting tests.

Now, try the bending ones. Stand straight with your heels and the back of your knees close to a wall. Bend at the waist to see if you can touch your toes without bending your knees (Illustration 13-7). Turn around now, facing the wall, bending backward at the waist. Do so slowly (Illustration 13-8). You should have some flexibility in the backward leaning position. With your back to the wall again, bend from the waist sideways, letting your hand reach as low on your leg as you can. You should be able to easily reach your knee on each side (Illustration 13-9).

Stretching tests for your spine require the help of someone to mark your contracting height to compare with your stretching height. Stand with your back against a wall and without bending your waist, knees, or neck make yourself as short as you can; have someone mark your height. Now, without standing on tiptoes, stretch as tall as you can. There should be an inch or more difference. Record your scores (Illustration 13-10).

When you test your flexibility and gracefulness in slow motion, note carefully where the strain or lack of strength is in your body. Pinpoint and identify which muscle mass seems not to function as it should. If you are inflexible,

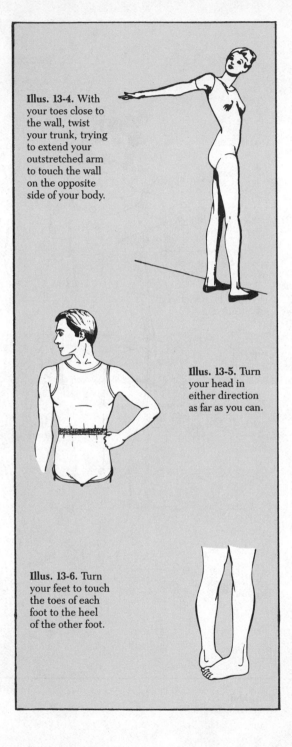

Illus. 13-4. With your toes close to the wall, twist your trunk, trying to extend your outstretched arm to touch the wall on the opposite side of your body.

Illus. 13-5. Turn your head in either direction as far as you can.

Illus. 13-6. Turn your feet to touch the toes of each foot to the heel of the other foot.

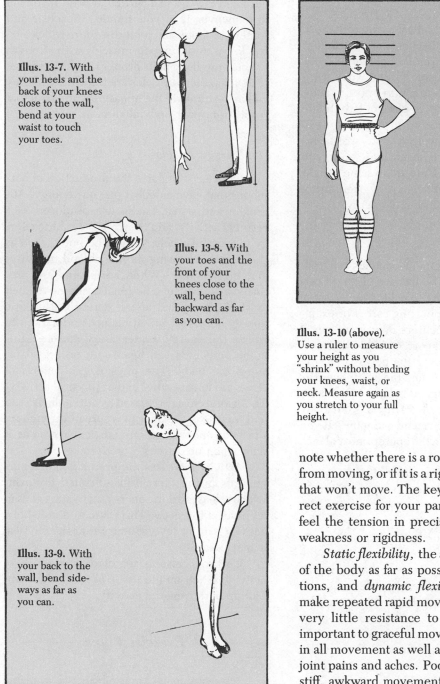

Illus. 13-7. With your heels and the back of your knees close to the wall, bend at your waist to touch your toes.

Illus. 13-8. With your toes and the front of your knees close to the wall, bend backward as far as you can.

Illus. 13-9. With your back to the wall, bend sideways as far as you can.

Illus. 13-10 (above). Use a ruler to measure your height as you "shrink" without bending your knees, waist, or neck. Measure again as you stretch to your full height.

note whether there is a roll of fat that keeps you from moving, or if it is a rigid spine or bone joint that won't move. The key to selecting the correct exercise for your particular problem is to feel the tension in precisely the area of your weakness or rigidness.

Static flexibility, the ability to stretch parts of the body as far as possible in various directions, and *dynamic flexibility*, the ability to make repeated rapid movements at a joint with very little resistance to the movement, are important to graceful movement in walking and in all movement as well as in the prevention of joint pains and aches. Poor flexibility results in stiff, awkward movement.

Efficiency

Exercise makes mechanical movement more efficient. Just as a car becomes more efficient when it requires less gasoline per mile, your movement becomes more efficient when it requires less energy for movement. The development of muscles in place of fatty tissue brings about such efficiency by replacing dead weight with working weight. Fatty tissue increases body weight, requiring more energy to maneuver it. Muscle tissue at the same weight contributes to the efficiency by facilitating movement with a minimum of energy.

Body Alignment

Proper body alignment depends on well-developed muscles. The balance of your body depends on your ability to center each part of your body over its supporting part. For example, the pelvic area centers over your legs if your center of gravity is correct. In like manner, the rib cage centers over the pelvic area; the neck, over the sternum; and the head, over the neck area. All are designed to form a particular line so that the center of gravity for your body provides balance as you stand and move. If you are not able to maintain the appropriate balance because of weak muscles in your back, abdomen, shoulders, or neck, you put undue pressure on areas not designed to support parts of your body. If your head projects forward, the neck and backbone, which were uniquely designed to support your head, do not bear its weight. Your front neck muscles rather than the vertebrae and muscles in your back support your head. You may, as a result, suffer muscular pain in your upper back because the muscles are constantly stretched to allow your head to assume its unnatural forward position.

If your pelvic area tilts forward, the muscles in your back near your waist will be stretched and vertebrae which should be straight will be curved, resulting in back pain. Your body is designed to work in a particular way. If you fail to maneuver it as you should, muscular and sometimes bone and joint disorders will occur. It takes well-developed muscles with strength to hold your body in its proper shape. Exercises to develop these muscles are available and they will help you avoid the uneasiness and pain that result from poor body alignment.

Energy Levels

Exercise stimulates the production of hormones that have an effect on your energy. Adrenalin and nonadrenalin are produced as a result of activity, and they release caloric energy to particular cells within the body, such as the heart, increasing its rate, blood pressure, and blood sugar. When adrenalins are produced as a result of emotional excitement, such as stress, fear, and anger, a resulting caloric energy occurs. If activity is not undertaken to utilize the energy, unnecessary muscle tightening and increased heart rate occurs, damaging the body. The physiological effects of stress are lessened by regular physical activity. The caloric energy released by adrenalin is used and the use of the energy is spread throughout the body, not taxing one particular area as it does when no activity is undertaken.

Activity increases the production of a hormone from the thyroid gland called thyroxin, which releases caloric energy, activating cells in all parts of the body. This increased metabolic activity lasts for several hours after the physical activity ceases.

Cortisone also is secreted as a result of activity. It acts on the tissue of the brain, stimulating better mental activity.

——————— Exercise Plans ———————

There are many kinds of exercise available for shaping the form of the body and developing muscular control. Isotonic calisthenics and isometrics are two of the finest. *Isotonic exercise* usually employs movement of muscles and joints, and sometimes the use of weights such as barbells, slant boards, and aids to increase the tension put on muscles exercised. *Isometric exercise* pits one muscle of the body against another for a certain period of time. Both kinds of exercise are very good. Weight training is good for developing specific muscle masses.

The calisthenic form of exercise requires movement of the body by stretching, bending, pushing, pulling, twisting, and lifting. Usually it is done privately or in an exercise class. Isometric exercise requires little movement beyond pushing, pulling, or the conscious contracting of a muscle for a certain period of time. Both are designed to strengthen and tone the muscles involved. However, calisthenics, because of the movement, tend to be more beneficial in developing flexibility and suppleness. The advantages of exercise along with the principles to be employed are important.

Isometric Exercise

Isometric exercises are simple and produce quick results. They require little time and no equipment. Frequently they can be done while you are sitting at your desk with no one noticing. This kind of exercise requires no particular type of clothing, and it causes little fatigue and no perspiring. It must, however, be accompanied by other kinds of exercise since it makes no contribution to cardiovascular endurance and little to flexibility.

Isometric Principles

Some guidelines to follow if you select an isometric program are:

- Select exercises that work all the major muscle groups that need strengthening.

- Hold each contraction for six to eight seconds.
- Use maximum effort for each contraction.
- Complete your entire group of exercises each day.
- Vary the exercises weekly so that different points in the muscle group are exercised on a weekly basis. Changing the angle of the flexion will accomplish this.
- Ordinarily, the breath is inhaled before the contraction, held during the contraction, and exhaled after the contraction.

Isometric Exercises

You may select from these exercises to strengthen particular muscles and use calisthenics to exercise other muscles, or you may select one from each category and omit calisthenic exercise except for developing flexibility. Both isometric and calisthenic exercises are to be done in addition to your recreative exercise. Begin by performing each exercise you choose once each day. Work up to two repetitions, then three repetitions. Remember to vary your exercises from week to week.

1. Neck — Upright position (sitting or standing), place palm side of interlaced fingers against forehead. Push forward with your head and resist with your hands (Exercise 1).
2. Neck — Upright position, place palm side of interlaced fingers behind your head. Push head backward resisting with a forward pull of the hands (Exercise 2).
3. Neck — Upright position, place left hand palm on left side of head. Push with hand and resist with head. Repeat, using right hand and right side (Exercise 3).
4. Shoulders and Arms — Standing, back to a wall, palms against wall at your side. Keeping arms straight and body still, push against the wall (Exercise 4).

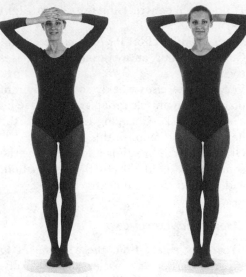

Exercise 1   Exercise 2

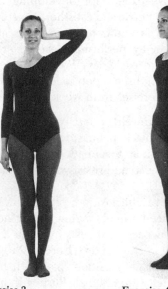

Exercise 3   Exercise 4

5. Shoulders and Arms — Sitting, grasp seat of chair at the sides. Pull on chair, resisting with buttocks and legs. Keep your spine straight (Exercise 5).

6. Shoulders and Arms — Sitting, place palms on chair seat at sides. Keep spine straight and push with hands (Exercise 6).

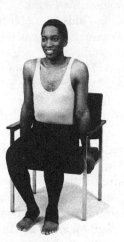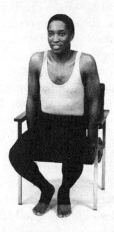

Exercise 5   Exercise 6

7. Shoulders and Arms — Upright position. Extend elbows to side at shoulder level. Place fist of one hand in palm of other hand. Push with fist and resist with palm. Reverse hands, and repeat (Exercise 7).

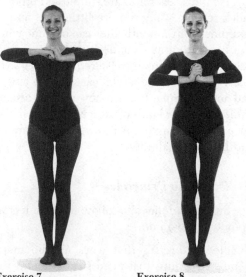

Exercise 7   Exercise 8

8. Chest and Arms — Upright position. Hands close to chest, palms clasped together. Push with right hand; resist with left. Reverse hands (Exercise 8).

9. Abdomen — Upright position. Pull stomach in toward backbone as far as possible, using only stomach muscles (Exercise 9).

10. Abdomen — Lying, face-up position, knees bent, feet flat on floor 8 to 10 inches from buttocks, hands on hips. Raise trunk to half-way sitting position and hold (Exercise 10).

11. Abdomen and Back — Standing. Heels 3 to 5 inches from wall, back to wall, knees bent slightly. Using gluteal and abdominal muscles, push as much as you can of your back against the wall. As strength is gained, move heels closer to wall and straighten knees. This exercise is your major posture building aid for the pelvic area (Exercise 11).

12. Back — Lying face-up position. Draw knees to chest, tightening abdominal muscles. Grasp legs below knees and pull them toward head (Exercise 12).

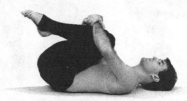

Exercise 12

13. Back — Prone (face-down) position. Place lower legs under heavy bed or sofa. Knees straight, push heel against sofa or bed above (Exercise 13).

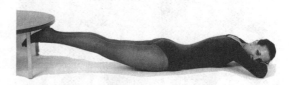

Exercise 13

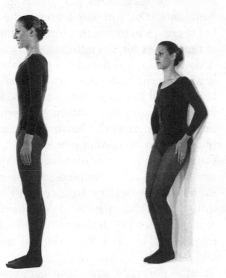

Exercise 9 (above)
Exercise 10 (below)   **Exercise 11 (above)**

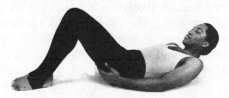

14. Legs — Sitting position. Knees 10 inches apart. Extend arms, palms against outer sides of knees. Press with hands; resist with thigh muscles (Exercise 14).

15. Legs — Sitting position. Knees 10 inches apart. Extend arms, palms against inner sides of knees. Press outward with hands; resist with thigh muscles (Exercise 15).

16. Legs — Sitting position. Ankles pressed against outside of chair legs. Pull legs toward one another against the resistance of the chair (Exercise 16).

17. Legs — Sitting position. Ankles pressed against inside of chair legs. Push legs away

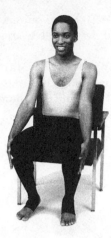
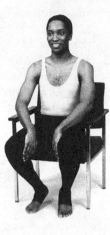

Exercise 14   Exercise 15

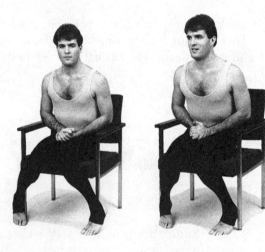

Exercise 16   Exercise 17

from one another against the resistance of the chair (Exercise 17).

Isotonic Exercise

A good calisthenic program includes exercises to develop flexibility, coordination, muscular strength and endurance, muscle tone, and good body lines.

Isotonic Principles

To achieve desired results, certain principles must be followed.

- Exercise groups equally on each side to insure balanced development and body symmetry.
- Select the appropriate exercise and number of repetitions to meet your specific goals. Strength is best developed by repeating two or three groups of ten to fifteen repetitions; whereas endurance is developed by increasing the repetitions to twenty or twenty-five but performing them without a break. Until you attain some strength, perform only one group of repetitions at a low number. Later, you may increase the number of repetitions per group to attain endurance. Or, you may increase the number of groups to two or three at a low number of repetitions for strength.
- A slow rhythmical pattern is preferable to a jerky pattern. After strength is developed, however, additional resistance can be added by speeding up the pattern somewhat. It must remain smooth, however, to accomplish the strengthening power.
- Correct form is necessary to achieve the desired results. The complete motion of the exercise is necessary to incorporate flexibility into the results. Poor form may strain muscles not designed to perform and may result in poor flexibility in muscles and joints.
- Breathe normally when you exercise. The basic rule is to exhale when you exert and inhale when you relax. This procedure may be reversed, though, when the exercise calls for expanding the rib cage while exerting.
- Plan to exercise regularly. Without regularity, more harm than good may be done. A Monday-Wednesday-Friday schedule is better than a slipshod schedule, but it is not

as good as a Monday through Friday schedule. You may find exercise so invigorating and the results so encouraging that taking the weekends off may not be appealing.

Isotonic Exercises

Select from the calisthenic exercises the ones that fit your needs of flexibility, strength, endurance, or body shaping. Aids such as barbells (or homemade substitutes of plastic bottles filled with sand to a specified weight), slant boards, and weights may be used in many cases to increase the tension of the muscle mass being exercised. Aids usually produce faster results but certainly are not necessary to an effective program. The exercises for flexibility, strength, and body shaping will be similar. Those for endurance will simply be more repetitions so that the muscle increases its ability to withstand longer periods of tension.

18. Neck — Lying, face-up position with head hanging off a bed or couch. Arms alongside body. Curl chin upward to chest, using neck muscles. Lower slowly. Vary exercise by turning head to right or left and raise head. 15 to 25 repetitions (Exercise 18).

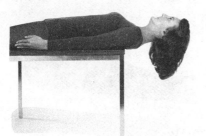

Exercise 18

19. Neck and Abdomen — Lying, face-up position, hands at sides. Using tightened abdominal muscles and neck and chest muscles, curl head and shoulders off the floor. Hold this position for five to eight seconds. Return head to floor slowly. 10 to 15 repetitions (Exercise 19).

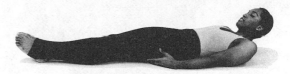

Exercise 19

20. Shoulders and Chest — Standing position, feet shoulder-width apart, arms at shoulder level extended sideward, palms up. Moving arms upward to the back, make large circles. Turn palms down and reverse the circle. 15 to 25 each way. Weights may be used (Exercise 20).

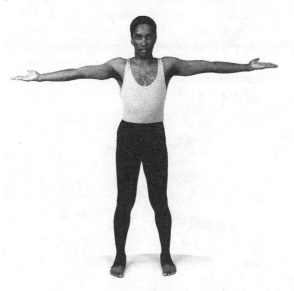

Exercise 20

21. Shoulders, Arms, and Chest — Prone (face-down) position, knees bent, feet raised from the floor, hands palm down placed under shoulders. Push body off floor fully extending arms. Keep

spine straight. Men may do push ups with straight legs. 10 to 15 repetitions (Exercise 21).

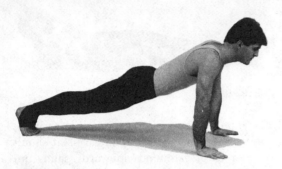

Exercise 21

22. Abdomen—Lying, face-up position, arms extended sideward, palms down, knees drawn to chest. Keeping knees together, touch left knee to floor to left of your body, bring back to starting position, then touch right knee to floor on right side of body, return to starting position. 10 repetitions (Exercise 22).

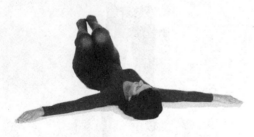

Exercise 22

23. Abdomen—Lying, face-up position, legs straight, arms at sides. Keep small of back on floor, bring knees to chest, extend legs upward, return knees to chest, straighten legs on floor. 10 to 15 repetitions (Exercise 23).

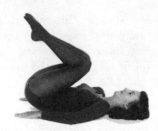

Exercise 23

24. Abdomen—Lying, face-up position, legs straight, arms crossed, hands grasping opposite arms. Roll up to a sitting position, lower yourself to lying position. 15 to 25 repetitions. This exercise may be varied by changing the arm position: arms may be extended above the head; arms may be above head with fingers laced behind head. Knees may be bent at a 45 degree angle. The more tension placed on the abdominal muscle mass, the quicker the results. Weights may be used in the extended arm position (Exercise 24).

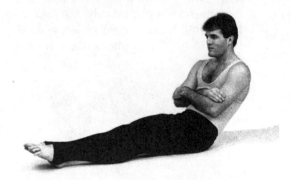

Exercise 24

25. Back—Standing position, feet close together. Slowly bend, reaching with your fingertips to touch your toes. Keep your knees straight. 20 to 25 repetitions. Weights may be used (Exercise 25).

26. Back—Standing position, feet shoulder-width apart, arms extended to the side at shoulder level. Bend and twist, touching right hand to left toe. Return to starting position. Bend and twist, touching left hand to right toe. 15 to 25 repetitions. Weights may be used (Exercise 26).

27. Sides—Standing position, feet shoulder-width apart, hands laced behind or above your head. Bend sideways as far as you can to the left, return to starting position, bend to the right, return to starting position. 10 to 15 repetitions each side. A weight may be held in the interlaced fingers (Exercise 27).

28. Side—Lying, face-up position, arms extended sideways, shoulder high, palms down, legs straight. Raise right leg to vertical position; keeping it straight, lower it to the floor on your left side. Arms, head, and shoulders are kept flat on the floor. Return leg to starting position. Repeat with left leg to right side. 15 to 20 repetitions (Exercise 28).

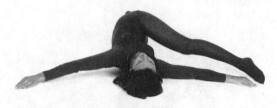

Exercise 28

29. Buttocks—Standing position, feet together, one hand on chair at side. Swing leg farthest from chair forward and up. Return leg to starting position, swing leg backward and up. Keep knee straight. Return to

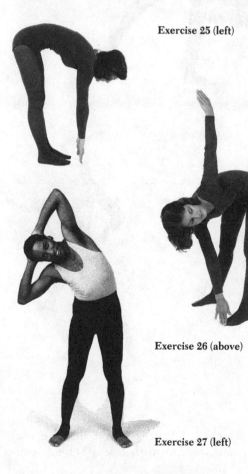

Exercise 25 (left)

Exercise 26 (above)

Exercise 27 (left)

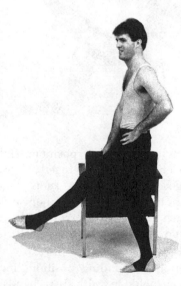

Exercise 29

starting position. Turn to brace yourself with your other hand and repeat for the other leg. 15 to 25 each side (Exercise 29).

30. Buttocks — Kneel on all fours (knees and hands). Attempt to touch left knee to head under body, then simultaneously raise head and extend leg back and up, arching back. Return to starting position. Repeat with other leg. 15 to 25 repetitions each leg (Exercise 30).

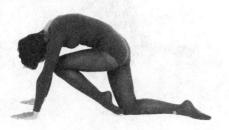

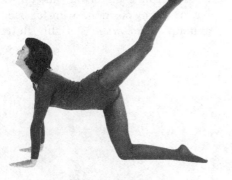

Exercise 30 (above and below)

31. Thighs — Standing position, right hand on chair, feet close together. Swing left leg sideward and up as far as you can. Return to starting position. Repeat 20 times. Turn to brace yourself with your left hand. Repeat with your right leg 20 times (Exercise 31).

32. Thighs — Standing position, feet wider than shoulder-width apart, hands on hips. Stretch to right, bending right leg, extend-

ing left leg. Return to starting position. Stretch to left bending left leg, extending right leg. 5 to 15 repetitions each side (Exercise 32).

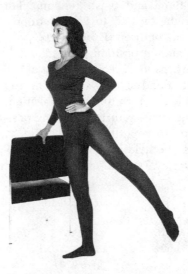

Exercise 31

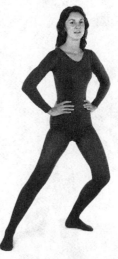

Exercise 32

33. Thighs — Sitting position, leaning backward, bracing with hands behind, palms

down, knees bent, feet lifted from floor. Alternately straighten each leg and return to bent position. 15 to 25 repetitions each leg (Exercise 33).

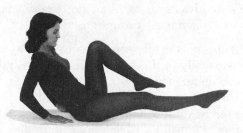

Exercise 33

34. Legs — Lying in side position, head resting on hand, elbow on floor. Lift top leg sideward as high as you can. Lower to starting position. Repeat 20 to 30 times each leg (Exercise 34).

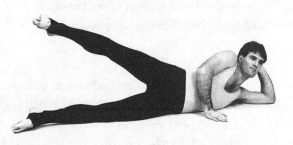

Exercise 34

35. Calves — Standing position, feet together, hands on hips. Raise body on toes. Lower to starting position. This exercise can be varied by standing with the toe half of the foot on a thick book and alternately lowering and raising from the level position. 20 to 25 repetitions (Exercise 35).

36. Calves — Standing position, hands on hips, knees half bent. Raise heels from the floor, balancing weight on toes. Lower heels to starting position. 15 to 20 repetitions (Exercise 36).

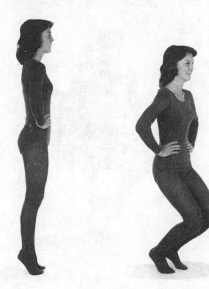

Exercise 35   **Exercise 36**

37. Feet — Sitting position, legs extended, hands palm down behind body to brace you. Point toes as far as possible, return to upright position, curl toes toward body as far as possible, return to upright position. 15 to 20 repetitions (Exercise 37).

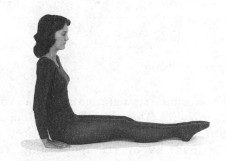

Exercise 37

38. Feet — Sitting position, feet resting on towel. Alternately with each foot pick up towel with toes and hold for 5 to 8 seconds. Release towel. 15 to 20 repetitions (Exercise 38).

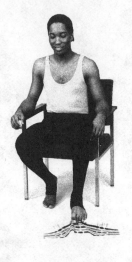

Exercise 38

Any of the isotonic exercises performed with the hands and arms free may be done with weights for added tension on the muscles. Use either barbells, dumbells, or homemade weights. Plastic bottles, either of a curved shape or with a handle, may be filled with sand to a two and one-half to five pound weight and used effectively. Ankle and wrist weights that can be strapped on are inexpensive but effective.

Weight Training

You can build strength and endurance with resistive devices. The principle of such training is that the body adapts to stresses placed on it (overload) by overcompensating. You progressively increase the intensity of effort and gain in strength and/or endurance. For weight training you will need equipment designed for that purpose. Many schools have such equipment in their physical education departments but most often it is available in spas and body building centers which will charge you to use the equipment.

Cautions

Resistive exercise equipment is best used by young athletes to build strength. Most adults do not need it to keep physically fit. There are some disadvantages to using the equipment, especially if you are unsupervised:

1. It does not develop cardiovascular fitness. It helps only in the areas of muscle strength and endurance.
2. Unless you move the weights and do the exercises throughout the full range of motion, you will lose flexibility and produce a muscle-bound appearance.
3. You will not improve your coordination, timing, or motor skills with weight training.
4. If you do not breathe properly and hold your breath during heavy exercise, you can become dizzy and faint and put undue stress on your heart.
5. Improper body alignment during lifting can cause back injuries.

Benefits

Progressive resistance weight training does produce benefits when performed correctly:

1. For developing strength, weight training is the best approach.
2. Specific muscles can be developed effectively.
3. For developing the physique (broad shoulders, large chests, better developed calves and thighs), weight training can produce results more quickly than other exercise programs.

Programs

Most weight training programs are based on the three-set, ten-repetition procedure. When modifications are made, they usually are in the total number of repetitions performed.

The weight is increased with each set. For example, if the most weight you can lift is 60 pounds, your first set of ten repetitions would be at one-half that weight or 30 pounds; after a pause of thirty seconds or so, your second set of repetitions would be at three-quarters of your maximum or 45 pounds; and your last set of repetitions would be at your maximum of 60 pounds. The term *progressive resistance* thus describes the increasing weight. Variations of this program are sets of six repetitions instead of 10. Other variations are:

1. One set of five to fifteen repetitions at maximum effort (the most weight that you can lift).
2. Ten sets performed beginning with maximum weight and decreasing weight with each set of ten repetitions.

Your Exercise

The key to achieving results with exercise is to choose correctly the exercises you need and to perform them faithfully. Go back to your tests of strength (graceful, slow motion movements) and flexibility and to your shape analysis. Note exactly what you want to improve and the shape you want to achieve. Select the appropriate exercises for those goals.

Remember that muscle strengthening (toning) can be done either with isometrics or isotonics. The more resistance you place on a muscle, the quicker results you will get. Therefore, the use of weights may provide faster results than you will get without them. The isometric form of exercise often is good to use at your desk or while you are watching television. It is a good resolution to make to yourself that for any thirty-minute period you spend in a sitting or lying position watching television, three minutes will be spent simultaneously in isometric or isotonic exercise. Concentrate in every case on putting tension in exactly the spot where you have determined there was inflexibility or weakness.

Exercise slowly. The longer tension is applied to the muscles being conditioned, the more conditioning effect takes place. When you bend, for example, bend slowly, forcing the weak muscles in your back and legs to control your body as you bend. In raising your body, require the same slow tension of the muscles in the opposite direction.

Stretching exercises improve both static and dynamic flexibility. A slow to moderate pace is required for both. Quick or jerky movements can negate the effect of the exercise and can pull muscles and possibly tear them.

Aids

Many people like to exercise to music. The rhythm of the music contributes to the rhythm of the exercise. Records to exercise by are on the market, and you may find them useful.

Joining a television performer in an exercise show is often a good way to exercise. The encouraging words the performer gives you tend to spur you on when you are tired. The regularity of the show helps to keep you exercising regularly.

Non-Aids

Because exercise takes energy and many people resist expending energy, short-cuts are constantly being advertised and sold. Most of the time they do more for your morale than for your body. Machines that shake, rub, bounce, and heat your body while you relax will do very little to turn fatty tissue to muscle tissue. They neither strengthen muscles nor make you flexible. Mainly, they increase surface circulation somewhat but not as well as recreative exercise does. The roughness of some machines can bruise and break small vessels causing unsightly discolorations in your skin.

A massage can be very relaxing to the muscles and provide stimulation to the skin. Pounding and kneading tissue, though, does not build strength and flexibility unless there is corresponding resistance which is not provided during massage.

Sauna baths can be very relaxing and can produce perspiring, which temporarily lowers body weight by dehydrating it. (A sponge without water weighs less than one with water.) Saunas have been shown to produce side effects, however, that may be damaging to the heart if the baths are taken immediately after exercise. Steam baths and whirlpools both can be very relaxing and are good for that purpose. They do not do any muscle building or body shaping.

Questions for Chapter 13

1. Why should the tissue under your skin be mostly muscle rather than fat?
2. Ideal proportions mean that the chest is how much larger than the waist on women? on men?
3. If you cannot move gracefully, what can you do about it?
4. What is the difference between static and dynamic flexibility?
5. Why does replacing fat tissue with muscle tissue increase your body's efficiency?
6. How can exercise increase your energy?
7. What are the benefits of a good calisthenic program?
8. What are the guidelines to follow for isometric exercising?
9. What are the principles for isotonic exercising?
10. What are some benefits of weight training?

Chapter 14

Special Body Care

Chapter Objectives

After studying this chapter, you should be able to:

1. Protect your skin from the sun.
2. Protect yourself from body odors.
3. Control unwanted body hair.
4. Groom your nails and hands appropriately for business.
5. Groom your feet and toenails for health and comfort.

Skin and nail problems vary from person to person. The sun destroys some skins and seems to make other skins glow. Discolorations result from both exposure to sun and simple aging. Some people have no trouble with body odor while others struggle constantly to combat it. Fragrances on some people enhance their presence and on others they detract. Women struggle sometimes with dark or heavy hair growth on their faces and legs while for others hair growth is not a problem. The information in this chapter should help you if you have special body care problems. Some grooming procedures for nails and skin that will give you a polished finish for your professional appearance are included.

Skin

Taking care of your skin is important more for your health than your appearance, although both are involved. Protection from damage by knowing what the sun can do to you is one important health consideration that must be balanced against the sun-tanned appearance many people seek. Recognizing whether discolorations need attention or not may involve both health and appearance considerations. Dealing with odors, fragrances, and hair usually is important to appearance.

Sun Damage

Deliberate exposure of the skin to the sun, specifically to its ultraviolet rays, is quite possibly the most damaging activity undertaken by people in the name of beauty. Although suntanning and sunbathing are popularly associated with beauty and health, they actually should be considered as a period of time you set aside to age your skin.

Tanned skin is the result of a permanent chemical change in the cells of the skin. With exposure to the sun, the blood vessels dilate, turning the skin red. The blood produces a substance in these dilated vessels that forms blisters and swelling. The tan that finally occurs in some people is a protective barrier the skin forms to prevent further damage to its cells.

Additional exposure adds damage to damage, and the chemistry of the cell can never be restored. The outermost cells are sloughed off in the normal course of time and replaced by new, normal ones. Deep sunburning though, alters cells deep within the skin that affect the texture, making it thick, rough, inelastic, lined, and leathery. Nothing can change it, and it will not heal. This kind of damage from the sun is permanent.

You can probably see some effects of the sun on your skin already. Compare an area like the back of your hand that is routinely exposed to sun to an area of your body that has never been exposed. There are ways to delay the aging effects of the sun. Shade yourself as often as you can from direct sunlight. When you cannot shade yourself, use a sunblock which can be obtained at your drug store. Sunblocks are different from suntan lotions. Sunblocks, if they do the job properly, do not allow sun rays to penetrate the barrier they make; suntan lotions do allow the rays to penetrate.

You can have tanned skin safely with the use of skin bronzers. There are two kinds. One is temporary, like makeup, and can be washed off. The other is more permanent. While it becomes lighter with bathing, all of it does not disappear until the cells of the skin die and flake off. Both of these preparations are satisfactory and easy ways of obtaining a tan without damaging your skin.

Skin Discolorations

Dark areas of skin on your face, neck, and hands can be a problem. Often these discolorations are caused by exposure to sunlight. If you curtail that exposure, sometimes the dark areas fade to their natural color. They also occur often as a result of chemical changes in the body during pregnancy or as a result of taking a birth

Illus. 14-1. Exposure to the sun can permanently damage your skin.

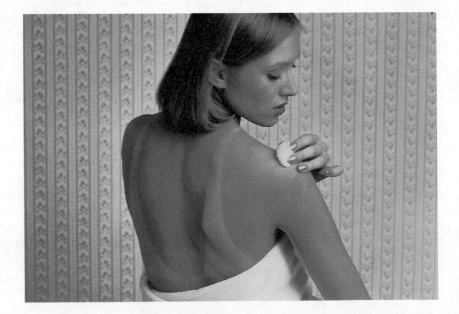

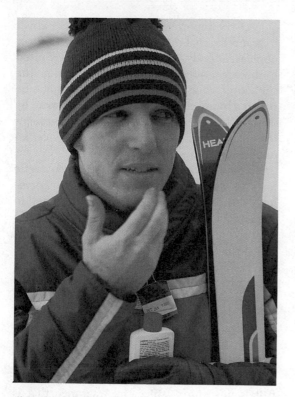

Illus. 14-2. Protect yourself with sunblocks when you are exposed to sunlight.

control pill. Usually the skin returns to normal after pregnancy or when the use of the pill has been discontinued. Dark, rough, or ashy areas can occur because of dry skin.

Bleach creams have been formulated to treat these isolated discolored areas, but the preparations available for home use rarely have a lasting effect. The easiest way for women to treat the discolored areas, if they are not too bad, is to use a concealing cream beneath make-up. Although temporary, this procedure is satisfactory for most people. If yours is a particularly bothersome problem and none of the home remedies seem to correct it to your satisfaction, consult a dermatologist.

Body Odors

It is unrealistic to consider yourself well-groomed if you have a body odor. Most body odors are caused by perspiration under your arms and in the genital area. The bacteria present on your skin most of the time are the cause of many body odors. They thrive in damp, warm places, decomposing body secretions such as perspiration, and causing the characteristic odors that are so offensive. You can easily control ordinary body odors with products available today, frequent bathing, and some special tips.

Perspiration is a secretion that forms on the surface of your skin to maintain your body at a constant temperature by evaporative cooling. Like other secretions and excretions, though, if it remains on your skin, it can harbor odor-producing bacteria. Bathing is the only way to control the bacterial odor after it has occurred. Once the bacterial decomposition of perspiration has taken place, producing the resulting odor, scented creams and sprays will not work. Only a bath will eliminate the odor.

There are two ways to avoid underarm perspiration odor: antiperspirants and deodorants. Both the amount of perspiration you produce and the number of bacteria on your skin can be reduced considerably with these products.

You can reduce the number of bacteria present under your arms by using a deodorant that kills bacteria. Bacteria grow easily, however, and deodorants must be applied frequently to keep the bacteria growth under control. Perspiration causes a major problem other than odor; it circles your clothing. The best way to control the amount of perspiration you secrete is to use an antiperspirant. Antiperspirants actually are astringents that reduce the amount of perspiration you secrete for several hours. It is possible now to purchase products which are an antiperspirant and deodorant combined. With these, most people can easily control the amount of perspiration and the growth of bacteria in the underarm area completely avoiding underarm odor. For the most effective protection, the products should be applied immediately after you bathe. If you have shaved your underarms during your bath, however, and your skin is tender or nicked, wait a few hours before applying your antiperspirant.

If you have a problem of excess underarm perspiration that cannot be controlled with an antiperspirant, your doctor may be able to help you. Tension sometimes increases perspiration, and foods with strong odors are said to influence the odor of perspiration as well as that of your breath.

Fragrances

Fragrances applied to your person are designed to enhance your grooming. It is possible to detract from your grooming with indiscriminate use of fragrance. Omitting it entirely deprives you of a little extra that can be a very enjoyable part of your grooming.

Fragrances are available in many forms: for women, perfume, cologne, and eau de toilette; for men, cologne, and after-shave. They vary in strength and should be used in different amounts to achieve the same degree of fragrance.

Perfume is the most concentrated of the forms. Incidentally, too, it is the most costly. A very small amount of perfume is required to impart a lasting fragrance.

Cologne is less concentrated and less expensive, but it takes more of it to achieve the same lasting fragrance as perfume. Cologne can be splashed or sprayed on large areas of your body without overdoing the fragrance.

Eau de toilette and after-shave are less concentrated. They usually are applied after your bath or shave, sometimes before you towel, so that the surface water spreads the fragrance over the surface of your skin.

A very important point to remember about fragrances is that they are not designed to cover unpleasant body odors. Body odors are caused by bacteria which decompose debris on the surface of your skin. These odors cannot be covered by anything. They must be removed by washing to eliminate them. Use your fragrances to enhance your clean body, never to cover an undesirable odor.

Almost everything you buy in cosmetic lines is scented with some fragrance. Fortunately, these scents are specifically designed to evaporate rapidly so that they do not compete with the one you select and apply in the form of a perfume, cologne, eau de toilette, or after-shave. If you find a scented product, such as a hairspray, lotion, or cream, that does seem to compete with the fragrance you select for yourself, look around for an unscented substitute. Frequently, unscented products are the same as the scented ones except for the added fragrance. Be prepared to distinguish any natural scent of the chemical makeup of the product, if it is unscented, since the fragrance that is normally added serves to disguise the less appealing odors of the natural substances of the product.

Perfumes, colognes, eau de toilette, and after-shave products are formulated for long-lasting emission of the fragrance with which they are scented. They are available in an infinite variety of mixtures including flowers, fruits, woods, and foods. There are heavy, light, smooth, sharp, gentle, and strong scents. Each person will find that a scent will be a little different when mixed with personal natural body oils and body scent. When you select a fragrance for yourself, take care to suit it to yourself, the occasions for which you plan to wear it, and, of course, to your budget.

At the fragrance counter, try only one or two fragrances at a time. Spray each lightly on your hand or arm and allow it to evaporate. It is a good idea to walk around the store and shop for a while before you decide that you want to purchase the fragrance. The scent may change somewhat with exposure to your body chemistry.

You can actually find scents that suit your personality—there are some fragrances that seem to complement a bright, loquacious person, while others enhance a subdued, thoughtful personality. Most people have many moods and find that a fragrance contributes to the enjoyment of a particular mood if it seems to fit. One thing you should be aware of is that when you are indoors, working closely with people, strong fragrances are offensive. Stick to the very subtle, light fragrances when you are working closely with people in offices or other enclosed areas. Save the strong, pronounced ones for outdoors or when you are in a large area, such as a large ballroom. Too strong a fragrance is as offensive as a strong body odor.

Women's Leg and Underarm Hair

There are several ways to remove body hair, and the method you choose depends upon how much effort and money you are willing to put into the process.

Shaving is probably the most commonly used method of hair removal for underarms and legs. Either a safety razor or an electric one will do the job. If you use a safety razor, lather the surface with soap or shaving cream carefully. Draw the razor across the surface against the grain of the growth of the hair. Rinse the razor frequently to clean the blade. This kind of shaving probably is most easily done in the shower or bath.

If you use an electric razor, the surface should be dry. You can prepare the skin surface for more efficient shaving by using a pre-shave lotion that makes electric shaving easier. Electric shaving is more effective if you draw the shaver across the surface in a direction opposite to the growth pattern of the hair. Usually, legs

are shaved from the ankles to only a few inches above the knee. If you have dark hair higher on your leg that shows when you wear a bathing suit, it probably will be more comfortable to bleach the hair than to shave it unless your complexion is quite dark making bleached hair noticeable.

Waxing and tweezing are two more ways to remove hair. Both pull the hair out by its roots and usually are not used to remove underarm hair. In waxing, heated, softened wax is spread over the surface and allowed to dry. The wax is then peeled off the skin, pulling the hairs out, leaving a smooth surface free of hair. This can be painful, somewhat like tweezing. Tweezing, though, is too tedious to use on large areas and usually is confined to your eyebrows, where only a few hairs are removed at a time.

Chemical depilatories are available for removing hair, but you should test these chemical substances on a small area of your skin before you use them on a large one. A test consists of covering a one-inch area of the skin according to the manufacturer's directions, rinsing it, and waiting 24 hours. If there is no redness or irritation after 24 hours, the product is safe for your skin, and you can use it over the entire hair surface. Chemical depilatories dissolve the hair to just below the surface of the skin. The skin is rinsed, taking off the depilatory and the dissolved hair. Hair regrowth takes a little longer with depilatories than with shaving.

Women's Facial Hair

Shaving, waxing, and depilatories can be used for underarm and leg hair. They should not ordinarily be used on your face. Facial hair can be removed professionally by electrolysis, or you can do it by tweezing, although this method sometimes causes irritation. Facial hair other than eyebrows can also be trimmed close to the skin with sharp fingernail scissors or it can be bleached. Facial depilatories may be used after careful testing if other methods are unsatisfactory.

Electrolysis is the permanent removal of hair with the use of electricity. You cannot do it yourself; it must be done professionally. It is about 80 percent effective the first time. Therefore, you will need to repeat about 20 percent of the treatment for complete removal of the unwanted hair. Electrolysis can be used for hairlines, eyebrows, other facial hair, and any body hair you desire removed permanently. Compared to other procedures, this one is more expensive.

Bleaching should not be done around the eyes. Other facial hair, however, can be bleached as well as body hair. Peroxide that is somewhat stronger than that used for cleansing minor cuts and wounds must be used. Scalp hair bleaching products may also be used, provided you test them first and follow the directions very carefully. There are also products specifically made for bleaching face and body hair.

—— *Fingernail and Hand Care* ——

Your hands are practically always in view. Their grooming or lack of it are almost as often noticed as your face and hair. The procedures for grooming hands are simple and can easily become habit if you conscientiously work at them.

The Nail Itself

Your fingernails and your success in having well-groomed ones are the result of many factors. Your inherited characteristics certainly have an impact on your nails, just as they do on other personal physical characteristics. Factors you can control are the effects that your personal habits and practices have on your nails.

The characteristics of the nail itself are important for you to understand. The hard,

epidermal cells that form the nail are called the nail plate. The chemical makeup of the nail plate is very much like that of your skin and hair. Nails are influenced by your overall health as your skin and hair are. Just as well-cared-for hair and skin contribute to your overall appearance, so do well-cared-for fingernails improve your appearance.

There are variations among people's nails, as there are among their other physical characteristics. There are even variations among the different nails on a person's hand. Some differences are inherited; some are the result of injury to the nail bed—that area beneath the cuticle where the nail plate is formed. Just as some hair will be thicker and coarser, some nails will be thicker and stronger for no reason other than simple differences in people. Just as you adjust your hair care procedures to accommodate the kind of hair you have, you adjust your nail care procedures to accommodate the kind of nails you have.

Environment has a definite effect on the nature of the nails. Skin subjected to harsh detergents day after day becomes dry and flaky. Nails subjected to the same abuse suffer injury also. Very cold weather, chemical solvents, wax, and hard blows all affect the skin; they affect the nails also. The difference between caring for your skin and your nails lies mainly in the time it takes to effect improvement or to correct damage that has been done.

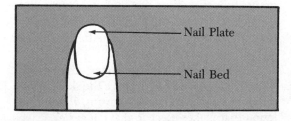

Illus. 14-3. You can damage your nail permanently if you injure the nail bed.

Skin is constantly flaking off and replacing itself, resulting in a shedding of abused skin on the outermost layer every twenty-six days. Therefore, if you have chapped, burned, or just flaky skin, lotions applied for about a month seem to correct your problem, provided, of course, your skin is not repeatedly subjected to the same abuse. Nails, however, do not completely replace themselves so quickly. It takes about six months for the part of the nail closest to your cuticle to grow to the end of your nail and to be filed, clipped, or, unfortunately, broken off. This means that when a nail is damaged, you must live with it much longer.

Even more important is damage to the nail bed. Excessive pressure due to a blow to the finger, such as shutting it accidentally in a drawer or squeezing a pencil constantly too hard against the side of the nail bed, can permanently damage the area where the nail is formed. This damage results in ridges, thickening, and weakened areas of the nail and cannot be cured. You can learn to live with it, though, by developing techniques to groom it.

Because, from beginning to end, the nail is on the tip of your finger for approximately six months, it has much greater potential for injury than your skin does. During their six-month lifetime, consider how many times nails are exposed to soap and water, which are drying agents, and how often they are subjected to

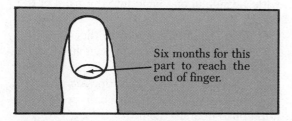

Illus. 14-4. It takes approximately six months for the nail forming in the nail bed to reach the tip of your finger.

chemicals, such as household cleaners, or to hair preparations, such as permanent solutions and coloring agents. Then, wonder how they survive as well as they do; and decide to take better care of your nails before you complain again of brittleness, flaking, peeling, chipping, or just plain poor nails.

Problem Nails

There are bodily impairments that affect your nails. Skin diseases such as psoriasis and fungus can affect your nails and should be treated by a physician. Diseases such as anemia and insufficient thyroid secretions can contribute to nail problems. Certainly, these kinds of complications must be treated by a qualified physician before you can hope to achieve healthy, well-groomed nails.

Some stopgap measures are available to help you have presentable hands while you are seeking more permanent solutions. It is important to keep in mind that good, strong nails are developed in the nail bed of each finger. Other means of achieving satisfactory results are temporary and offer no lasting results.

It has been commonly believed by many that increased intake of protein improves nails, because they, like hair and skin, are dependent upon protein for replacement of dead cells that are continuously shed. The common practice has been to consume gelatin daily, either in capsule form or mixed in fruit juice. The truth of the effectiveness of this kind of treatment depends upon the reason for your nail problems. If you have weak nails because your diet is low in protein, increasing the intake of protein should, of course, effect an improvement in your nails (and incidentally, in your skin and hair). Check back in the nutrition section of this book. Analyze your intake of daily protein and the suggested daily allowance to determine if protein deficiency could be the cause of nail problems before you decide to prescribe increased intake for yourself in the form of gelatin.

If, in fact, your diet is not low in protein and you add protein in the form of gelatin to your diet, you may well effect only a weight gain. Excess protein, like excess fat and carbohydrate, is stored by the body as fat if it is not burned as energy. If you are low in protein and choose to correct the condition by consuming gelatin or any other protein-rich food, do not expect immediate results. Remember that good nails are formed in the nail bed and that it takes six months for the nail being formed today to cover the entire nail plate of your finger. Any benefit from improving your health and diet will take approximately six months to show before completely replacing the entire nail plate with a healthier surface.

In the meantime, there are chemical substances you can use to strengthen your nail plate. Two basic kinds are available. One is a substance, mainly formaldehyde, that actually acts to harden the protein surface of the nail plate upon contact. The other is a preparation, containing fibers such as nylon in a clear, thick liquid, that, when dry, supports the nail with a strong film.

Formaldehyde has the tendency to cause allergic skin reactions and is not made available by cosmetic companies in nail preparations because of numerous such complaints. Many drug stores, however, have such preparations, and you may be able to obtain them by prescription from your dermatologist.

The fiber-type hardeners sometimes leave a rough, unattractive surface on your nails. Frequently, however, women can use colored nail enamel over the hardener to achieve a better appearance. Nail enamel applied over any of the hardeners may not wear well, though.

There are other hardeners that are said to work because they contain protein substances that strengthen the nail upon contact. It is doubtful that protein applied to the surface of either the nail or the hair has any beneficial effect on the strength or quality of either one. Studies are not conclusive in this area, and you should beware of spending resources and time on a process that may be worthless.

Soft nails that do not respond to good diet, precautionary care, and temporary help may be best groomed by keeping them short so that they are less vulnerable to tearing and snagging. It is better, by far, to have short, well-groomed nails than long, ragged ones.

Preventive Care

Some protective practices you can cultivate to protect nails are easy to develop. Unlike hair that has been neglected for weeks and can be spectacularly conditioned and groomed within two or three hours, nails require continuous care if they are to look good every day.

Begin your route to healthy nails by reviewing how you treat them daily. If your nervous times are relieved by picking at your cuticle or by biting your nail plate, you must concentrate on some other release of tension—one that is not destructive to your physical structure.

Try to develop habits like dialing the telephone with the rubber end of a pencil; picking up a piece of paper by using the straightened fingers to gently pinch an uncreased fold in it to lift it; and sweeping coins, clips, and pins off with the side of one hand into the palm of the other.

Obtain a letter opener or other device to force stubborn latches open. Switch lights on and off with your knuckle or the side of your thumb instead of your fingertip. Avoid clasps and closures that snag your nails when you attempt to operate them.

Use cleaning brushes with handles that allow you to keep your hands out of the water and cleaning solvents. Wear rubber gloves when you must put your hands in hot water. If you

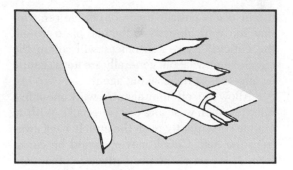

Illus. 14-5. Learn to pick up items in a way that does not damage your nails.

have strong nails, keep them a length that is practical for the tasks you are expected to perform with your hands.

During periods of extreme exposure, such as to cold weather or to harsh solvents, conscientiously keep your nails well lubricated with creams. If you find that you must perform a very messy job and for some reason you cannot wear protective gloves, scrape your nails across a bar of soap to deposit soap under your nails and apply a heavy coat of lubricating cream before you start. That will prevent ugly stains from discoloring the skin beneath the tip of your nail and will make it much easier to clean that area when you are through with the messy job.

Manicuring

A weekly manicure is an excellent preventive care practice as well as a grooming technique for your nails. There seems to be more incentive to preserve a well-groomed nail than to protect a ragged, stubby one. There is a set routine to follow in manicuring your nails.

It is necessary to start with clean nails. This is best achieved with gentle washing with soap and water and a soft fingernail brush. Avoid using pointed, sharp objects beneath the nail to clean it. You can separate the nail plate from

your skin before it is ready and damage the nail. Gentle brushing removes the dirt and debris without damaging the area where the nail is joined to your skin. Next, clean any buffing wax or nail enamel off the surface of the nail plate.

Nail enamel remover is specially formulated to dissolve and remove chemicals applied to the nail, but it must be used carefully. It is never wise to dip your nail into the remover. Use, instead, a cotton ball saturated with remover, applied to the surface of the nail only. Usually enamel and wax are effectively and gently removed if you allow the saturated cotton ball to rest for a few seconds on the nail plate to dissolve the chemicals. Then, with only very light pressure, wipe the surface clean. The area near the cuticle should be cleaned very gently and can be most effectively cleaned with a cotton-tipped stick or an orange stick that is wrapped in cotton and saturated with remover. The more effectively you keep the remover away from the cuticle and your skin, the better. It is the strong solvent in remover that is not good for your skin. Because the solvent is very drying, the shorter the time the remover is on the nail plate itself, the better.

After you have wiped the enamel and buffing wax from the surface of the nail, rinse your nails quickly to remove any remover that may have been deposited on your skin.

Dry your nails carefully but gently, and you are ready to shape them. Shaping can be done with either an emery board or a metal file. Many people feel that a metal file is destructive to the nail plate. If you seem to have more trouble with your nails when you use the metal file, switch to the fiber emery one, which generally is gentler to your nails.

Filing is done in one direction only — from the side to the center of the nail. The file is held at a slight angle so that it files the underside of the end of the nail first. A back-and-forth sawing tears the fingernail by pulling it against the grain near the outer corners.

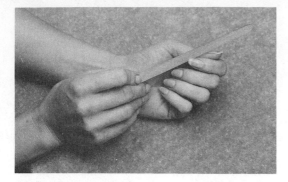

Illus. 14-6. Filing is done in one direction only—from the side to the center of the nail.

The shape of your nail is very important to its strength. The sides of the nail must be allowed to grow to the top of your finger. That means that you should not file down into the corners of the nail since to do so severely weakens it.

It is generally considered very hard on nails to clip or cut them. The layers forming the nail plate tend to split and separate when they are subjected to cutting or clipping, thus weakening the tip of the nail, making it vulnerable to snags and splits.

Nails are shaped before they are soaked because the plate itself becomes somewhat pliable when it is soaked, making a smooth surface difficult to achieve with a file or emery board. After shaping has been effected, though, it is an excellent procedure to soak your nails in warm water, to which you can add mild soap or a cuticle softening agent made especially for soaking nails. The purpose of the soaking is to loosen cuticle from the nail plate so that the cuticle can be pushed back with a minimum of effort. Very gentle handling of the cuticle is vital because the nail bed can be permanently damaged if you use too much pressure or force the cuticle away from the plate before the nail is fully developed.

If you do not have time to soak your nails, use instead a cuticle cream or cuticle remover that you apply directly to the nail plate around the cuticle. These substances will soften the cuticle somewhat but generally are not as gentle or effective as the soaking agent.

Allow the softening agent to work about five minutes; then wash and dry your nails. With an orange stick, gently push the cuticle back away from the nail. Cuticle never should be cut or torn. It is part of the protective area that contributes to the formation of new nail plate. Abusing it leads to weakened nail plates. It is far better to push too little cuticle back than to push too much. Your goal is to allow the nail plate that is matured to be exposed.

When you have followed the regular practice of softening and pushing your cuticle back with an orange stick for a few months, it probably will not be necessary to continue to do it weekly. Simply pushing the cuticle back with the towel on which you dry your nails each day will be enough to contain the growth of cuticle on the nail plate.

Cuticle sheds itself regularly, just as the surface of all your skin does. Occasionally, due to dryness or harsh treatment, the shedding may produce a jagged area that snags your clothing. If that happens, carefully clip the snag, but do not attempt to cut the semicircle of the entire cuticle off the nail. Your nails have a far better chance of growing strong with the protective band of cuticle intact than without it.

After nails are cleaned and shaped and the cuticle has been pushed back from the nail plate, you are ready either to apply nail enamel or to buff the nails. Most men and many women like the smooth finish buffing gives the nail plate.

Buffing

Buffing is done with a soft chamois and buffing wax. After you have cleaned and shaped

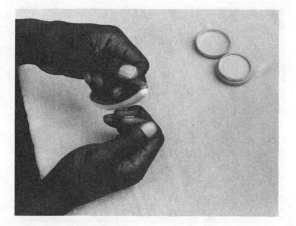

Illus. 14-7. Buffing
is done with a soft
chamois and buffing wax.

your nails and have pushed back the cuticle, buffing wax is applied sparingly to the nail plate and allowed to dry. Some wax may be applied to the buffing chamois also and allowed to dry. The buffer is drawn across the nail plate in one direction only. Lift the buffer for each stroke and avoid roughing the cuticle or placing pressure on the unsupported tip of the nail. A few strokes are usually all that is needed to achieve a shine on the nail that lasts for several days. Using a sawing motion with the buffer creates too much heat on the nail plate and can damage it. Be careful not to buff with too much pressure or too much vigor since either may damage the nail plate.

When the nail plate is as smooth as you desire, clean the surface of the buffer with an orange stick and wash and dry your nails. After buffing is an excellent time for applying rich lubricants to dry, rough surfaces that may appear around your nails.

Enameling

If you want to use enamel, a clear coat for men or women is appropriate for business.

Women may also wear unobtrusive pastel colors to work.

The procedure which produces the longest-wearing enamel follows. First, be sure that the nail-plate surface is clean and free from oil or debris. If you have used cream or oil to remove the cuticle, it will be necessary to cleanse the nail plate of the substance. Soap and water with your soft fingernail brush are effective. Some people find nail enamel remover useful for this cleaning. However, the enamel remover is very hard on the nail plate, and the less time you allow it to stay on the nail surface, the better.

The nail plate should be completely dry. Be especially careful to dry the area around the cuticle where water may deposit itself. A base coat usually is applied first to the clean nail plate. Its purpose is to provide a smooth surface for the enamel and in many cases to provide a buffer for the nail plate from the enamel, which may be formulated with chemicals that are hard on the nail itself. The base coat usually enhances the wearability of the enamel if it is applied not only to the upper surface of the nail plate but also to the under edge of the tip of the nail.

The correct procedure for applying base coat, enamel, and top coat to the nail is first to dip the brush in the fluid, wiping one side of the brush against the top edge of the bottle. Then apply the full side of the brush to the base of the center of the nail and lightly brush to the tip of the center of the nail. Quickly follow with one sweep from the base of the nail plate to the tip on each side. Those three sweeps should cover the nail entirely with a very thin layer of liquid. Additional strokes should not be used at this point. Redip the brush anew for each nail. Additional coats after the first one has dried thoroughly will fill in any gaps that may be left. Very thin applications that are allowed to dry thoroughly before the next application provide a more durable surface than thick coats do.

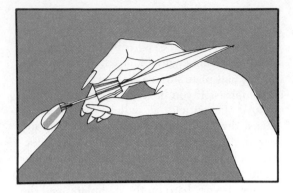

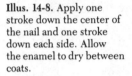

Illus. 14-8. Apply one stroke down the center of the nail and one stroke down each side. Allow the enamel to dry between coats.

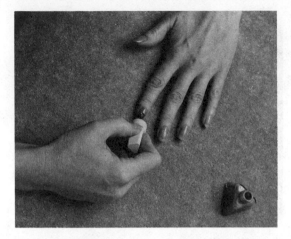

Illus. 14-9. The number of coats of enamel you apply depends upon the color of the enamel.

The first application is a base coat. The next application is an enamel of the color you desire. Nail enamel colors for women change with the dictates of fashion. It is always in fashion and always presents a well-groomed hand, though, if you select enamel according to the way it looks with the color of your skin. Usually a light tint of either muted pink, beige, brownish orange, or one of the infinite mixtures is suitable for women in business. It is, of course, not necessary to use color at all. Clear enamel is never out of style and can present a very well-groomed hand, in good taste for any occasion.

The number of coats of the enamel depends upon the color of the enamel. Very light colors usually require three very thin coats for maximum shine and durability. Darker colors may be satisfactory with only two coats.

When the enamel has dried completely, a top coat is applied. It is a clear coat, the purpose of which is to take the abuse of wear without showing chips that would appear if the color were exposed to abuse. The top coat is best applied in very thin layers from the base of the nail to the tip and under the tip, just as the base coat was. Two top coats are usually sufficient for

protection. Many people apply one coat of top coat daily to provide protection for the colored enamel.

A good quality, fresh product is essential to a successful manicure. Base coat, enamel, or top coat that has thickened will never be satisfactory. Any of the three that are not fresh can reduce the wearability of the manicure. Nail enamel solvents are available but usually do not produce very good results. It is better to buy one versatile color in the smallest bottle you can find, use it regularly as long as you wish, and plan to discard whatever may be left when it becomes thick.

Hand Care

Well-cared-for nails are the beginning of attractive hands. Hands become unattractive sometimes because of dry skin and abuse. The procedures for caring for your hands are simple and easy to learn.

The skin on your hands is the most abused skin area of your body. It is exposed to more soap, water, weather, and offending substances than any other area. It is small wonder that hands dry out and age so easily. They need special care in moisturizing, and you should be aware that they will be the first part of your body to reflect abuse.

Some precautions and remedies that you can take to protect your hard-working hands are to keep hand lotion in several places at your home and in your place of work. Try to keep a bottle of hand lotion near every sink where you wash your hands—kitchen, bathroom, utility room, and garage. Try to keep a bottle or tube of hand lotion in desk drawers and bedside table drawers. Use it every time you wet hands that are dry, handle papers excessively, or expose your hands to extreme temperatures.

If you notice dryness, apply a heavy coat of lotion or petroleum jelly to your hands.

Hardened skin surfaces on your hands, both in the palm and on your fingers, can be treated so that your hands stay soft. Use a fine emery board to file the hardened surface in one direction only. You can see the direction in which the skin grows, as it will be smoother when you file in one direction than in the other. File in the direction that smoothes the skin. Often the hardened skin occurs alongside the nail on your thumb and first finger. Carefully emery-file those areas while they are dry; then apply cream to soften the newly exposed skin. Be careful when you are filing away the hardened, dead skin not to file into the nail along the side because you may weaken it.

Warts on your hands usually are believed to be caused by viruses. Although there are many superstitions about how to remove them, the most reliable process is to have a dermatologist perform the job. It is a painless, relatively inexpensive procedure to be rid of the unsightly imperfection, and well worth the week or two you are required to wear a small bandage. Picking at a wart yourself or trying to cut it off with a razor or other sharp instrument

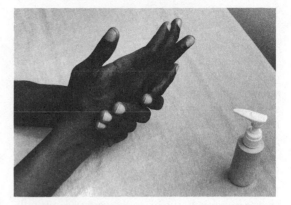

Illus. 14-10. Apply hand lotion frequently throughout the day.

is definitely not recommended. It is possible to spread the virus to other parts of your skin as well as to subject the area to an infection. Such risks are not justified since it is a very simple matter to have the job done by a dermatologist once and for all.

As some people age, small brown spots appear on their hands. These spots can be bleached if they are offensive or make you feel self-conscious. Creams designed especially for lightening these spots are available, but the creams are designed to be used daily. Actually the spots are harmless and usually are not noticeable. Unless they are serious enough to make you feel uncomfortable about the appearance of your hands, you may ignore them.

Toenail and Foot Care

Caring for your feet often is the last thing you think about in grooming yourself. Actually it may have the greatest impact on that elusive quality of warmth and glow that shines in your face; for if your feet hurt, it shows on the face, allowing little else to be reflected.

Foot Care

Care for your feet is simple and can be incorporated easily into your bath and hand-care routines. Protection of your feet includes wearing shoes that allow movement within the shoe and arranging your activities so that your feet are not suffering from restricted circulation for hours at a time.

The ordinary pull of gravity is hard on your feet. Pumping blood that carries waste from them to organs in the upper part of your body that rid your body of such waste is difficult against the pull of gravity. Therefore, you need to be aware of promoting such flow of waste-carrying blood from your feet to the upper part of your body by sitting so that there is no pressure at any point along the leg. Do not tightly cross your knees, hang your knees over a ridge at the edge of a chair, or tightly cross your ankles. Also, whenever you can, in the privacy of your home, you should elevate your feet somewhat as you are sitting. A small footstool beneath your desk also can provide some relief during the day if it is not noticeable and if it can be used so that the remainder of your body alignment is not distorted. You can select shoes that allow enough room for your toes to move and for your arch to slide in and out without pinching. Changing the position of your feet often as you sit seems to provide relief to restricted blood flow.

Poor circulation in your feet leads to numerous problems. Besides pain and numbness resulting from blood-starved, waste-harboring muscles, the skin on the feet is starved of nutrients carried by blood. You may notice hardened areas of the skin, and general dry skin resulting from abuse to the feet. The hardened areas are destructive to clothing and can be smoothed with a pumice stone, an emery board, or a specially designed rough-skin remover. Corns and calluses can be smoothed on the surface with the same appliances, but they should not be trimmed with a razor or other sharp instrument. Corns and calluses generally are caused by pressure on a particular area of the foot and will never be cured as long as the pressure exists. If they become painful, a podiatrist or dermatologist may surgically remove them, but you may expect them to reappear if the pressure is not corrected.

Another surface problem that may occur on your feet is warts. They are called plantar warts when they occur on the soles of your feet, but they are believed to be caused by the same virus as warts on your hands. The difference is that they grow inward because of pressure on your feet instead of outward as they do on the hands. These warts may be extremely painful, and the only known successful treatment is to have them removed surgically.

If the circulation is poor in your feet, it probably is poor in your legs. The skin on the lower part of the leg may become scaly and develop a rash if it does not receive enough nourishment. The best treatment, of course, is to promote good circulation by elevating the feet and avoiding sitting and standing positions that deter good circulation. Treatment of the affected skin can be undertaken by using good creams and lotions each night and morning on the scaly areas of skin.

Some good practices in caring for your feet are to buy shoes that are large enough, to wash your feet thoroughly and often, to dry them carefully, and to purchase hosiery that is properly sized.

Shoes should be bought late in the day so that you can fit your feet when they are at their largest. Most feet tend to swell somewhat during the day. If shoes are bought to fit your morning size rather than your afternoon size, they will pinch all afternoon, severely restricting the circulation of the blood and affecting your disposition. Most people's feet vary somewhat in size from foot to foot. Learn which of your feet is larger, and be sure the shoes you buy are comfortable for both the larger and smaller foot. Stand in shoes and walk in them before you buy them. If you are in doubt about whether or not they fit, put off buying them at the moment. Come back later and try them again. A poorly fitting shoe at any price is a very bad bargain.

When you wash your feet, carefully wash the area around your toes. Most fungus, athlete's foot, and other debris collect in that area and are apt to flourish if the area is not clean and dry. Powder may be sprinkled lightly between your toes if you have a tendency to perspire in this area. Moisture is a prime breeding ground for diseases of the skin on your feet. Be careful, however, not to cake the powder on your feet. Caked powder may absorb moisture, stay wet, and breed its own bacteria.

Be sure your hosiery allows your toes unrestricted movement. Because hosiery seems so flexible, you may think it cannot cramp your toes. It can, and it will if you wear a size too small for you.

Because of poor circulation, the skin on your feet may be very dry. If you notice such a problem, treat it somewhat as you treat dry skin on your hands. Apply a heavy coat of cream, lotion, or petroleum jelly overnight. In the morning, you should notice considerably improved skin on your feet. This procedure may be repeated as often as you wish to improve the skin on your feet.

After your bath, you may find it helpful, also, to rub baby or mineral oil over the skin on your feet and legs and rinse lightly before you dry. The very thin coating of oil is protective, but it is not heavy enough to soil your clothing.

Toenail Grooming

Toenails are treated somewhat like fingernails. The desirable shape of the toenail is one that is squared across the end, extending no further than the fleshy part of your toe.

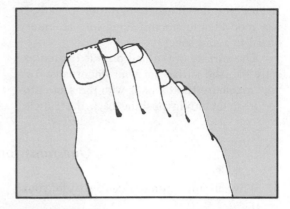

Illus. 14-11. Toenails should be squared off at the end of your toes.

It is especially important in shaping the toenail, as it is in shaping the fingernail, not to file or cut into the side of the nail. Although you need not worry about weakening the toenail when the sides are cut, you will suffer the risk of painful ingrown nails as the nail replaces itself during regular growth. As long as there is a straight surface along the side of the nail that replaces itself with regular growth, there is little possibility of the nail cutting into your toe, developing the ingrown nail. However, if there is a corner where the side has been cut, that pointed edge may easily penetrate the skin and cause you much pain before you are able to correct the situation.

Toenails may be filed or clipped. Clipping may promote separation of the layers of the nail, as it does with more fragile fingernails. Often however, toenails are so tough that they do not succumb to filing and must be clipped. Try to find clippers or scissors that enable you to get a straight edge across the end of your toe. Curved clippers may invite ingrown nails. Gently filing your toenails often gives the most satisfactory surface since there is little chance of a rough edge resulting in torn stockings or catching other surfaces and tearing the nail.

Even if you do choose to clip your toenails, it is a good idea to smooth them with an emery board to avoid snags.

The surface of the nail plate is treated exactly like the surface of your fingernails. You may manicure the toenails with the same procedures, including pushing back the cuticle, buffing, and applying enamel. The skin around your toenails is very tender, however, and you should use very gentle touches in manicuring them if you are to avoid soreness. Enamel is more easily applied if the toes are separated with cotton balls or laced with a folded tissue to expose the entire surface of each nail.

Questions for Chapter 14

1. Why can suntanning be dangerous for your skin?
2. What can you do to avoid the aging effects of the sun?
3. What causes body odors?
4. What is the difference between a deodorant and an antiperspirant?
5. What fragrances are best for when you are working closely with people?
6 What choices do women have in removing unwanted hair?
7. How long does it take for nail plate formation to grow to the tip of your finger?
8. What are some preventive measures you can take to protect your fingernails?
9. How do you treat the cuticle around your fingernails?
10. What does buffing do for fingernails?
11. How can you treat hardened surfaces on your hands?
12. What should you do about warts on your hands?
13. How should you care for the skin on your feet?

Chapter 15

Eating for Well-Being

Chapter Objectives

After studying this chapter, you should be able to:

1. *Evaluate the nutrients you need for good nutrition.*
2. *Identify and avoid foods which contribute little nutrition to your diet.*
3. *Plan a diet that meets your nutritional needs.*
4. *Plan a nutritional diet that allows you to lose or gain weight.*

The state of your nutrition depends upon your knowledge and your habits. You will spend a great amount of your time throughout your life eating, and often it will serve mainly a social function rather than a biological one. The effects of consuming food are the same regardless of your reasons. To make nutritious choices, you need to understand your personal needs for nutrients; but eating is more than making choices. It is an activity that is governed by habit.

Besides knowing which foods to eat, you must form habits of selecting them and consuming an appropriate amount. You will not find this difficult, provided the eating habits you have already acquired are good. However, if your present habits are less than adequate for good nutrition, you must be very determined as well as knowledgeable to correct them.

Analyzing Nutrition

A nutritious diet is readily available today, but the problem is that frequently you don't eat to nurture your body; you eat for a number of other reasons. The guides for good nutrition are easy to understand and to follow. If they conflict with your eating habits, though, your body shows it. It shows in your weight, your energy, and often in your attitude. Since these areas form the basis of your personal development in many ways, analyzing your nutrition is vital in your program of personal development.

The Nutrients

In addition to altering your eating habits, decide why you eat at all. You eat to live, not live to eat! In order to survive, your body needs

Illus. 15-1. Analyzing your nutrition is vital in your program of personal development.

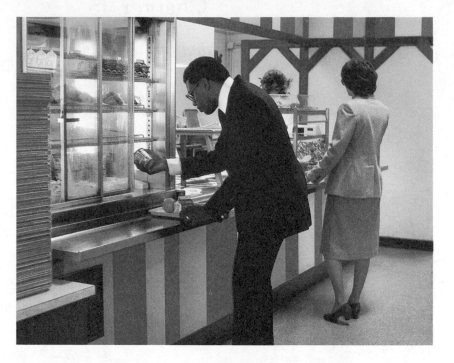

a balance of nutrients: protein, carbohydrates, fat, vitamins, and minerals. In general terms, protein is needed to repair body tissue, carbohydrates are needed for energy, and fat is needed for energy, insulation, and certain body functions, such as elimination. Any of these three nutrients can be changed by your body to energy. If the energy is not used, it will be stored as fat.

Various vitamins and minerals are also necessary to your health. Some of the effects you can see and measure yourself. Vitamin A provides for night vision and skin development; C and D, for bones and teeth; and K, for digestion. The B vitamins affect your digestion, mental state, nerves, and skin. The effects of minerals are not easily seen but are dramatic. They control such areas as muscle contractions (heart rhythm) and the chemical balances necessary for absorbing and using the other nutrients. The recommended daily dietary allowances in

Illustration 15-2 show the approximate amount of food nutrients your body requires.

Find your category by sex and age. Follow the column down, and you will see how many calories, grams of protein, and units of minerals and vitamins you need on the average per day.

You will balance your needs if you tailor your food intake according to the report issued by the Select Committee on Nutrition and Human Needs entitled *Dietary Goals for the United States* which suggested:

1. Increase the consumption of complex carbohydrates (starches) and "naturally occurring sugars" (in fruits) from 28 percent of daily total calories to 48 percent.
2. At the same time, halve the amount of refined sugar eaten every day, from 18 percent of daily calories to 10 percent.
3. Eat less fat (from 40 percent of daily calories to 30 percent).

Age, years	Males					Females				
	11-14	15-18	19-22	23-50	51+	11-14	15-18	19-22	23-50	51+
Weight, kg (lbs)	45 (99)	66 (145)	70 (154)	70 (154)	70 (154)	46 (101)	55 (120)	55 (120)	55 (120)	55 (120)
Height, cm (ins)	157 (62)	176 (69)	177 (70)	178 (70)	178 (70)	157 (62)	163 (64)	163 (64)	163 (64)	163 (64)
Protein, g	45	56	56	56	56	46	46	44	44	44
Vitamin A, µg R.E.[2]	1,000	1,000	1,000	1,000	1,000	800	800	800	800	800
Vitamin D, µg[3]	10	10	7.5	5	5	10	10	7.5	5	5
Vitamin E, mg αT.E.[4]	8	10	10	10	10	8	8	8	8	8
Vitamin C, mg	50	60	60	60	60	50	60	60	60	60
Thiamin, mg	1.4	1.4	1.5	1.4	1.2	1.1	1.1	1.1	1.0	1.0
Riboflavin, mg	1.6	1.7	1.7	1.6	1.4	1.3	1.3	1.3	1.2	1.2
Niacin, mg N.E.[5]	18	18	19	18	16	15	14	14	13	13
Vitamin B6, mg	1.8	2.0	2.2	2.2	2.2	1.8	2.0	2.0	2.0	2.0
Folacin,[6] g	400	400	400	400	400	400	400	400	400	400
Vitamin B12, µg	3.0	3.0	3.0	3.0	3.0	3.0	3.0	3.0	3.0	3.0
Calcium, mg	1,200	1,200	800	800	800	1,200	1,200	800	800	800
Phosphorus, mg	1,200	1,200	800	800	800	1,200	1,200	800	800	800
Magnesium, mg	350	400	350	350	350	300	300	300	300	300
Iron, mg	18	18	10	10	10	18	18	18	18	10
Zinc, mg	15	15	15	15	15	15	15	15	15	15
Iodine, µg	150	150	150	150	150	150	150	150	150	150

[1] Revised 1980. The allowances are intended to provide for individual variations among most normal persons as they live in the United States under usual environmental stresses. Diets should be based on a wide variety of common foods in order to provide other nutrients for which human requirements have been less well defined. Amounts may differ for children and pregnant or lactating women.

[2] Retinol equivalents. 1 Retinol equivalent = 1 µg retinol or 6 µg βcarotine.

[3] As cholecalciferol. 10 µg cholecalciferol = 400 I.U. vitamin D.

[4] α-tocopherol equivalents. 1 mg d-α-tocopherol = 1 α T.E.

[5] 1 N.E. (niacin equivalent) is equal to 1 mg of niacin or 60 mg of dietary tryptophan.

[6] The folacin allowances refer to dietary sources as determined by Lactobacilus casei assay after treatment with enzymes (conjugases) to make polyglutamyl forms of the vitamin available to the test organism.

Source: Food and Nutrition Board, National Academy of Sciences–National Research Council.

Illus. 15-2. Recommended Dietary Allowances[1]

4. Balance the kinds of fats eaten so that 10 percent of daily calories are saturated fats (such as butter); and another 10 percent are polyunsaturated fats (such as safflower and corn oil).
5. Hold daily cholesterol consumption to 300 milligrams a day (slightly less than the amount in one egg yolk).
6. Eat no more than 5 grams of table salt a day.

Use the Appendix (pages 238-271) to determine the amounts of various nutrients in the foods you eat. Use Illustration 15-3 to learn how your total calories per day should break down nutrient by nutrient.

Empty Calories

You've known for years that candy bars and colas weren't "good" for you, but you may not have known why. They are "empty" calories, meaning that they have few, if any, nutrients.

The calories you consume in these foods are converted to energy by your body, and your hunger is satisfied. You have energy for increased activity; but you have no protein for body repair and growth; no vitamins for radiant skin, beautiful teeth, and chemical changes for digestion of foods; no bulk for elimination; and no minerals for other body functions. All you get is energy, which, by the way, if it isn't used, is stored as *fat*. Because these empty calories satisfy your hunger, you are not inclined to eat the foods that do provide the nutrients your body needs.

Nutritious Food

A study was made by a Senate Select Committee to determine what Americans really need nutritionally. General guidelines came from that study. They apply to everyone in the United States except people with diseases or conditions that interfere with normal nutrition.

Illus. 15-3. Relationship of Nutrients in Daily Diets (Based on *Dietary Goals for the United States*)

Calories per Day	Nutrients as a Percent of Daily Calories			
	Carbohydrate 48%	Refined Sugar 10%*	Fat 30%	Protein 12%*
1,600	768	112*	480	240*
1,800	864	156*	540	240*
2,000	960	200	600	240
2,050	984	205	615	246
2,100	1,008	210	630	252
2,200	1,056	220	660	264
2,400	1,152	240	720	288
2,700	1,296	270	810	324
2,800	1,344	280	840	336
2,900	1,392	290	870	348

* Adults need approximately 60 grams of protein per day (240 calories). When 12 percent of the total calories is less than 240, sugar and carbohydrate must be reduced to compensate.

Based on a report issued by a U. S. Senate Select Committee on Nutrition and Human Needs.

They are intended for people who are already healthy, and they include things to do and things to avoid doing:

1. Eat a variety of foods.
2. Eat foods with adequate starch and fiber.
3. Avoid too much sugar.
4. Avoid too much fat, saturated fat, and cholesterol.
5. Avoid too much sodium.
6. If you drink alcohol, do so in moderation.
7. Maintain ideal weight.

Variety

The first guideline specifies a variety of foods. Because you need about 40 different nutrients to stay healthy, no single food item will meet all your needs.

Vitamins, minerals, amino acids (from proteins), essential fatty acids (from vegetable oils and animal fats), and sources of energy (calories from carbohydrates, proteins, and fats) make up the nutrients you need. To assure that you get all these nutrients, you should eat daily selections from these groups:

- Fruits
- Whole grain and enriched breads, cereals, and grain products
- Legumes (dry peas and beans)
- Vegetables
- Milk, cheese, and yogurt
- Meats, poultry, fish, and eggs

Except in special situations, such as that of women during childbearing years, or women who are either pregnant or breast-feeding, people who eat this daily variety of food usually do not need supplemental vitamins.

Starch and Fiber

Because the major sources of energy in the American diet are carbohydrates and fats, and because too much fat may cause health problems, you should be sure to eat foods with adequate starch and fiber. Some of the starchy foods are better than others.

Sugars provide energy calories but very few other nutrients. *Complex* carbohydrates such as beans, peas, nuts, seeds, fruits, vegetables, whole grain breads, cereals, and cereal products contain the starch and many of the nutrients you need. These complex carbohydrates have other advantages:

- Complex carbohydrates contain dietary fiber; sugars do not.
- Complex carbohydrates contain less than half the calories per ounce that fats contain.

Sugar

The main health hazard in eating sugar is tooth decay. The amount of sugar is not as important as the frequency with which you eat sugar in risking tooth decay.

A second hazard is substituting sugar for more nutritious foods in meeting your energy needs. Sugar does supply energy calories. It does not supply other nutrients. If you eat most of your daily calorie allotment in sugar, you will have plenty of energy but not enough nutrients for repair and maintenance of your body: You will starve many parts of your body.

To avoid excessive sugars:

- Use less of all sugars, including white sugar, brown sugar, raw sugar, honey, and syrups.
- Eat less of foods containing these sugars, such as candy, soft drinks, ice cream, cakes, and cookies.
- Select fresh fruits or fruits canned without sugar or in light syrup rather than fruits canned in heavy syrup.
- Read food labels for clues on sugar content—if sucrose, glucose, maltose, dextrose, lactose, fructose, or syrups appear first, then there is a large amount of sugar.

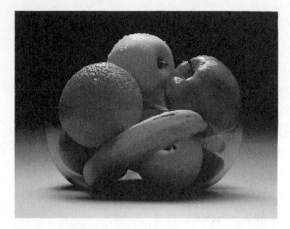

Illus. 15-4. Select fresh fruits to avoid excessive sugars.

- Remember, how often you eat sugar is as important as how much sugar you eat.

Fat and Cholesterol

You risk having high blood cholesterol, which is related to heart attack, if you consume too much fat. While you are young and very active, your risks are reduced; however, the eating habits you acquire while you are young are those you will have when you are older when your risks are greater. Therefore, learning to eat less fat, saturated fat, and cholesterol is important no matter what age you may be.

To avoid too much fat, saturated fat, and cholesterol:

- Choose lean meat, fish, poultry, dry beans, and peas as your protein sources.
- Moderate your use of eggs and organ meats such as liver.
- Limit your intake of butter, cream, hydrogenated margarines, shortenings, and coconut oil, and foods made from such products.

- Trim excess fat off meats.
- Broil, bake, or boil rather than fry.
- Read labels carefully to determine both the amount and types of fat contained in foods.

Sodium

Your most serious risk in consuming too much sodium is its effect on your blood pressure. Because sodium is hidden in many processed foods, you may be getting more than you know about. Table salt is an important source of sodium; however, sodium is also commonly found in condiments, sauces, pickled foods, salty snacks, sandwich meats, baking soda, baking powder, monosodium glutamate (MSG), soft drinks, and antacids.

To avoid too much sodium:

- Learn to enjoy the unsalted flavors of foods.
- Cook with only small amounts of added salt.
- Add little or no salt to food at the table.
- Limit your intake of salty foods such as potato chips, pretzels, salted nuts, popcorn, condiments (soy sauce, steak sauce, garlic salt), cheese, pickled foods, and cured meats.
- Read food labels carefully to determine the amounts of sodium in processed foods and snack items.

Alcohol

The risks in consuming alcohol are numerous. You probably know about many of them. Those related to your health and diet are:

- Alcoholic beverages tend to be high in calories and low in other nutrients.
- Heavy drinkers may lose their appetites for foods containing essential nutrients.
- Alcohol alters the absorption and use of essential nutrients.
- Consumption of alcohol by pregnant women has caused birth defects.

- Cirrhosis of the liver and some neurological disorders are linked to heavy drinking.
- Cancer of the throat and neck is much more common in people who drink and smoke than in people who don't.

Weight

The most obvious and most easily seen indicator of your eating habits is your weight. It reflects whether you eat too much, too little, or a proper amount. Maintaining your weight within the recommended range is vital to your health as well as to your appearance.

Weight is, of course, related to the structure, height, and condition of your body. A chart showing desirable weights related to height (Illustration 15-5 on page 232) will help you find the proper range of weight for yourself. The relative size of your frame will probably be medium unless you are very much larger or smaller than the majority of people. The height-weight chart is designed so that your height is without shoes, and your weight is what you weigh in the morning nude before you have eaten breakfast.

Your weight is directly related to how much you eat. In very simple terms, for every 3,500 calories consumed (be it from carrots, meat, or candy), one pound of fat is stored unless the calories are burned as energy. Burning the 3,500 calories requires a great deal of activity—walking approximately 36 miles, playing tennis approximately 7½ hours, or playing golf 10½ hours. While activity has an important place in your life, it will not bear the burden of overeating—your shape will!

Find your ideal weight range on the height-weight chart. If you are not in good condition; that is, if most of the padding is fatty tissue rather than muscle tissue, aim for the lower figure of the weight range. A pound of fatty tissue is several times larger than a pound of muscle tissue. Also, fatty tissue rarely deposits

itself in an attractive array on your body, whereas, muscle tissue develops in a systematic pattern which improves your form. Without an extensive conditioning program designed for muscle building, you are not likely to develop excessive muscle tissue. However, with only occasional overeating, you can accumulate excessive fatty tissue—in the most unattractive places.

If you are in doubt as to whether you are padded with fat or muscle, take a good look at yourself nude in a full-length mirror. Using your thumb and forefinger, take the skin-fold test by pinching up a fold of skin and subcutaneous tissue just below your navel. You are too fat if the distance between your thumb and forefinger is 1½ inches or more.

If you pass the skin-fold test and are not too fat, you are ahead of many of your friends; but you should be knowledgeable and vigilant about controlling your weight. A critical period of weight control for young people is at about 22 years of age. Full growth is reached, and there is usually a decrease in activity at that time. Unfortunately, the slowdown in metabolism begun during the teen years continues, and fewer and fewer calories per pound are needed to maintain weight, as shown in Illustration 15-6 on page 233. Activities accompanying school years cease at about this time and people often switch from light work to sedentary life-styles. Inactivity and the slowdown in metabolism must be offset and accompanied by a decreased caloric intake if weight is to be controlled. Decreasing the calories consumed takes a great deal of self-control and willpower because eating habits acquired over the last 20 or so years have to be altered. This is a difficult task.

Forming Habits

If you don't like what your eating habits have done to your weight, energy, and attitude,

Feet	Inches	Small Frame	Medium Frame	Large Frame
For Men...				
5	1	104-112	110-121	118-133
5	2	107-115	113-125	121-136
5	3	110-118	116-128	124-140
5	4	113-121	119-131	127-144
5	5	116-125	122-135	130-148
5	6	120-129	126-139	134-153
5	7	124-133	130-144	139-158
5	8	128-137	134-148	143-162
5	9	132-142	138-152	147-166
5	10	136-146	142-157	151-171
5	11	140-150	146-162	156-176
6	0	144-154	150-167	160-181
6	1	148-159	154-172	165-186
6	2	152-163	159-177	170-191
6	3	156-167	164-182	174-196
For Women...				
4	8	87-93	91-102	99-114
4	9	89-96	93-105	101-117
4	10	91-99	96-108	104-120
4	11	94-102	99-111	107-123
5	0	97-105	102-114	110-126
5	1	100-108	105-117	113-129
5	2	103-111	108-121	116-133
5	3	106-114	111-125	120-137
5	4	109-118	113-130	124-141
5	5	113-122	119-134	128-145
5	6	117-126	123-138	132-149
5	7	121-130	127-142	136-153
5	8	125-133	131-146	140-158
5	9	129-139	135-150	144-163
5	10	133-143	139-154	148-168

* Between the ages of 18 and 25, subtract 1 pound for each year under 25.
** Modified from figures published by the Metropolitan Life Insurance Company. Their figures
included shoes and indoor clothing. Figures in this table have been calculated by subtracting 1
inch from men's height and 2 inches from women's height. It was assumed that men's indoor
clothing weighs 8 pounds and that women's indoor clothing weighs 5 pounds.

you can do something about it. To find exactly
where you are going wrong, analyze your
present habits by keeping a chart for a few days
of what you eat and the time of day you eat it.
An analysis of what you are eating can be made
by using a chart showing nutritive values of
food (see the Appendix, pages 238-271) and
comparing what you eat with your recommended daily dietary allowances (see Illustration 15-2 on page 227).

Illus. 15-6. Calories Needed to Maintain One Pound of Weight for Persons Engaged in Light Work

Age	Daily Calories	÷ Weight	= Calories Per Pound
For Men...			
11-14	2700	99	27
15-18	2800	145	19
19-22	2900	154	18
23-50	2700	154	17
51-75	2400	154	15
76+	2050	154	13
For Women...			
11-14	2200	101	21
15-18	2100	120	17
19-22	2100	120	17
23-50	2000	120	16
51-75	1800	120	15
76+	1600	120	13

You can further analyze your eating habits by observing the time of day you are eating. Some patterns to observe are: Do I frequently snack shortly before meals? Do I snack as a result of advertising or the suggestion of food on television or in a magazine? Do I eat when I am bored? Do I eat to delay doing things I don't like to do?

If your weight and eating habits are not what they should be, resolve this minute (not tomorrow or next Monday) to begin correcting them. Maintaining your ideal weight brings such rewards as a longer life expectancy, confidence in your self-discipline, and a reflection in the mirror you can be proud of. It takes consistent and determined effort to form good eating habits, but the rewards are worth it.

Behavior Modification

Changing habits that are detrimental to your good health is behavior modification. To correct poor habits in eating, you will have to recognize them first, then select the modification that will make you slim and fit. A

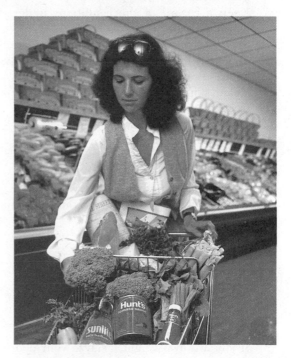

Illus. 15-7. It takes consistent and determined effort to form good eating habits.

list of suggestions from which you can choose may help:

1. Keep food out of sight and keep on hand only those foods that require preparation time.
2. Deliberately overeat your favorite food until you are disgusted with it.
3. Learn to relax.
4. Substitute an activity for eating. When you feel the urge to eat a piece of cake, go for a walk instead.
5. If you must eat something or die, reach for celery.
6. Practice self-control in small ways. Eat only when you are sitting down; stop eating for three minutes in the middle of a meal; limit the time you will eat at each meal.
7. Keep a record of the conditions under which you eat.
8. Record what you plan to eat before you eat.
9. Shop only from a list, only after eating, and never for snacks.
10. Never skip a meal completely, especially breakfast.
11. Do nothing else when you eat, and eat always in the same place.
12. Set your fork down between every other bite.
13. Never finish what you are served.
14. Go without snacks for a few days and record your cravings.
15. Record every feeling you have when you are hungry.
16. Make a list of safe snack foods, that is, those low in calories.

Losing Weight

If you are overweight, analyze your poor eating habits and begin correcting them today. Excess weight contributes to a number of health problems and often affects your personal out-look as well as the way people respond to you. Resolve now to form habits that will enable you to live the rest of your life at your ideal weight.

Counting Calories

In order to lose weight, you must, in addition to forming new habits, consume fewer calories daily than you use. Your recommended daily dietary allowance (Illustration 15-2) assures you of good health and normal energy. Before you undertake to routinely consume less than that which is normal for your age and height, you should consult a physician.

To lose one pound of fat, you must cut your food intake by 3,500 calories. Obviously this isn't done in a day. The speed with which weight can be lost depends upon how many calories you cut out daily. If your recommended daily allowance is 2,200 calories, you can lose approximately 2 pounds per week on 1,200 calories per day. The calculations are:

7 days @ 2,200
    calories/day = 15,400 calories/week
7 days @ 1,200
    calories/day =   8,400 calories/week
The difference =   7,000 calories (2 lbs.)

If your recommended daily allowance is 2,000 calories, you will need to cut to 1,000 per day to lose 2 pounds per week. Two pounds per week is considered safe for most people.

By using Illustration 15-8 and the Appendix (pages 238-271) you can devise an eating plan for yourself that meets your needs and your goals. Remember that any successful plan for a lifetime of healthful eating must:

- provide all necessary nutrients in sufficient amounts.
- be palatable.
- be available to you.
- provide the desired number of calories to meet your goal.

Illus. 15-8. Relationship of Nutrients in Low-Calorie Diets (Based on *Dietary Goals for the United States*)

| Calories per Day | Nutrients as a Percent of Daily Calories | | | |
	Carbohydrate 48%*	Refined Sugar 10%*	Fat 30%	Protein 12%*
800**	320	0	240	240
900**	390	0	270	240
1,000**	440	0	300	240
1,200	576	24	360	240
1,500	720	90	450	240

* Adults need approximately 60 grams of protein per day (240 calories). When 12 percent of the total calories is less than 240, sugar and carbohydrate must be reduced to compensate.
** People consuming fewer than 1,200 calories per day usually need a vitamin supplement for good nutrition.

Based on a report issued by a U. S. Senate Select Committe on Nutrition and Human Needs.

Good Diets

If you need to lose weight but don't want to devise your own plan, you can see your physician, or with your physician's approval you can try one of the following diets which have been evaluated by Theodore Berland and the editors of *Consumer Guide*[1] as meeting average nutritional requirements:

Weight Watchers Diet
LaCosta Spa Diet
New York City Department of Health Diet
Diet Workshop Diet
Prudent Diet
Trims Club, Inc. Diet
Dr. Blackburn's Balanced Deficit Diet
Royal Swedish Diet
Meditation Diet
Joy of Dieting
Live Longer Diet
Redbook's Wise Woman's Diet

---

[1]Theodore Berland and the Editors of *Consumer Guide®*, *Rating the Diets* (New York: Beekman House, a Division of Crown Publishers, Inc., 1980), pp. 236-237.

Dr. Glenn's Once and For All Diet
Astronaut Diet
Bazaar's Second Nine-Day Wonder Diet
Planned Vegetarian Diets
The Wine Diet
The Yogurt Diet
Helena Rubenstein's 1938 Food for Beauty Diet

Fad Diets

Because changing lifelong eating habits is very difficult, it is tempting to resort to a temporary solution, such as a fad diet, to adjust your weight. It is possible to lose weight on a fad diet, of course; but if the eating habits that made you too fat in the first place are resumed when you reach your desired weight, you will begin gaining weight as soon as you get off the fad diet. Allowing your weight to fluctuate up and down is considered detrimental to your overall health.

Many fad diets are based on consuming large amounts of water or eggs or grapefruit or all-in-one liquids or a special combination of

Illus. 15-9. Energy Expenditure by a 150-Pound Person in Various Activities

Activity	Gross Energy Cost-Cal/Hr[1].
A. Rest and Light Activity	**50-200**
Lying down or sleeping	80
Sitting	100
Driving an Automobile	120
Standing	140
Domestic work	180
B. Moderate Activity	**200-350**
Bicycling (5½ mph)	210
Walking (2½ mph)	210
Gardening	220
Canoeing (2½ mph)	230
Golf	250
Lawn mowing (power mower)	250
Bowling	270
Lawn mowing (hand mower)	270
Fencing	300
Rowboating (2½ mph)	300
Swimming (¼ mph)	300
Walking (3¾ mph)	300
Badminton	350
Horseback riding (trotting)	350
Square dancing	350
Volleyball	350
Roller skating	350
C. Vigorous Activity	**over 350**
Table tennis	360
Ditch digging (hand shovel)	400
Ice skating (10 mph)	400
Wood chopping or sawing	400
Tennis	420
Water skiing	480
Hill climbing (100 ft./hr.)	490
Skiing (10 mph)	600
Squash and handball	600
Cycling (13 mph)	660
Scull rowing (race)	840
Running (10 mph)	900

[1] The standards represent a compromise between those proposed by the British Medical Association (1950), Christensen (1953), and Wells, Balke, and Van Fossan (1956). Where available, actual measured values have been used; for other values, a "best guess" was made.

Prepared by Robert E. Johnson, M. D., Ph.D., and Colleagues, Department of Physiology and Biophysics, University of Illinois, August, 1967. Reprinted from: *Exercise and Weight Control*, The President's Council on Physical Fitness and Sports, Washington, D. C. 20201 (Washington: U. S. Government Printing Office, 1976).

foods. Although you can lose weight temporarily either by chemical changes or because you are taking in fewer calories, you are not correcting the real problem — the eating habits that made you fat in the first place. Once you resume those old eating habits, you will regain your lost weight.

Dietetic Foods

Beware of dietetic candy and desserts. They have little food value, and they frequently contain many calories. If you use them as a substitute for regular candy and desserts as a regular part of your diet, you are admitting that you cannot afford to consume the calories in candy and desserts, but you are not changing your eating habits. As a matter of habit, you will continue to include these kinds of foods in your diet and thus delay adopting the sorely needed new eating habits.

Activity

Like a fad diet, another ploy to delay changing your eating habits is to increase activity to burn up the excessive calories you consume. Regular exercise is good for your body, but it can't compensate for poor eating habits. Illustration 15-9 shows how many calories per hour various activities burn up for a person weighing 150 pounds. People weighing less burn fewer calories per hour. You can see that burning an extra 1,000 calories per day for your 2-pound-per-week recommended weight loss would require a taxing amount of vigorous activity.

Gaining Weight

If your are underweight, it will be necessary for you to consume 3,500 calories more than you use for each pound you wish to gain. Your habits, though, are what you must correct if you are to maintain normal weight. Be guided by the proportions of carbohydrates, refined sugar, fat, and protein in Illustration 15-3 for basic lifelong nutrition. In addition, you can add a liquid supplement or some very high-calorie foods to your daily diet while you are gaining weight. Check the nutritive values on the food chart (Appendix, pages 238-271), and select foods you like that are high in calories. In addition, eat regularly, chew your food well, and get plenty of rest while you are trying to gain weight. You can be consoled by the fact that as you grow older, fewer and fewer calories are needed to maintain ideal weight.

Questions for Chapter 15

1. According to the Select Committee on Nutrition and Human Needs, what should be the dietary goals for people in the United States?
2. According to Illustration 15-2, how many grams of protein do most adults need daily?
3. What are the guidelines established by the Senate Select Committee concerning nutritious food?
4. How do complex carbohydrates differ from simple sugars?
5. What happens to metabolism as you age?
6. How do calories relate to losing weight?
7. How many hours would a 150-pound person have to roller-skate to burn 3,500 calories?

APPENDIX

NUTRITIVE VALUES OF THE EDIBLE PART OF FOODS

Source: "Nutritive Value of Foods," Home and Garden Bulletin No. 72, published by U.S. Department of Agriculture.

[Dashes in the columns for nutrients show that no suitable value could be found although there is reason to believe that a measurable amount of the nutrient may be present]

Milk, Cheese, Cream, Imitation Cream; Related Products

	FOOD, APPROXIMATE MEASURE, AND WEIGHT (IN GRAMS)		WATER	FOOD ENERGY	PRO-TEIN	FAT	SATU-RATED (TOTAL)	UNSATURATED OLEIC	LIN-OLEIC	CARBO-HY-DRATE	CAL-CIUM	IRON	VITA-MIN A VALUE	THIA-MIN	RIBO-FLAVIN	NIACIN	ASCOR-BIC ACID
			Grams Percent	Calories	Grams	Grams	Grams	Grams	Grams	Grams	Milli-grams	Milli-grams	Inter-national units	Milli-grams	Milli-grams	Milli-grams	Milli-grams
	Milk: Fluid:																
1	Whole, 3.5% fat	1 cup	244 87	160	9	9	5	3	Trace	12	288	.1	350	.07	.41	.2	2
2	Nonfat (skim)	1 cup	245 90	90	9	Trace				12	296	.1	10	.09	.44	.2	2
3	Partly skimmed, 2% nonfat milk solids added.	1 cup	246 87	145	10	5	3	2	Trace	15	352	.1	200	.10	.52	.2	2
4	Canned, concentrated, undiluted: Evaporated, unsweetened.	1 cup	252 74	345	18	20	11	7	1	24	635	.3	810	.10	.86	.5	3
5	Condensed, sweetened.	1 cup	306 27	980	25	27	15	9	1	166	802	.3	1,100	.24	1.16	.6	3
6	Dry, nonfat instant: Low-density (1⅓ cups needed for reconstitution to 1 qt.).	1 cup	68 4	245	24	Trace				35	879	.4	¹20	.24	1.21	.6	5
7	High-density (⅞ cup needed for reconstitution to 1 qt.).	1 cup	104 4	375	37	1				54	1,345	.6	¹30	.36	1.85	.9	7

No.	Food	Measure	Grams	Water (%)	Food energy (cal.)	Protein (g)	Fat (g)	Saturated (total) (g)	Oleic (g)	Linoleic (g)	Carbohydrate (g)	Calcium (mg)	Iron (mg)	Vitamin A (I.U.)	Thiamine (mg)	Riboflavin (mg)	Niacin (mg)	Ascorbic acid (mg)
	Buttermilk:																	
8	Fluid, cultured, made from skim milk.	1 cup	245	90	90	9	Trace				12	296	.1	10	.10	.44	.2	2
9	Dried, packaged	1 cup	120	3	465	41	6				60	1,498	.7	260	.31	2.06	1.1	....
	Cheese:																	
	Natural:																	
	Blue or Roquefort type:																	
10	Ounce	1 oz.	28	40	105	6	9	5	3	Trace	Trace	89	.1	350	.01	.17	.3	0
11	Cubic inch	1 cu. in.	17	40	65	4	5	3	2	Trace	Trace	54	.1	210	.01	.11	.2	0
12	Camembert, packaged in 4-oz. pkg. with 3 wedges per pkg.	1 wedge	38	52	115	7	9	5	3	Trace	1	40	.2	380	.02	.29	.3	0
	Cheddar:																	
13	Ounce	1 oz.	28	37	115	7	9	5	3	Trace	1	213	.3	370	.01	.13	Trace	0
14	Cubic inch	1 cu. in.	17	37	70	4	6	3	2	Trace	Trace	129	.2	230	.01	.08	Trace	0
	Cottage, large or small curd:																	
	Creamed:																	
15	Package of 12-oz., net wt.	1 pkg.	340	78	360	46	14	8	5	Trace	10	320	1.0	580	.10	.85	.3	0
16	Cup, curd pressed down.	1 cup	245	78	260	33	10	6	3	Trace	7	230	.7	420	.07	.61	.2	0
	Uncreamed:																	
17	Package of 12-oz., net wt.	1 pkg.	340	79	290	58	1	1	Trace	Trace	9	306	1.4	30	.10	.95	.3	0
18	Cup, curd pressed down.	1 cup	200	79	170	34	1	Trace	Trace	Trace	5	180	.8	20	.06	.56	.2	0
	Cream:																	
19	Package of 8-oz., net wt.	1 pkg.	227	51	850	18	86	48	28	3	5	141	.5	3,500	.05	.54	.2	0
20	Package of 3-oz., net wt.	1 pkg.	85	51	320	7	32	18	11	1	2	53	.2	1,310	.02	.20	.1	0
21	Cubic inch.	1 cu. in.	16	51	60	1	6	3	2	Trace	Trace	10	Trace	250	Trace	.04	Trace	0
	Parmesan, grated:																	
22	Cup, pressed down.	1 cup	140	17	655	60	43	24	14	1	5	1,893	.7	1,760	.03	1.22	.3	0
23	Tablespoon	1 tbsp.	5	17	25	2	2	1	Trace	Trace	Trace	68	Trace	60	Trace	.04	Trace	0
24	Ounce	1 oz.	28	17	130	12	9	5	3	Trace	1	383	.1	360	.01	.25	.1	0
	Swiss:																	
25	Ounce	1 oz.	28	39	105	8	8	4	3	Trace	Trace	262	.3	320	Trace	.11	Trace	0
26	Cubic inch.	1 cu. in.	15	39	55	4	4	2	1	Trace	Trace	139	.1	170	Trace	.06	Trace	0
	Pasteurized processed cheese:																	
	American:																	
27	Ounce.	1 oz.	28	40	105	7	9	5	3	Trace	1	198	.3	350	.01	.12	Trace	0
28	Cubic inch.	1 cu. in.	18	40	65	4	5	3	2	Trace	Trace	122	.2	210	Trace	.07	Trace	0
	Swiss:																	
29	Ounce.	1 oz.	28	40	100	8	8	4	3	Trace	1	251	.3	310	Trace	.11	Trace	0
30	Cubic inch.	1 cu. in.	18	40	65	5	5	3	2	Trace	Trace	159	.2	200	Trace	.07	Trace	0
	Pasteurized process cheese food, American:																	
31	Tablespoon.	1 tbsp.	14	43	45	3	3	2	1	Trace	1	80	.1	140	Trace	.08	Trace	0
32	Cubic inch.	1 cu. in.	18	43	60	4	4	2	1	Trace	1	100	.1	170	Trace	.10	Trace	0
33	Pasteurized process cheese spread, American.	1 oz.	28	49	80	5	6	3	2	Trace	2	160	.2	250	Trace	.15	Trace	0
	Cream:																	
34	Half-and-half (cream and milk).	1 cup	242	80	325	8	28	15	9	1	11	261	.1	1,160	.07	.39	.1	2
35		1 tbsp.	15	80	20	1	2	1	1	Trace	1	16	Trace	70	Trace	.02	Trace	Trace

NUTRITIVE VALUES OF THE EDIBLE PART OF FOODS — Continued

[Dashes in the columns for nutrients show that no suitable value could be found although there is reason to believe that a measurable amount of the nutrient may be present]

MILK, CHEESE, CREAM, IMITATION CREAM; RELATED PRODUCTS — Continued:

No.	FOOD, APPROXIMATE MEASURE, AND WEIGHT (IN GRAMS)	Weight (Grams)	WATER (Percent)	FOOD ENERGY (Calories)	PROTEIN (Grams)	FAT (Grams)	FATTY ACIDS SATURATED (TOTAL) (Grams)	FATTY ACIDS UNSATURATED OLEIC (Grams)	FATTY ACIDS UNSATURATED LINOLEIC (Grams)	CARBOHYDRATE (Grams)	CALCIUM (Milligrams)	IRON (Milligrams)	VITAMIN A VALUE (International units)	THIAMIN (Milligrams)	RIBOFLAVIN (Milligrams)	NIACIN (Milligrams)	ASCORBIC ACID (Milligrams)
	Cream, Continued:																
36	Light, coffee or table. 1 cup	240	72	505	7	49	27	16	1	10	245	.1	2,020	.07	.36	.1	2
37	1 tbsp.	15	72	30	1	3	2	1	Trace	1	15	Trace	130	Trace	.02	Trace	Trace
38	Sour. 1 cup	230	72	485	7	47	26	16	1	10	235	.1	1,930	.07	.35	.1	2
39	1 tbsp.	12	72	25	Trace	2	1	1	Trace	1	12	Trace	100	Trace	.02	Trace	Trace
40	Whipped topping (pressurized). 1 cup	60	62	155	2	14	8	5	Trace	6	67	—	570	—	.04	—	—
41	1 tbsp.	3	62	10	Trace	1	Trace	Trace	Trace	Trace	3	—	30	—	Trace	—	—
	Whipping, unwhipped (volume about double when whipped):																
42	Light. 1 cup	239	62	715	6	75	41	25	2	9	203	.1	3,060	.05	.29	.1	2
43	1 tbsp.	15	62	45	Trace	5	3	2	Trace	1	13	Trace	190	Trace	.02	Trace	Trace
44	Heavy. 1 cup	238	57	840	5	90	50	30	3	7	179	.1	3,670	.05	.26	.1	2
45	1 tbsp.	15	57	55	Trace	6	3	2	Trace	1	11	Trace	230	Trace	.02	Trace	Trace
	Imitation cream products (made with vegetable fat):																
	Creamers:																
46	Powdered. 1 cup	94	2	505	4	33	31	1	0	52	21	.6	² 200	0	0	Trace	—
47	1 tsp.	2	2	10	Trace	1	Trace	Trace	0	1	1	Trace	² Trace	0	0	—	—
48	Liquid (frozen). 1 cup	245	77	345	3	27	25	1	0	25	29	—	² 100	0	0	—	—
49	1 tbsp.	15	77	20	Trace	2	1	Trace	0	2	2	.1	² 10	0	0	—	—
50	Sour dressing (imitation sour cream) made with nonfat dry milk. 1 cup	235	72	440	9	38	35	1	Trace	17	277	—	20	.07	.38	.2	1
51	1 tbsp.	12	72	20	Trace	2	2	Trace	Trace	1	14	Trace	Trace	Trace	Trace	Trace	Trace
	Whipped topping:																
52	Pressurized. 1 cup	70	61	190	1	17	15	1	0	9	5	—	² 340	0	0	—	Trace
53	1 tbsp.	4	61	10	Trace	1	1	Trace	0	Trace	Trace	—	² 20	0	0	—	—
54	Frozen. 1 cup	75	52	230	1	20	18	Trace	0	15	5	—	² 560	0	0	—	—
55	1 tbsp.	4	52	10	Trace	1	1	Trace	0	1	Trace	—	² 30	0	0	—	—
56	Powdered, made with whole milk. 1 cup	75	58	175	3	12	10	1	Trace	15	62	Trace	² 330	.02	.08	.1	Trace
57	1 tbsp.	4	58	10	Trace	1	1	Trace	Trace	1	3	Trace	² 20	Trace	Trace	Trace	Trace

No.	Food	Amount	Grams	Water (%)	Food energy	Protein	Fat	Saturated	Oleic	Linoleic	Carbohydrate	Calcium	Iron	Vitamin A	Thiamin	Riboflavin	Niacin	Ascorbic acid
	Milk beverages:																	
58	Cocoa, homemade.	1 cup	250	79	245	10	12	7	4	Trace	27	295	1.0	400	.10	.45	.5	3
59	Chocolate-flavored drink made with skim milk and 2% added butterfat.	1 cup	250	83	190	8	6	3	2	Trace	27	270	.5	210	.10	.40	.3	3
60	Malted milk: Dry powder, approximately 3 heaping teaspoons per ounce.	1 oz.	28	3	115	4	2				20	82	.6	290	.09	.15	.1	0
61	Beverage.	1 cup	235	78	245	11	10				28	317	.7	590	.14	.49	.2	2
	Milk desserts:																	
62	Custard, baked	1 cup	265	77	305	14	15	7	5	1	29	297	1.1	930	.11	.50	.3	1
63	Ice cream: Regular (approx. 10% fat).	½ gal.	1,064	63	2,055	48	113	62	37	3	221	1,553	.5	4,680	.43	2.23	1.1	11
64		1 cup	133	63	255	6	14	8	5	Trace	28	194	.1	590	.05	.28	.1	1
65		3 fl. oz. cup	50	63	95	2	5	3	2	Trace	10	73	Trace	220	.02	.11	.1	1
66	Rich (approx. 16% fat).	½ gal.	1,188	63	2,635	31	191	105	63	6	214	927	.2	7,840	.24	1.31	1.2	12
67		1 cup	148	63	330	4	24	13	8	1	27	115	Trace	980	.03	.16	.1	1
	Ice milk:																	
68	Hardened.	½ gal.	1,048	67	1,595	50	53	29	17	2	235	1,635	1.0	2,200	.52	2.31	1.0	10
69		1 cup	131	67	200	6	7	4	2	Trace	29	204	.1	280	.07	.29	.1	1
70	Soft-serve.	1 cup	175	67	265	8	9	5	3	Trace	39	273	.2	370	.09	.39	.2	2
	Yogurt:																	
71	Made from partially skimmed milk.	1 cup	245	89	125	8	4	2	1	Trace	13	294	.1	170	.10	.44	.2	2
72	Made from whole milk.	1 cup	245	88	150	7	8	5	3	Trace	12	272	.1	340	.07	.39	.2	2

Eggs

No.	Food	Amount	Grams	Water (%)	Food energy	Protein	Fat	Saturated	Oleic	Linoleic	Carbohydrate	Calcium	Iron	Vitamin A	Thiamin	Riboflavin	Niacin	Ascorbic acid
	Eggs, large, 24 ounces per dozen: Raw or cooked in shell or with nothing added:																	
73	Whole, without shell.	1 egg	50	74	80	6	6	2	3	Trace	Trace	27	1.1	590	.05	.15	Trace	0
74	White of egg.	1 white	33	88	15	4	Trace				Trace	3	Trace	0	Trace	.09	Trace	0
75	Yolk of egg.	1 yolk	17	51	60	3	5	2	2	Trace	Trace	24	.9	580	.04	.07	Trace	0
76	Scrambled with milk and fat.	1 egg	64	72	110	7	8	3	3	Trace	1	51	1.1	690	.05	.18	Trace	0

NUTRITIVE VALUES OF THE EDIBLE PART OF FOODS — Continued

[Dashes in the columns for nutrients show that no suitable value could be found although there is reason to believe that a measurable amount of the nutrient may be present]

	FOOD, APPROXIMATE MEASURE, AND WEIGHT (IN GRAMS)		WATER	FOOD ENERGY	PROTEIN	FAT	FATTY ACIDS SATURATED (TOTAL)	UNSATURATED OLEIC	UNSATURATED LINOLEIC	CARBOHYDRATE	CALCIUM	IRON	VITAMIN A VALUE	THIAMIN	RIBOFLAVIN	NIACIN	ASCORBIC ACID
		Grams	Percent	Calories	Grams	Grams	Grams	Grams	Grams	Grams	Milligrams	Milligrams	International units	Milligrams	Milligrams	Milligrams	Milligrams
77	**Bacon,** (20 slices per lb. raw), broiled or fried, crisp. 2 slices	15	8	90	5	8	3	4	1	1	2	.5	0	.08	.05	.8	

Meat, Poultry, Fish, Shellfish; Related Products

	FOOD, APPROXIMATE MEASURE, AND WEIGHT (IN GRAMS)		WATER	FOOD ENERGY	PROTEIN	FAT	FATTY ACIDS SATURATED (TOTAL)	UNSATURATED OLEIC	UNSATURATED LINOLEIC	CARBOHYDRATE	CALCIUM	IRON	VITAMIN A VALUE	THIAMIN	RIBOFLAVIN	NIACIN	ASCORBIC ACID
	Beef,[3] cooked:																
	Cuts braised, simmered, or pot-roasted:																
78	Lean and fat. 3 ounces	85	53	245	23	16	8	7	Trace	0	10	2.9	30	.04	.18	3.5	
79	Lean only. 2.5 ounces	72	62	140	22	5	2	2	Trace	0	10	2.7	10	.04	.16	3.3	
	Hamburger (ground beef), broiled:																
80	Lean. 3 ounces	85	60	185	23	10	5	4	Trace	0	10	3.0	20	.08	.20	5.1	
81	Regular. 3 ounces	85	54	245	21	17	8	8	Trace	0	9	2.7	30	.07	.18	4.6	
	Roast, oven-cooked, no liquid added:																
	Relatively fat, such as rib:																
82	Lean and fat. 3 ounces	85	40	375	17	34	16	15	1	0	8	2.2	70	.05	.13	3.1	
83	Lean only. 1.8 ounces	51	57	125	14	7	3	3	Trace	0	6	1.8	10	.04	.11	2.6	
	Relatively lean, such as heel of round:																
84	Lean and fat. 3 ounces	85	62	165	25	7	3	3	Trace	0	11	3.2	10	.06	.19	4.5	
85	Lean only. 2.7 ounces	78	65	125	24	3	1	1	Trace	0	10	3.0	Trace	.06	.18	4.3	
	Steak, broiled:																
	Relatively fat, such as sirloin:																
86	Lean and fat. 3 ounces	85	44	330	20	27	13	12	1	0	9	2.5	50	.05	.16	4.0	
87	Lean only. 2.0 ounces	56	59	115	18	4	2	2	Trace	0	7	2.2	10	.05	.14	3.6	
	Relatively lean, such as round:																
88	Lean and fat. 3 ounces	85	55	220	24	13	6	6	Trace	0	10	3.0	20	.07	.19	4.8	
89	Lean only. 2.4 ounces	68	61	130	21	4	2	2	Trace	0	9	2.5	10	.06	.16	4.1	

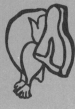

No.	Food	Measure	Grams	Water (%)	Food energy (cal.)	Protein (g)	Fat (g)	Saturated	Oleic	Linoleic	Carbohydrate (g)	Calcium (mg)	Iron (mg)	Vitamin A (I.U.)	Thiamin (mg)	Riboflavin (mg)	Niacin (mg)	Ascorbic acid (mg)
	Beef, canned:																	
90	Corned beef	3 ounces	85	59	185	22	10	5	4	Trace	0	17	3.7	20	.01	.20	2.9	
91	Corned beef hash	3 ounces	85	67	155	7	10	5	4	Trace	9	11	1.7		.01	.08	1.8	
92	**Beef, dried or chipped.**	2 ounces	57	48	115	19	4	2	2	Trace	0	11	2.9		.04	.18	2.2	
93	**Beef and vegetable stew.**	1 cup	235	82	210	15	10	5	4	Trace	15	28	2.8	2,310	.13	.17	4.4	15
94	**Beef potpie, baked, 4¼-inch diam., weight before baking about 8 ounces.**	1 pie	227	55	560	23	33	9	20	2	43	32	4.1	1,860	.25	0.27	4.5	7
	Chicken, cooked:																	
95	Flesh only, broiled.	3 ounces	85	71	115	20	3	1	1	1	0	8	1.4	80	.05	.16	7.4	
	Breast, fried, ½ breast:																	
96	With bone	3.3 ounces	94	58	155	25	5	1	2	1	1	9	1.3	70	.04	.17	11.2	
97	Flesh and skin only.	2.7 ounces	76	58	155	25	5	1	2	1	1	9	1.3	70	.04	.17	11.2	
	Drumstick, fried:																	
98	With bone.	2.1 ounces	59	55	90	12	4	1	2	1	Trace	6	.9	50	.03	.15	2.7	
99	Flesh and skin only.	1.3 ounces	38	55	90	12	4	1	2	1	Trace	6	.9	50	.03	.15	2.7	
100	**Chicken, canned, boneless.**	3 ounces	85	65	170	18	10	3	4	2	0	18	1.3	200	.03	.11	3.7	3
101	**Chicken potpie, baked, 4¼-inch diam., weight before baking about 8 ounces.**	1 pie	227	57	535	23	31	10	15	3	42	68	3.0	3,020	.25	.26	4.1	5
	Chili con carne, canned:																	
102	With beans.	1 cup	250	72	335	19	15	7	7	Trace	30	80	4.2	150	.08	.18	3.2	
103	Without beans.	1 cup	255	67	510	26	38	18	17	1	15	97	3.6	380	.05	.31	5.6	
104	**Heart, beef, lean, braised.**	3 ounces	85	61	160	27	5				1	5	5.0	20	.21	1.04	6.5	1
105	**Lamb,[3] cooked:** Chop, thick, with bone, broiled.	1 chop, 4.8 ounces	137	47	400	25	33	18	12	1	0	10	1.5		.14	.25	5.6	
106	Lean and fat.	4.0 ounces	112	47	400	25	33	18	12	1	0	10	1.5		.14	.25	5.6	
107	Lean only.	2.6 ounces	74	62	140	21	6	3	2	Trace	0	9	1.5		.11	.20	4.5	
	Leg, roasted:																	
108	Lean and fat.	3 ounces	85	54	235	22	16	9	6	Trace	0	9	1.4		.13	.23	4.7	
109	Lean only.	2.5 ounces	71	62	130	20	5	3	2	Trace	0	9	1.4		.12	.21	4.4	
	Shoulder, roasted:																	
110	Lean and fat.	3 ounces	85	50	285	18	23	13	8	1	0	9	1.0		.11	.20	4.0	
111	Lean only.	2.3 ounces	64	61	130	17	6	3	2	Trace	0	8	1.0		.10	.18	3.7	
112	**Liver, beef, fried.**	2 ounces	57	57	130	15	6				3	6	5.0	30,280	.15	2.37	9.4	15
113	**Pork, cured, cooked:** Ham, light cure, lean and fat, roasted.	3 ounces	85	54	245	18	19	7	8	2	0	8	2.2	0	.40	.16	3.1	
	Luncheon meat:																	
114	Boiled ham, sliced.	2 ounces	57	59	135	11	10	4	4	1	0	6	1.6	0	.25	.09	1.5	
115	Canned, spiced or unspiced.	2 ounces	57	55	165	8	14	5	6	1	1	5	1.2	0	.18	.12	1.6	
116	**Pork, fresh,[3] cooked:** Chop, thick, with bone.	1 chop, 3.5 ounces	98	42	260	16	21	8	9	2	0	8	2.2	0	.63	.18	3.8	
117	Lean and fat.	2.3 ounces	66	42	260	16	21	8	9	2	0	8	2.2	0	.63	.18	3.8	
118	Lean only.	1.7 ounces	48	53	130	15	7	2	3	1	0	7	1.9	0	.54	.16	3.3	

NUTRITIVE VALUES OF THE EDIBLE PART OF FOODS — Continued

[Dashes in the columns for nutrients show that no suitable value could be found although there is reason to believe that a measurable amount of the nutrient may be present]

	FOOD, APPROXIMATE MEASURE, AND WEIGHT (IN GRAMS)	Weight	WATER	FOOD ENERGY	PRO-TEIN	FAT	FATTY ACIDS SATU-RATED (TOTAL)	UNSATURATED OLEIC	UNSATURATED LIN-OLEIC	CARBO-HY-DRATE	CAL-CIUM	IRON	VITA-MIN A VALUE	THIA-MIN	RIBO-FLAVIN	NIACIN	ASCOR-BIC ACID
		Grams	Percent	Calories	Grams	Grams	Grams	Grams	Grams	Grams	Milli-grams	Milli-grams	Inter-national units	Milli-grams	Milli-grams	Milli-grams	Milli-grams

MEAT, POULTRY, FISH, SHELLFISH; RELATED PRODUCTS — Continued:

	FOOD, APPROXIMATE MEASURE, AND WEIGHT	Weight	WATER	FOOD ENERGY	PRO-TEIN	FAT	SATU-RATED (TOTAL)	OLEIC	LIN-OLEIC	CARBO-HY-DRATE	CAL-CIUM	IRON	VITA-MIN A	THIA-MIN	RIBO-FLAVIN	NIACIN	ASCOR-BIC ACID
	Pork, Fresh,³ cooked — Continued:																
	Roast, oven-cooked, no liquid added:																
119	Lean and fat. 3 ounces	85	46	310	21	24	9	10	2	0	9	2.7	0	.78	.22	4.7	
120	Lean only. 2.4 ounces	68	55	175	20	10	3	4	1	0	9	2.6	0	.73	.21	4.4	
	Cuts simmered:																
121	Lean and fat. 3 ounces	85	46	320	20	26	9	11	2	0	8	2.5	0	.46	.21	4.1	
122	Lean only. 2.2 ounces	63	60	135	18	6	2	3	1	0	8	2.3	0	.42	.19	3.7	
	Sausage:																
123	Bologna, slice, 3-in. Diam. by ⅛ inch. 2 slices	26	56	80	3	7				Trace	2	.5		.04	.06	.7	
124	Braunschweiger, slice 2-in. diam. by ¼ inch. 2 slices	20	53	65	3	5				Trace	2	1.2	1,310	.03	.29	1.6	
125	Deviled ham, canned. 1 tablespoon.	13	51	45	2	4	2			0	1	.3		.02	.01	.2	
126	Frankfurter, heated (8 per lb. purchased package). 1 frank	56	57	170	7	15		2	Trace	1	3	.8		.08	.11	1.4	
127	Pork links, cooked (16 links per lb. raw). 2 links	26	35	125	5	11	4	5	1	Trace	2	.6	0	.21	.09	1.0	
128	Salami, dry type. 1 ounce	28	30	130	7	11				Trace	4	1.0		.10	.07	1.5	
129	Salami, cooked. 1 ounce	28	51	90	5	7				Trace	3	.7		.07	.07	1.2	
130	Vienna, canned (7 sausages per 5-ounce can). 1 sausage	16	63	40	2	3				Trace	1	.3		.01	.02	.4	
	Veal, medium fat, cooked, bone removed:																
131	Cutlet. 3 ounces	85	60	185	23	9	5	4	Trace	0	9	2.7		.06	.21	4.6	
132	Roast. 3 ounces	85	55	230	23	14	7	6	Trace		10	2.9		.11	.26	6.6	
	Fish and shellfish:																
133	Bluefish, baked with table fat. 3 ounces	85	68	135	22	4				0	25	.6	40	.09	.08	1.6	
	Clams:																
134	Raw, meat only. 3 ounces	85	82	65	11	1				2	59	5.2	90	.08	.15	1.1	
135	Canned, solids and liquid. 3 ounces	85	86	45	7	1				2	47	3.5		.01	.09	.9	8

No.	Food	Measure	Grams	Water (%)	Food energy (cal)	Protein (g)	Fat (g)	Saturated (g)	Oleic (g)	Linoleic (g)	Carbohydrate (g)	Calcium (mg)	Iron (mg)	Vitamin A (IU)	Thiamin (mg)	Riboflavin (mg)	Niacin (mg)	Ascorbic acid (mg)
136	Crabmeat, canned.	3 ounces	85	77	85	15	2	—	—	—	1	38	.7	—	.07	.07	1.6	—
137	Fish sticks, breaded, cooked, frozen: stick 3¾ by 1 by ½ inch.	10 sticks or 8 oz. pkg.	227	66	400	38	20	5	4	10	15	25	.9	—	.09	.16	3.6	2
138	Haddock, breaded, fried.	3 ounces	85	66	140	17	5	—	—	—	5	34	1.0	—	.03	.06	2.7	—
139	Ocean perch, breaded, fried.	3 ounces	85	59	195	16	11	—	—	—	6	28	1.1	—	.08	.09	1.5	—
140	Oysters, raw, meat only (13–19 med. selects).	1 cup	240	85	160	20	4	—	—	—	8	226	13.2	740	.33	.43	6.0	—
141	Salmon, pink, canned.	3 ounces	85	71	120	17	5	1	1	Trace	0	[4]167	.7	60	.03	.16	6.8	—
142	Sardines, Atlantic, canned in oil, drained solids.	3 ounces	85	62	175	20	9	—	—	—	0	372	2.5	190	.02	.17	4.6	—
143	Shad, baked with table fat and bacon.	3 ounces	85	64	170	20	10	—	—	—	0	20	.5	20	.11	.22	7.3	—
144	Shrimp, canned, meat.	3 ounces	85	70	100	21	1	—	—	—	1	98	2.6	50	.01	.03	1.5	—
145	Swordfish, broiled with butter or margarine.	3 ounces	85	65	150	24	5	—	—	—	0	23	1.1	1,750	.03	.04	9.3	—
146	Tuna, canned in oil, drained solids.	3 ounces	85	61	170	24	7	—	—	—	0	7	1.6	70	.04	.10	10.1	—

Mature Dry Beans and Peas, Nuts, Peanuts; Related Products

No.	Food	Measure	Grams	Water (%)	Food energy (cal)	Protein (g)	Fat (g)	Saturated (g)	Oleic (g)	Linoleic (g)	Carbohydrate (g)	Calcium (mg)	Iron (mg)	Vitamin A (IU)	Thiamin (mg)	Riboflavin (mg)	Niacin (mg)	Ascorbic acid (mg)
147	Almonds, shelled, whole kernels.	1 cup	142	5	850	26	77	6	52	15	28	332	6.7	0	.34	1.31	5.0	Trace
	Beans, dry: Common varieties as Great Northern, navy, and others: Cooked, drained:																	
148	Great Northern.	1 cup	180	69	210	14	1	—	—	—	38	90	4.9	0	.25	.13	1.3	0
149	Navy (pea).	1 cup	190	69	225	15	1	—	—	—	40	95	5.1	0	.27	.13	1.3	0
	Canned, solids and liquid: White with —																	
150	Frankfurters (sliced).	1 cup	255	71	365	19	18	—	—	—	32	94	4.8	330	.18	.15	3.3	Trace
151	Pork and tomato sauce.	1 cup	255	71	310	16	7	—	—	—	49	138	4.6	330	.20	.08	1.5	5
152	Pork and sweet sauce.	1 cup	255	66	385	16	12	—	—	—	54	161	5.9	—	.15	.10	1.3	—
153	Red kidney.	1 cup	255	76	230	15	1	—	—	—	42	74	4.6	10	.13	.10	1.5	—
154	Lima, cooked, drained.	1 cup	190	64	260	16	1	—	—	—	49	55	5.9	—	.25	.11	1.3	—
155	Cashew nuts, roasted.	1 cup	140	5	785	24	64	11	45	4	41	53	5.3	140	.60	.35	2.5	—
	Coconut, fresh, meat only:																	
156	Pieces, approximately 2 by 2 by ½ inch.	1 piece	45	51	155	2	16	14	1	Trace	4	6	.8	0	.02	.01	.2	1
157	Shredded or grated, firmly packed.	1 cup	130	51	450	5	46	39	3	Trace	12	17	2.2	0	.07	.03	.7	4

NUTRITIVE VALUES OF THE EDIBLE PART OF FOODS — Continued

[Dashes in the columns for nutrients show that no suitable value could be found although there is reason to believe that a measurable amount of the nutrient may be present]

FOOD, APPROXIMATE MEASURE, AND WEIGHT (IN GRAMS)	WATER	FOOD ENERGY	PROTEIN	FAT	FATTY ACIDS SATURATED (TOTAL)	UNSATURATED OLEIC	LINOLEIC	CARBOHYDRATE	CALCIUM	IRON	VITAMIN A VALUE	THIAMIN	RIBOFLAVIN	NIACIN	ASCORBIC ACID
	Grams · Percent	Calories	Grams	Grams	Grams	Grams	Grams	Grams	Milligrams	Milligrams	International units	Milligrams	Milligrams	Milligrams	Milligrams
MATURE DRY BEANS AND PEAS, NUTS, PEANUTS; RELATED PRODUCTS — Continued:															
158 Cowpeas or blackeye peas, dry, cooked. 1 cup 248	80	190	13	1				34	42	3.2	20	.41	.11	1.1	Trace
159 Peanuts, roasted, salted, halves. 1 cup 144	2	840	37	72	16	31	21	27	107	3.0		.46	.19	24.7	0
160 Peanut butter. 1 tablespoon 16	2	95	4	8	2	4	2	3	9	.3		.02	.02	2.4	0
161 Peas, split, dry, cooked. 1 cup 250	70	290	20	1				52	28	4.2	100	.37	.22	2.2	
162 Pecans, halves. 1 cup 108	3	740	10	77	5	48	15	16	79	2.6	140	.93	.14	1.0	2
163 Walnuts, black or native, chopped. 1 cup 126	3	790	26	75	4	26	36	19	Trace	7.6	380	.28	.14	.9	
Vegetables and Vegetable Products															
Asparagus, green: Cooked, drained:															
164 Spears, ½-in. diam. at base. 4 spears 60	94	10	1	Trace				2	13	.4	540	.10	.11	.8	16
165 Pieces, 1½ to 2-inch lengths. 1 cup 145	94	30	3	Trace				5	30	.9	1,310	.23	.26	2.0	38
166 Canned, solids and liquid. 1 cup 244	94	45	5	1				7	44	4.1	1,240	.15	.22	2.0	37

Item No.	Food, approximate measure, and weight	Measure	Grams	Water (%)	Food energy (cal.)	Protein (g)	Fat (g)	Sat.	Oleic	Linoleic	Carboh. (g)	Calcium (mg)	Iron (mg)	Vit. A (I.U.)	Thiamin (mg)	Riboflavin (mg)	Niacin (mg)	Ascorbic acid (mg)
	Beans:																	
167	Lima, immature seeds, cooked, drained.	1 cup	170	71	190	13	1				34	80	4.3	480	.31	.17	2.2	29
	Snap:																	
	Green:																	
168	Cooked, drained.	1 cup	125	92	30	2	Trace				7	63	.8	680	.09	.11	.6	15
169	Canned, solids and liquid.	1 cup	239	94	45	2	Trace				10	81	2.9	690	.07	.10	.7	10
	Yellow or wax:																	
170	Cooked, drained.	1 cup	125	93	30	2	Trace				6	63	0.8	290	.09	.11	.6	16
171	Canned, solids and liquid.	1 cup	239	94	45	2	1				10	81	2.9	140	.07	.10	.7	12
172	Sprouted mung beans, cooked, drained.	1 cup	125	91	35	4	Trace				7	21	1.1	30	.11	.13	.9	8
	Beets:																	
	Cooked, drained, peeled:																	
173	Whole beets, 2-in. diam.	2 beets	100	91	30	1	Trace				7	14	.5	20	.03	.04	.3	6
174	Diced or sliced.	1 cup	170	91	55	2	Trace				12	24	.9	30	.05	.07	.5	10
175	Canned, solids and liquid.	1 cup	246	90	85	2	Trace				19	34	1.5	20	.02	.05	.2	7
176	Beet greens, leaves and stems, cooked, drained.	1 cup	145	94	25	3	Trace				5	144	2.8	7,400	.10	.22	.4	22
	Blackeye peas. See Cowpeas.																	
	Broccoli, cooked, drained:																	
177	Whole stalks, medium size.	1 stalk	180	91	45	6	1				8	158	1.4	4,500	.16	.36	1.4	162
178	Stalks cut into ½-in. pieces.	1 cup	155	91	40	5	1				7	136	1.2	3,880	.14	.31	1.2	140
179	Chopped, yield from 10-oz. frozen pkg.	1⅜ cups	250	92	65	7	1				12	135	1.8	6,500	.15	.30	1.3	143
180	Brussels sprouts, 7-8 sprouts (1¼ to 1½ in. diam.) per cup, cooked.	1 cup	155	88	55	7	1				10	50	1.7	810	.12	.22	1.2	135
	Cabbage:																	
	Common varieties:																	
	Raw:																	
181	Coarsely shredded or sliced.	1 cup	70	92	15	1	Trace				4	34	.3	90	.04	.04	.2	33
182	Finely shredded or chopped.	1 cup	90	92	20	1	Trace				5	44	.4	120	.05	.05	.3	42
183	Cooked.	1 cup	145	94	30	2	Trace				6	64	.4	190	.06	.06	.4	48
184	Red, raw, coarsely shredded.	1 cup	70	90	20	1	Trace				5	29	.6	30	.06	.04	.3	43
185	Savoy, raw, coarsely shredded.	1 cup	70	92	15	2	Trace				3	47	.6	140	.04	.06	.2	39
186	Cabbage, celery or Chinese, raw, cut in 1-in. pieces.	1 cup	75	95	10	1	Trace				2	32	.5	110	.04	.03	.5	19
187	Cabbage, spoon (or pakchoy), cooked.	1 cup	170	95	25	2	Trace				4	252	1.0	5,270	.07	.14	1.2	26

NUTRITIVE VALUES OF THE EDIBLE PART OF FOODS — Continued

[Dashes in the columns for nutrients show that no suitable value could be found although there is reason to believe that a measurable amount of the nutrient may be present]

VEGETABLES AND VEGETABLE PRODUCTS — Continued:

	FOOD, APPROXIMATE MEASURE, AND WEIGHT (IN GRAMS)	WATER	FOOD ENERGY	PROTEIN	FAT	FATTY ACIDS SATURATED (TOTAL)	UNSATURATED OLEIC	LINOLEIC	CARBOHYDRATE	CALCIUM	IRON	VITAMIN A VALUE	THIAMIN	RIBOFLAVIN	NIACIN	ASCORBIC ACID
	(Grams)	Percent	Calories	Grams	Grams	Grams	Grams	Grams	Grams	Milligrams	Milligrams	International units	Milligrams	Milligrams	Milligrams	Milligrams
	Carrots: Raw:															
188	Whole, 5½ by 1 inch, (25 thin strips). 1 carrot, 50	88	20	1	Trace				5	18	.4	5,500	.03	.03	.3	4
189	Grated. 1 cup, 110	88	45	1	Trace				11	41	.8	12,100	.06	.06	.7	9
190	Cooked, diced. 1 cup, 145	91	45	1	Trace				10	48	.9	15,220	.08	.07	.7	9
191	Canned, strained or chopped (baby food). 1 ounce, 28	92	10	Trace	Trace				2	7	.1	3,690	.01	.01	.1	1
192	**Cauliflower, cooked, flowerbuds.** 1 cup, 120	93	25	3	Trace				5	25	.8	70	.11	.10	.7	66
	Celery, raw:															
193	Stalk, large outer, 8 by about 1½ inches, at root end. 1 stalk, 40	94	5	Trace	Trace				2	16	.1	100	.01	.01	.1	4
194	Pieces, diced. 1 cup, 100	94	15	1	Trace				4	39	.3	240	.03	.03	.3	9
195	**Collards, cooked.** 1 cup, 190	91	55	5	1				9	289	1.1	10,260	.27	.37	2.4	87
	Corn sweet:															
196	Cooked, ear 5 by 1¾ inches.[5] 1 ear, 140	74	70	3	1				16	2	.5	[6] 310	.09	.08	1.0	7
197	Canned, solids and liquid. 1 cup, 256	81	170	5	2				40	10	1.0	[6] 690	.07	.12	2.3	13
198	**Cowpeas, cooked, immature seeds.** 1 cup, 160	72	175	13	1				29	38	3.4	560	.49	.18	2.3	28
	Cucumbers, 10-ounce; 7½ by about 2 inches:															
199	Raw, pared. 1 cucumber, 207	96	30	1	Trace				7	35	.6	Trace	.07	.09	.4	23
200	Raw, pared, center slice ⅛-inch thick. 6 slices, 50	96	5	Trace	Trace				2	8	.2	Trace	.02	.02	.1	6
201	**Dandelion greens, cooked.** 1 cup, 180	90	60	4	1				12	252	3.2	21,060	.24	.29	......	32

No.	Food	Measure	Grams	Water (%)	Food energy (cal.)	Protein (g)	Fat (g)	Saturated	Oleic	Linoleic	Carbohydrate (g)	Calcium (mg)	Iron (mg)	Vitamin A (I.U.)	Thiamine (mg)	Riboflavin (mg)	Niacin (mg)	Ascorbic acid (mg)
202	Endive, curly (including escarole).	2 ounces	57	93	10	1	Trace				2	46	1.0	1,870	.04	.08	.3	6
203	Kale, leaves including stems, cooked.	1 cup	110	91	30	4	1				4	147	1.3	8,140				68
	Lettuce, raw:																	
204	Butterhead, as Boston types; head, 4-inch diameter.	1 head	220	95	30	3	Trace				6	77	4.4	2,130	.14	.13	.6	18
205	Crisphead, as Iceburg; head, 4¾-inch diameter.	1 head	454	96	60	4	Trace				13	91	2.3	1,500	.29	.27	1.3	29
206	Looseleaf, or bunching varieties, leaves.	2 large	50	94	10	1	Trace				2	34	.7	950	.03	.04	.2	9
207	Mushrooms, canned, solids and liquid.	1 cup	244	93	40	5	Trace				6	15	1.2	Trace	.04	.60	4.8	4
208	Mustard greens, cooked.	1 cup	140	93	35	3	1				6	193	2.5	8,120	.11	.19	.9	68
209	Okra, cooked, pod 3 by ⅝ inch.	8 pods	85	91	25	2	Trace				5	78	.4	420	.11	.15	.8	17
	Onions: Mature:																	
210	Raw, onion 2½-inch diameter.	1 onion	110	89	40	2	Trace				10	30	.6	40	.04	.04	.2	11
211	Cooked.	1 cup	210	92	60	3	Trace				14	50	.8	80	.06	.06	.4	14
212	Young green, small, without tops.	6 onions	50	88	20	1	Trace				5	20	.3	Trace	.02	.02	.2	12
213	Parsley, raw, chopped.	1 tablespoon	4	85	Trace	Trace	Trace				Trace	8	.2	340	Trace	.01	Trace	7
214	Parsnips, cooked.	1 cup	155	82	100	2	1				23	70	.9	50	.11	.12	.2	16
	Peas, green:																	
215	Cooked.	1 cup	160	82	115	9	1				19	37	2.9	860	.44	.17	3.7	33
216	Canned, solids and liquid.	1 cup	249	83	165	9	1				31	50	4.2	1,120	.23	.13	2.2	22
217	Canned, strained (baby food).	1 ounce	28	86	15	1	Trace				3	3	.4	140	.02	.02	.4	3
218	Peppers, hot, red, without seeds, dried (ground chili powder, added seasonings).	1 tablespoon	15	8	50	2	2				8	40	2.3	9,750	.03	.17	1.3	2
	Peppers, sweet:																	
219	Raw, about 5 per pound: Green pod without stem and seeds.	1 pod	74	93	15	1	Trace				4	7	.5	310	.06	.06	.4	94
220	Cooked, boiled, drained.	1 pod	73	95	15	1	Trace				3	7	.4	310	.05	.05	.4	70
221	Potatoes, medium (about 3 per pound raw): Baked, peeled after baking.	1 potato	99	75	90	3	Trace				21	9	.7	Trace	.10	.04	1.7	20
	Boiled:																	
222	Peeled after boiling.	1 potato	136	80	105	3	Trace				23	10	.8	Trace	.13	.05	2.0	22
223	Peeled before boiling.	1 potato	122	83	80	2	Trace				18	7	.6	Trace	.11	.04	1.4	20

NUTRITIVE VALUES OF THE EDIBLE PART OF FOODS — Continued

[Dashes in the columns for nutrients show that no suitable value could be found although there is reason to believe that a measurable amount of the nutrient may be present]

FOOD, APPROXIMATE MEASURE, AND WEIGHT (IN GRAMS)	WATER	FOOD ENERGY	PROTEIN	FAT	FATTY ACIDS SATURATED (TOTAL)	UNSATURATED OLEIC	UNSATURATED LINOLEIC	CARBOHYDRATE	CALCIUM	IRON	VITAMIN A VALUE	THIAMIN	RIBOFLAVIN	NIACIN	ASCORBIC ACID
	Grams	Percent	Calories	Grams	Grams	Grams	Grams	Grams	Grams	Milligrams	Milligrams	International units	Milligrams	Milligrams	Milligrams	Milligrams

VEGETABLES AND VEGETABLE PRODUCTS — Continued:

FOOD, APPROXIMATE MEASURE, AND WEIGHT (IN GRAMS)	WATER	FOOD ENERGY	PROTEIN	FAT	SATURATED (TOTAL)	OLEIC	LINOLEIC	CARBOHYDRATE	CALCIUM	IRON	VITAMIN A VALUE	THIAMIN	RIBOFLAVIN	NIACIN	ASCORBIC ACID
Potatoes, Medium — Continued:															
French-fried, piece 2 by ½ by ½ inch:															
224 Cooked in deep fat. 10 pieces	57	45	155	2	2	2	4	20	9	.7	Trace	.07	.04	1.8	12
225 Frozen, heated. 10 pieces	57	53	125	2	1	1	2	19	5	1.0	Trace	.08	.01	1.5	12
Mashed:															
226 Milk added. 1 cup	195	83	125	4	1			25	47	.8	50	.16	.10	2.0	19
227 Milk and butter added. 1 cup	195	80	185	4	8	4	3	Trace	24	47	.8	330	.16	.10	1.9	18
228 Potato chips, medium, 2-inch diameter. 10 chips	20	2	115	1	8	2	2	4	10	8	.4	Trace	.04	.01	1.0	3
229 Pumpkin, canned. 1 cup	228	90	75	2	1			18	57	.9	14,590	.07	.12	1.3	12
230 Radishes, raw, small, without tops. 4 radishes	40	94	5	Trace	Trace			1	12	.4	Trace	.01	.01	.1	10
231 Sauerkraut, canned, solids and liquid. 1 cup	235	93	45	2	Trace			9	85	1.2	120	.07	.09	.4	33
Spinach:															
232 Cooked. 1 cup	180	92	40	5	1			6	167	4.0	14,580	.13	.25	1.0	50
233 Canned, drained solids. 1 cup	180	91	45	5	1			6	212	4.7	14,400	.03	.21	.6	24
Squash:															
Cooked:															
234 Summer, diced. 1 cup	210	96	30	2	Trace			7	52	.8	820	.10	.16	1.6	21
235 Winter, baked, mashed. 1 cup	205	81	130	4	1			32	57	1.6	8,610	.10	.27	1.4	27
Sweetpotatoes:															
Cooked, medium, 5 by 2 inches, weight raw about 6 ounces:															
236 Baked, peeled after baking. 1 sweetpotato.	110	64	155	2	1			36	44	1.0	8,910	.10	.07	.7	24

No.	Food	Measure	Grams	Water %	Cal.	Prot.	Fat	Sat.	Oleic	Lino.	Carb.	Ca	Fe	Vit. A	Thiam.	Ribo.	Niacin	Asc.
237	Boiled, peeled after boiling.	1 sweetpotato	147	71	170	2	1				39	47	1.0	11,610	.13	.09	.9	25
238	Candied, 3½ by 2¼ inches.	1 sweetpotato	175	60	295	2	6	2	3	1	60	65	1.6	11,030	.10	.08	.8	17
239	Canned, vacuum or solid pack.	1 cup	218	72	235	4	Trace				54	54	1.7	17,000	.10	.10	1.4	30
	Tomatoes:																	
240	Raw, approx. 3-in. diam. 2⅛ in. high; wt., 7 oz.	1 tomato	200	94	40	2	Trace				9	24	.9	1,640	.11	.07	1.3	42[7]
241	Canned, solids and liquid.	1 cup	241	94	50	2	1				10	14	1.2	2,170	.12	.07	1.7	41
	Tomato catsup:																	
242	Cup.	1 cup	273	69	290	6	1				69	60	2.2	3,820	.25	.19	4.4	41
243	Tablespoon.	1 tablespoon	15	69	15	Trace	Trace				4	3	.1	210	.01	.01	.2	2
	Tomato juice, canned:																	
244	Cup.	1 cup	243	94	45	2	Trace				10	17	2.2	1,940	.12	.07	1.9	39
245	Glass (6 fl. oz.).	1 glass	182	94	35	2	Trace				8	13	1.6	1,460	.09	.05	1.5	29
246	Turnips, cooked, diced.	1 cup	155	94	35	1	Trace				8	54	.6	Trace	.06	.08	.5	34
247	Turnip greens, cooked.	1 cup	145	94	30	3	Trace				5	252	1.5	8,270	.15	.33	.7	68

Fruits and Fruit Products

No.	Food	Measure	Grams	Water %	Cal.	Prot.	Fat	Sat.	Oleic	Lino.	Carb.	Ca	Fe	Vit. A	Thiam.	Ribo.	Niacin	Asc.
248	Apples, raw (about 3 per lb.).[5]	1 apple	150	85	70	Trace	Trace				18	8	.4	50	.04	.02	.1	3
249	Apple juice, bottled or canned.	1 cup	248	88	120	Trace	Trace				30	15	1.5	......	.02	.05	.2	2
	Applesauce, canned:																	
250	Sweetened	1 cup	255	76	230	1	Trace				61	10	1.3	100	.05	.03	.1	3[8]
251	Unsweetened or artificially sweetened.	1 cup	244	88	100	1	Trace				26	10	1.2	100	.05	.02	.1	2[8]
	Apricots:																	
252	Raw (about 12 per lb.).[5]	3 apricots	114	85	55	1	Trace				14	18	.5	2,890	.03	.04	.7	10
253	Canned in heavy sirup.	1 cup	259	77	220	2	Trace				57	28	.8	4,510	.05	.06	.9	10
254	Dried, uncooked (40 halves per cup).	1 cup	150	25	390	8	1				100	100	8.2	16,350	.02	.23	4.9	19
255	Cooked, unsweetened, fruit and liquid.	1 cup	285	76	240	5	1				62	63	5.1	8,550	.01	.13	2.8	8
256	Apricot nectar, canned.	1 cup	251	85	140	1	Trace				37	23	.5	2,380	.03	.03	.5	8[8]

NUTRITIVE VALUES OF THE EDIBLE PART OF FOODS — Continued

[Dashes in the columns for nutrients show that no suitable value could be found although there is reason to believe that a measurable amount of the nutrient may be present]

FRUITS AND FRUIT PRODUCTS — Continued:

	FOOD, APPROXIMATE MEASURE, AND WEIGHT (IN GRAMS)	WATER	FOOD ENERGY	PROTEIN	FAT	FATTY ACIDS SATURATED (TOTAL)	UNSATURATED OLEIC	UNSATURATED LINOLEIC	CARBOHYDRATE	CALCIUM	IRON	VITAMIN A VALUE	THIAMIN	RIBOFLAVIN	NIACIN	ASCORBIC ACID
		Percent	Calories	Grams	Grams	Grams	Grams	Grams	Grams	Milligrams	Milligrams	International units	Milligrams	Milligrams	Milligrams	Milligrams
257	Avocados, whole fruit, raw:[5] California (mid- and late-winter; diam. 3⅛ in.). 1 avocado 284	74	370	5	37	7	17	5	13	22	1.3	630	.24	.43	3.5	30
258	Florida (late summer, fall: diam. 3⅝ in.). 1 avocado 454	78	390	4	33	7	15	4	27	30	1.8	880	.33	.61	4.9	43
259	Bananas, raw, medium size.[5] 1 banana 175	76	100	1	Trace				26	10	.8	230	.06	.07	.8	12
260	Banana flakes. 1 cup 100	3	340	4	1				89	32	2.8	760	.18	.24	2.8	7
261	Blackberries, raw. 1 cup 144	84	85	2	1				19	46	1.3	290	.05	.06	.5	30
262	Blueberries, raw. 1 cup 140	83	85	1	1				21	21	1.4	140	.04	.08	.6	20
263	Cantaloups, raw; medium, 5-inch diameter about 1⅔ pounds.[5] ½ melon 385	91	60	1	Trace				14	27	.8	[9]6,540	.08	.06	1.2	63
264	Cherries, canned, red, sour, pitted, water pack. 1 cup 244	88	105	2	Trace				26	37	.7	1,660	.07	.05	.5	12
265	Cranberry juice cocktail, canned. 1 cup 250	83	165	Trace	Trace				42	13	.8	Trace	.03	.03	.1	[10]40
266	Cranberry sauce, sweetened, canned, strained. 1 cup 277	62	405	Trace	1				104	17	.6	60	.03	.03	.1	6
267	Dates, pitted, cut. 1 cup 178	22	490	4	1				130	105	5.3	90	.16	.17	3.9	0
268	Figs, dried, large, 2 by 1 in. 1 fig 21	23	60	1	Trace				15	26	.6	20	.02	.02	.1	0
269	Fruit cocktail, canned, in heavy sirup. 1 cup 256	80	195	1	Trace				50	23	1.0	360	.05	.03	1.3	5

No.	Food, approximate measure, and weight (in grams)	Grams	Water (%)	Food energy (cal.)	Protein (g)	Fat (g)				Carbohydrate (g)	Calcium (mg)	Iron (mg)	Vitamin A (I.U.)	Thiamine (mg)	Riboflavin (mg)	Niacin (mg)	Ascorbic acid (mg)
	Grapefruit:																
	Raw, medium, 3¾-in. diam.[5]																
270	White. ½ grapefruit	241	89	45	1	Trace				12	19	.5	10	.05	.02	.2	44
271	Pink or red. ½ grapefruit	241	89	50	1	Trace				13	20	.5	540	.05	.02	.2	44
272	Canned, sirup pack. 1 cup	254	81	180	2	Trace				45	33	.8	30	.08	.05	.5	76
	Grapefruit juice:																
273	Fresh. 1 cup	246	90	95	1	Trace				23	22	.5	(¹¹)	.09	.04	.4	92
	Canned, white:																
274	Unsweetened. 1 cup	247	89	100	1	Trace				24	20	1.0	20	.07	.04	.4	84
275	Sweetened. 1 cup	250	86	130	1	Trace				32	20	1.0	20	.07	.04	.4	78
	Frozen concentrate, unsweetened:																
276	Undiluted, can, 6 fluid ounces. 1 can	207	62	300	4	1				72	70	.8	60	.29	.12	1.4	286
277	Diluted with 3 parts water, by volume. 1 cup	247	89	100	1	Trace				24	25	.2	20	.10	.04	.5	96
278	Dehydrated crystals. 4 ounces	113	1	410	6	1				102	100	1.2	80	.40	.20	2.0	396
279	Prepared with water (1 pound yields about 1 gallon). 1 cup	247	90	100	1	Trace				24	22	.2	20	.10	.05	.5	91
	Grapes, raw:[5]																
280	American type (slip skin). 1 cup	153	82	65	1	1				15	15	.4	100	.05	.03	.2	3
281	European type (adherent skin). 1 cup	160	81	95	1	Trace				25	17	.6	140	.07	.04	.4	6
	Grapejuice:																
282	Canned or bottled. 1 cup	253	83	165	1	Trace				42	28	.8		.10	.05	.5	Trace
	Frozen concentrate, sweetened:																
283	Undiluted, can, 6 fluid ounces. 1 can	216	53	395	1	Trace				100	22	.9	40	.13	.22	1.5	(¹²)
284	Diluted with 3 parts water, by volume. 1 cup	250	86	135	1	Trace				33	8	.3	10	.05	.08	.5	(¹²)
285	Grapejuice drink, canned. 1 cup	250	86	135	Trace	Trace				35	8	.3		.03	.03	.3	(¹²)
286	Lemons, raw, 2⅛-in. diam., size 165.[5] Used for juice. 1 lemon	110	90	20	1	Trace				6	19	.4	10	.03	.01	.1	39
287	Lemon juice, raw. 1 cup	244	91	60	1	Trace				20	17	.5	50	.07	.02	.2	112
	Lemonade concentrate:																
288	Frozen, 6 fl. oz. per can. 1 can	219	48	430	Trace	Trace				112	9	.4	40	.04	.07	.7	66
289	Diluted with 4⅓ parts water, by volume. 1 cup	248	88	110	Trace	Trace				28	2	Trace	Trace	Trace	.02	.2	17
	Lime juice:																
290	Fresh. 1 cup	246	90	65	1	Trace				22	22	.5	20	.05	.02	.2	79
291	Canned, unsweetened. 1 cup	246	90	65	1	Trace				22	22	.5	20	.05	.02	.2	52
	Limeade concentrate, frozen:																
292	Undiluted, can, 6 fluid ounces. 1 can	218	50	410	Trace	Trace				108	11	.2	Trace	.02	.02	.2	26
293	Diluted with 4⅓ parts water, by volume. 1 cup	247	90	100	Trace	Trace				27	2	Trace	Trace	Trace	Trace	Trace	5

NUTRITIVE VALUES OF THE EDIBLE PART OF FOODS — Continued

[Dashes in the columns for nutrients show that no suitable value could be found although there is reason to believe that a measurable amount of the nutrient may be present]

FRUITS AND FRUIT PRODUCTS — Continued:

FOOD, APPROXIMATE MEASURE, AND WEIGHT (IN GRAMS)		WATER	FOOD ENERGY	PRO-TEIN	FAT	FATTY ACIDS SATU-RATED (TOTAL)	UNSATURATED OLEIC	LIN-OLEIC	CARBO-HY-DRATE	CAL-CIUM	IRON	VITA-MIN A VALUE	THIA-MIN	RIBO-FLAVIN	NIACIN	ASCOR-BIC ACID
		Percent	Calories	Grams	Grams	Grams	Grams	Grams	Grams	Milli-grams	Milli-grams	Inter-national units	Milli-grams	Milli-grams	Milli-grams	Milli-grams
294	Oranges, raw, 2⅝-in. diam., all commercial, varieties.[5]	1 orange	180	86	65	1	Trace				16	54	.5	260	.13	.05	.5	66
295	Orange juice, fresh, all varieties.	1 cup	248	88	110	2	Trace				26	27	.5	500	.22	.07	1.0	124
296	Canned, unsweetened.	1 cup	249	87	120	2	Trace				28	25	1.0	500	.17	.05	.7	100
297	Frozen concentrate: Undiluted, can, 6 fluid ounces.	1 can	213	55	360	5	Trace				87	75	.9	1,620	.68	.11	2.8	360
298	Diluted with 3 parts water, by volume.	1 cup	249	87	120	2	Trace				29	25	.2	550	.22	.02	1.0	120
299	Dehydrated crystals.	4 ounces	113	1	430	6	2				100	95	1.9	1,900	.76	.24	3.3	408
300	Prepared with water (1 pound yields about 1 gallon).	1 cup	248	88	115	2	1				27	25	.5	500	.20	.07	1.0	109
301	Orange-apricot juice drink.	1 cup	249	87	125	1	Trace				32	12	.2	1,440	.05	.02	.5	[10] 40
	Orange and grapefruit juice:																
302	Frozen concentrate: Undiluted, can, 6 fluid ounces.	1 cup	210	59	330	4	1				78	61	.8	800	.48	.06	2.3	302
303	Diluted with 3 parts water, by volume.	1 cup	248	88	110	1	Trace				26	20	.2	270	.16	.02	.8	102
304	Papayas, raw, ½-inch cubes.	1 cup	182	89	70	1	Trace				18	36	.5	3,190	.07	.08	.5	102
	Peaches: Raw:																
305	Whole, medium, 2-inch diameter, about 4 per pound.[5]	1 peach	114	89	35	1	Trace				10	9	.5	[13]1,320	.02	.05	1.0	7
306	Sliced.	1 cup	168	89	65	1	Trace				16	15	.8	[13]2,230	.03	.08	1.6	12

Item	Food, approximate measure	Measure	Grams	Water (%)	Food energy (cal)	Protein (g)	Fat (g)	Saturated	Oleic	Linoleic	Carbohydrate (g)	Calcium (mg)	Iron (mg)	Vitamin A (I.U.)	Thiamine (mg)	Riboflavin (mg)	Niacin (mg)	Ascorbic acid (mg)
	Canned, yellow-fleshed, solids and liquid: Sirup pack, heavy:																	
307	Halves or slices.	1 cup	257	79	200	1	Trace				52	10	.8	1,100	.02	.06	1.4	7
308	Water pack.	1 cup	245	91	75	1	Trace				20	10	.7	1,100	.02	.06	1.4	7
309	Dried, uncooked.	1 cup	160	25	420	5	1				109	77	9.6	6,240	.02	.31	8.5	28
310	Cooked, unsweetened, 10–12 halves and juice.	1 cup	270	77	220	3	1				58	41	5.1	3,290	.01	.15	4.2	6
	Frozen:																	
311	Carton, 12 ounces, not thawed.	1 carton	340	76	300	1	Trace				77	14	1.7	2,210	.03	.14	2.4	[14]135
	Pears:																	
312	Raw, 3 by 2½-inch diameter.[5]	1 pear	182	83	100	1	1				25	13	.5	30	.04	.07	.2	7
	Canned, solids and liquid: Sirup pack, heavy:																	
313	Halves or slices.	1 cup	255	80	195	1	1				50	13	.5	Trace	.03	.05	.3	4
	Pineapple:																	
314	Raw, diced.	1 cup	140	85	75	1	Trace				19	24	.7	100	.12	.04	.3	24
	Canned, heavy sirup pack, solids and liquid:																	
315	Crushed.	1 cup	260	80	195	1	Trace				50	29	.8	120	.20	.06	.5	17
316	Sliced, slices and juice.	2 small or 1 large	122	80	90	Trace	Trace				24	13	.4	50	.09	.03	.2	8
317	Pineapple juice, canned.	1 cup	249	86	135	1	Trace				34	37	.7	120	.12	.04	.5	[3]22
	Plums, all except prunes:																	
318	Raw, 2-inch diameter, about 2 ounces.[5]	1 plum	60	87	25	Trace	Trace				7	7	.3	140	.02	.02	.3	3
319	Canned, sirup pack (Italian prunes): Plums (with pits) and juice.[5]	1 cup	256	77	205	1	Trace				53	22	2.2	2,970	.05	.05	.9	4
	Prunes, dried, "softenized," medium:																	
320	Uncooked.[5]	4 prunes	32	28	70	1	Trace				18	14	1.1	440	.02	.04	.4	1
321	Cooked, unsweetened, 17–18 prunes and ⅓ cup liquid.[5]	1 cup	270	66	295	2	1				78	60	4.5	1,860	.08	.18	1.7	2
322	Prune juice, canned or bottled.	1 cup	256	80	200	1	Trace				49	36	10.5		.03	.03	1.0	[3]5
	Raisins, seedless:																	
323	Packaged, ½ oz. or 1½ tbsp. per pkg.	1 pkg.	14	18	40	Trace	Trace				11	9	.5	Trace	.02	.01	.1	Trace
324	Cup, pressed down.	1 cup	165	18	480	4	Trace				128	102	5.8	30	.18	.13	.8	2
	Raspberries, red:																	
325	Raw.	1 cup	123	84	70	1	1				17	27	1.1	160	.04	.11	1.1	31
326	Frozen, 10-ounce carton, not thawed.	1 carton	284	74	275	2	1				70	37	1.7	200	.06	.17	1.7	59
327	Rhubarb, cooked, sugar added.	1 cup	272	63	385	1	Trace				98	212	1.6	220	.06	.15	.7	17
	Strawberries:																	
328	Raw, capped.	1 cup	149	90	55	1	1				13	31	1.5	90	.04	.10	1.0	88
329	Frozen, 10-ounce carton, not thawed.	1 carton	284	71	310	1	1				79	40	2.0	90	.06	.17	1.5	150

NUTRITIVE VALUES OF THE EDIBLE PART OF FOODS — Continued

[Dashes in the columns for nutrients show that no suitable value could be found although there is reason to believe that a measurable amount of the nutrient may be present]

FOOD, APPROXIMATE MEASURE, AND WEIGHT (IN GRAMS)	WATER	FOOD ENERGY	PRO-TEIN	FAT	FATTY ACIDS SATU-RATED (TOTAL)	UNSATURATED OLEIC	UNSATURATED LIN-OLEIC	CARBO-HY-DRATE	CAL-CIUM	IRON	VITA-MIN A VALUE	THIA-MIN	RIBO-FLAVIN	NIACIN	ASCOR-BIC ACID
	Grams	Percent	Calories	Grams	Grams	Grams	Grams	Grams	Grams	Milli-grams	Milli-grams	Inter-national units	Milli-grams	Milli-grams	Milli-grams	Milli-grams

FRUITS AND FRUIT PRODUCTS — Continued:

FOOD, APPROXIMATE MEASURE, AND WEIGHT	WATER	FOOD ENERGY	PROTEIN	FAT	SATURATED (TOTAL)	OLEIC	LINOLEIC	CARBOHYDRATE	CALCIUM	IRON	VITAMIN A	THIAMIN	RIBOFLAVIN	NIACIN	ASCORBIC ACID
330 Tangerines, raw, medium, 2⅜-in. diam., size 176.[5] — 1 tangerine — 116	87	40	1	Trace	......			10	34	.3	360	.05	.02	.1	27
331 Tangerine juice, canned, sweetened. — 1 cup — 249	87	125	1	1	......		1	30	45	.5	1,050	.15	.05	.2	55
332 Watermelon, raw, wedge, 4 by 8 inches (1/16 of 10 by 16-inch melon, about 2 pounds with rind).[5] — 1 wedge — 925	93	115	2	1	......			27	30	2.1	2,510	.13	.13	.7	30

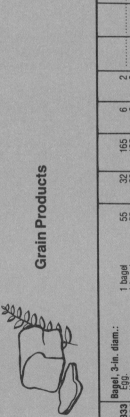

Grain Products

FOOD, APPROXIMATE MEASURE, AND WEIGHT	WATER	FOOD ENERGY	PROTEIN	FAT	SATURATED (TOTAL)	OLEIC	LINOLEIC	CARBOHYDRATE	CALCIUM	IRON	VITAMIN A	THIAMIN	RIBOFLAVIN	NIACIN	ASCORBIC ACID
333 Bagel, 3-in. diam.: Egg. — 1 bagel — 55	32	165	6	2		1	1	28	9	1.2	30	.14	.10	1.2	0
334 Water. — 1 bagel — 55	29	165	6	2		1	1	30	8	1.2	0	.15	.11	1.4	0
335 Barley, pearled, light, uncooked. — 1 cup — 200	11	700	16	2	Trace	1	1	158	32	4.0	0	.24	.10	6.2	0
336 Biscuits, baking powder from home recipe with enriched flour, 2-in. diam. — 1 biscuit — 28	27	105	2	5	1	2	1	13	34	.4	Trace	.06	.06	.1	Trace
337 Biscuits, baking powder from mix, 2-in. diam. — 1 biscuit — 28	28	90	2	3	1	1	1	15	19	.6	Trace	.08	.07	.6	Trace

No.	Food, description	Measure	Grams	Water (%)	Food energy (cal)	Protein (g)	Fat (g)	Saturated (g)	Oleic (g)	Linoleic (g)	Carbohydrate (g)	Calcium (mg)	Iron (mg)	Vitamin A (IU)	Thiamin (mg)	Riboflavin (mg)	Niacin (mg)	Ascorbic acid (mg)
338	**Bran flakes (40% bran), added thiamin and iron.**	1 cup	35	3	105	4	1				28	25	12.3	0	.14	.06	2.2	0
339	**Bran flakes with raisins, added thiamin and iron.**	1 cup	50	7	145	4	1				40	28	13.5	Trace	.16	.07	2.7	Trace
	Breads:																	
340	Boston brown bread, slice 3 by ¾ in.	1 slice	48	45	100	3	1				22	43	.9	0	.05	.03	.6	0
	Cracked-wheat bread:																	
341	Loaf, 1 lb.	1 loaf	454	35	1,190	40	10	2	5	2	236	399	5.0	Trace	.53	.41	5.9	Trace
342	Slice, 18 slices per loaf.	1 slice	25	35	65	2	1				13	22	.3	Trace	.03	.02	.3	Trace
	French or vienna bread:																	
343	Enriched, 1 lb. loaf.	1 loaf	454	31	1,315	41	14	3	8	2	251	195	10.0	Trace	1.27	1.00	11.3	Trace
344	Unenriched, 1 lb. loaf.	1 loaf	454	31	1,315	41	14	3	8	2	251	195	3.2	Trace	.36	.36	3.6	Trace
	Italian bread:																	
345	Enriched, 1 lb. loaf.	1 loaf	454	32	1,250	41	4	Trace	1	2	256	77	10.0	0	1.32	.91	11.8	0
346	Unenriched, 1 lb. loaf.	1 loaf	454	32	1,250	41	4	Trace	1	2	256	77	3.2	0	.41	.27	3.6	0
	Raisin bread:																	
347	Loaf, 1 lb.	1 loaf	454	35	1,190	30	13	3	8	2	243	322	5.9	Trace	.23	.41	3.2	Trace
348	Slice, 18 slices per loaf.	1 slice	25	35	65	2	1				13	18	.3	Trace	.01	.02	.2	Trace
	Rye bread: American, light (⅓ rye, ⅔ wheat):																	
349	Loaf, 1 lb.	1 loaf	454	36	1,100	41	5				236	340	7.3	0	.82	.32	6.4	0
350	Slice, 18 slices per loaf.	1 slice	25	36	60	2	Trace				13	19	.4	0	.05	.02	.4	0
351	Pumpernickel, loaf, 1 lb.	1 loaf	454	34	1,115	41	5				241	381	10.9	0	1.04	.64	5.4	0
	White bread, enriched:[15] Soft-crumb type:																	
352	Loaf, 1 lb.	1 loaf	454	36	1,225	39	15	3	8	2	229	381	11.3	Trace	1.13	.95	10.9	Trace
353	Slice, 18 slices per loaf.	1 slice	25	36	70	2	1				13	21	.6	Trace	.06	.05	.6	Trace
354	Slice, toasted.	1 slice	22	25	70	2	1				13	21	.6	Trace	.06	.05	.6	Trace
355	Slice, 22 slices per loaf.	1 slice	20	36	55	2	1				10	17	.5	Trace	.05	.04	.5	Trace
356	Slice, toasted.	1 slice	17	25	55	2	1				10	17	.5	Trace	.05	.04	.5	Trace
357	Loaf, 1½ lbs.	1 loaf	680	36	1,835	59	22	5	12	3	343	571	17.0	Trace	1.70	1.43	16.3	Trace
358	Slice, 24 slices per loaf.	1 slice	28	36	75	2	1				14	24	.7	Trace	.07	.06	.7	Trace
359	Slice, toasted.	1 slice	24	25	75	2	1				14	24	.7	Trace	.07	.06	.7	Trace
360	Slice, 28 slices per loaf.	1 slice	24	36	65	2	1				12	20	.6	Trace	.06	.05	.6	Trace
361	Slice, toasted.	1 slice	21	25	65	2	1				12	20	.6	Trace	.06	.05	.6	Trace
	Firm-crumb type:																	
362	Loaf, 1 lb.	1 loaf	454	35	1,245	41	17	4	10	2	228	435	11.3	Trace	1.22	.91	10.9	Trace
363	Slice, 20 slices per loaf.	1 slice	23	35	65	2	1				12	22	.6	Trace	.06	.05	.6	Trace
364	Slice, toasted.	1 slice	20	24	65	2	1				12	22	.6	Trace	.06	.05	.6	Trace
365	Loaf, 2 lbs.	1 loaf	907	35	2,495	82	34	8	20	4	455	871	22.7	Trace	2.45	1.81	21.8	Trace
366	Slice, 34 slices per loaf.	1 slice	27	35	75	2	1				14	26	.7	Trace	.07	.05	.6	Trace
367	Slice, toasted.	1 slice	23	35	75	2	1				14	26	.7	Trace	.07	.05	.6	Trace
	Whole-wheat bread, soft-crumb type:																	
368	Loaf, 1 lb.	1 loaf	454	36	1,095	41	12	2	6	2	224	381	13.6	Trace	1.36	.45	12.7	Trace

NUTRITIVE VALUES OF THE EDIBLE PART OF FOODS — Continued

[Dashes in the columns for nutrients show that no suitable value could be found although there is reason to believe that a measurable amount of the nutrient may be present]

GRAIN PRODUCTS — Continued:

	FOOD, APPROXIMATE MEASURE, AND WEIGHT (IN GRAMS)		WATER	FOOD ENERGY	PRO-TEIN	FAT	SATU-RATED (TOTAL)	UNSATURATED OLEIC	LIN-OLEIC	CARBO-HY-DRATE	CAL-CIUM	IRON	VITA-MIN A VALUE	THIA-MIN	RIBO-FLAVIN	NIACIN	ASCOR-BIC ACID
		Grams	Percent	Calories	Grams	Grams	Grams	Grams	Grams	Grams	Milli-grams	Milli-grams	Inter-national units	Milli-grams	Milli-grams	Milli-grams	Milli-grams
	Breads — Continued:																
369	Slice, 16 slices per loaf. 1 slice	28	36	65	3	1				14	24	.8	Trace	.09	.03	.8	Trace
370	Slice, toasted. 1 slice	24	24	65	3	1				14	24	.8	Trace	.09	.03	.8	Trace
	Whole-wheat bread, firm-crumb type:																
371	Loaf, 1 lb. 1 loaf	454	36	1,100	48	14	3	6	3	216	449	13.6	Trace	1.18	.54	12.7	Trace
372	Slice, 18 slices per loaf. 1 slice	25	36	60	3	1				12	25	.8	Trace	.06	.03	.7	Trace
373	Slice, toasted. 1 slice	21	24	60	3	1				12	25	.8	Trace	.06	.03	.7	Trace
374	Breadcrumbs, dry, grated. 1 cup	100	6	390	13	5	1	2	1	73	122	3.6	Trace	.22	.30	3.5	Trace
375	Buckwheat flour, light, sifted. 1 cup	98	12	340	6	1				78	11	1.0	0	.08	.04	.4	0
376	Bulgur, canned, seasoned. 1 cup	135	56	245	8	4				44	27	1.9	0	.08	.05	4.1	0
	Cakes made from cake mixes:																
	Angelfood:																
377	Whole cake. 1 cake	635	34	1,645	36	1				377	603	1.9	0	.03	.70	.6	0
378	Piece, 1/12 of 10-in. diam. cake. 1 piece	53	34	135	3	Trace				32	50	.2	0	Trace	.06	.1	0
	Cupcakes, small, 2½ in. diam.:																
379	Without icing. 1 cupcake	25	26	90	1	3	1	1	1	14	40	.1	40	.01	.03	.1	Trace
380	With chocolate icing. 1 cupcake	36	22	130	2	5	2	2	1	21	47	.3	60	.01	.04	.1	Trace
	Devil's food, 2-layer, with chocolate icing;																
381	Whole cake. cake	1,107	24	3,755	49	136	54	58	16	645	653	8.9	1,660	.33	.89	3.3	1
382	Piece, 1/16 of 9-in. diam. cake. 1 piece	69	24	235	3	9	3	4	1	40	41	.6	100	.02	.06	.2	Trace
383	Cupcake, small, 2½ in. diam. 1 cupcake	35	24	120	2	4	1	2	Trace	20	21	.3	50	.01	.03	.1	Trace
	Gingerbread:																
384	Whole cake. 1 cake	570	37	1,575	18	39	10	19	9	291	513	9.1	Trace	.17	.51	4.6	2
385	Piece, 1/9 of 8-in. square cake. 1 piece	63	37	175	2	4	1	2	1	32	57	1.0	Trace	.02	.06	.5	Trace

No.	Food, approximate measure	Grams	Water (%)	Food energy (cal.)	Protein (g)	Fat (g)	Saturated (g)	Oleic (g)	Linoleic (g)	Carbohydrate (g)	Calcium (mg)	Iron (mg)	Vitamin A (I.U.)	Thiamin (mg)	Riboflavin (mg)	Niacin (mg)	Ascorbic acid (mg)
	White, 2-layer, with chocolate icing:																
386	Whole cake. 1 cake	1,140	21	4,000	45	122	45	54	17	716	1,129	5.7	680	.23	.91	2.3	2
387	Piece, 1/16 of 9-in. diam. cake. 1 piece	71	21	250	3	8	3	3	1	45	70	.4	40	.01	.06	.1	Trace
	Cakes made from home recipes:[16]																
388	Boston cream pie; piece 1/12 of 8-in. diam. 1 piece	69	35	210	4	6	2	3	1	34	46	.3	140	.02	.08	.1	Trace
	Fruitcake, dark, made with enriched flour:																
389	Loaf, 1 lb. 1 loaf	454	18	1,720	22	69	15	37	13	271	327	11.8	540	.59	.64	3.6	2
390	Slice, 1/30 of 8-in. loaf. 1 slice	15	18	55	1	2	Trace	1	Trace	9	11	.4	20	.02	.02	.1	Trace
	Plain sheet cake: Without icing:																
391	Whole cake. 1 cake	777	25	2,830	35	108	30	52	21	434	497	3.1	1,320	.16	.70	1.6	2
392	Piece, 1/9 of 9-in. square cake. 1 piece	86	25	315	4	12	3	6	2	48	55	.3	150	.02	.08	.2	Trace
393	With boiled white icing, piece, 1/9 of 9-in. square cake. 1 piece	114	23	400	4	12	3	6	2	71	56	.3	150	.02	.08	.2	Trace
	Pound:																
394	Loaf, 8½ by 3½ by 3 in. 1 loaf	514	17	2,430	29	152	34	68	17	242	108	4.1	1,440	.15	.46	1.0	0
395	Slice, ½-in. thick. 1 slice	30	17	140	2	9	2	4	1	14	6	.2	80	.01	.03	.1	0
	Sponge:																
396	Whole cake. 1 cake	790	32	2,345	60	45	14	20	4	427	237	9.5	3,560	.40	1.11	1.6	Trace
397	Piece, 1/12 of 10-in. diam. cake. 1 piece	66	32	195	5	4	1	2	Trace	36	20	.8	300	.03	.09	.1	Trace
	Yellow, 2-layer, without icing:																
398	Whole cake. 1 cake	870	24	3,160	39	111	31	53	22	506	618	3.5	1,310	.17	.70	1.7	2
399	Piece, 1/16 of 9-in. diam. cake. 1 piece	54	24	200	2	7	2	3	1	32	39	.2	80	.01	.04	.1	Trace
	Yellow, 2-layer, with chocolate icing:																
400	Whole cake. 1 cake	1,203	21	4,390	51	156	55	69	23	727	818	7.2	1,920	.24	.96	2.4	Trace
401	Piece, 1/16 of 9-in. diam. cake. 1 piece	75	21	275	3	10	3	4	1	45	51	.5	120	.02	.06	.2	Trace
	Cake icings. See Sugars, Sweets.																
	Cookies:																
	Brownies with nuts:																
402	Made from home recipe with enriched flour. 1 brownie	20	10	95	1	6	1	3	1	10	8	.4	40	.04	.02	.1	Trace
403	Made from mix. 1 brownie	20	11	85	1	4	1	2	1	13	9	.4	20	.03	.02	.1	Trace
	Chocolate chip:																
404	Made from home recipe with enriched flour. 1 cookie	10	3	50	1	3	1	1	1	6	4	.2	10	.01	.01	.1	Trace
405	Commercial. 1 cookie	10	3	50	1	2	1	1	Trace	7	4	.2	10	Trace	Trace	Trace	Trace
406	Fig bars, commercial. 1 cookie	14	14	50	1	1	1	1		11	11	.2	20	Trace	.01	.1	Trace
407	Sandwich, chocolate or vanilla, commercial. 1 cookie	10	2	50	1	2	1	1	Trace	7	2	.1	0	Trace	Trace	.1	0
	Corn flakes, added nutrients:																
408	Plain. 1 cup	25	4	100	2	Trace				21	4	.4	0	.11	.02	.5	0
409	Sugar-covered. 1 cup	40	2	155	2	Trace				36	5	.4	0	.16	.02	.8	0
	Corn (hominy) grits, degermed, cooked:																
410	Enriched. 1 cup	245	87	125	3	Trace				27	2	.7	[17]150	.10	.07	1.0	0
411	Unenriched. 1 cup	245	87	125	3	Trace				27	2	.2	[17]150	.05	.02	.5	0

NUTRITIVE VALUES OF THE EDIBLE PART OF FOODS — Continued

[Dashes in the columns for nutrients show that no suitable value could be found although there is reason to believe that a measurable amount of the nutrient may be present]

FOOD, APPROXIMATE MEASURE, AND WEIGHT (IN GRAMS)			WATER	FOOD ENERGY	PRO-TEIN	FAT	FATTY ACIDS SATU-RATED (TOTAL)	UNSATURATED OLEIC	LIN-OLEIC	CARBO-HY-DRATE	CAL-CIUM	IRON	VITA-MIN A VALUE	THIA-MIN	RIBO-FLAVIN	NIACIN	ASCOR-BIC ACID
		Grams	Percent	Calories	Grams	Grams	Grams	Grams	Grams	Grams	Milli-grams	Milli-grams	Inter-national units	Milli-grams	Milli-grams	Milli-grams	Milli-grams
GRAIN PRODUCTS — Continued:																	
412	Cornmeal: Whole-ground, unbolted, dry.	1 cup	122	12	435	11	5	1	2	2	90	24	2.9	[17] 620	.46	.13	2.4	0
413	Bolted (nearly wholegrain) dry.	1 cup	122	12	440	11	4	Trace	1	2	91	21	2.2	[17] 590	.37	.10	2.3	0
	Degermed, enriched:																	
414	Dry form.	1 cup	138	12	500	11	2				108	8	4.0	[17] 610	.61	.36	4.8	0
415	Cooked.	1 cup	240	88	120	3	1				26	2	1.0	[17] 140	.14	.10	1.2	0
	Degermed, unenriched:																	
416	Dry form.	1 cup	138	12	500	11	2				108	8	1.5	[17] 610	.19	.07	1.4	0
417	Cooked.	1 cup	240	88	120	3	1				26	2	.5	[17] 140	.05	.02	.2	0
418	Corn muffins, made with enriched degermed cornmeal and enriched flour, muffin 2⅜-in. diam.	1 muffin	40	33	125	3	4	2	2	Trace	19	42	.7	[17] 120	.08	.09	.6	Trace
419	Corn muffins, made with mix, egg, and milk; muffin 2⅜-in. diam.	1 muffin	40	30	130	3	4	1	2	1	20	96	.6	100	.07	.08	.6	Trace
420	Corn, puffed, presweetened, added nutrients.	1 cup	30	2	115	1	Trace				27	3	.5	0	.13	.05	.6	0
421	Corn, shredded, added nutrients.	1 cup	25	3	100	2	Trace				22	1	.6	0	.11	.05	.5	0
	Crackers:																	
422	Graham, 2½-in. square.	4 crackers	28	6	110	2	3				21	11	.4	0	.01	.06	.4	0
423	Saltines.	4 crackers	11	4	50	1	1		1		8	2	.1	0	Trace	Trace	.1	0
424	Danish pastry, plain (without fruit or nuts): Packaged ring, 12 ounces.	1 ring	340	22	1,435	25	80	24	37	15	155	170	3.1	1,050	.24	.51	2.7	Trace

	Food	Measure	Grams	Water %	Calories	Protein (g)	Fat (g)	Sat. fat (g)	Oleic (g)	Linoleic (g)	Carb. (g)	Calcium (mg)	Iron (mg)	Vit. A (IU)	Thiamin (mg)	Riboflavin (mg)	Niacin (mg)	Asc. acid (mg)
425	Round piece, approx. 4¼-in. diam. by 1 in.	1 pastry	65	22	275	5	15	5	7	3	30	33	.6	200	.05	.10	.5	Trace
426	Ounce.	1 ounce	28	22	120	2	7	2	3	1	13	14	.3	90	.02	.04	.2	Trace
427	Doughnuts, cake type.	1 doughnut	32	24	125	1	6	1	4	1	16	13	[18].4	30	[18].05	[18].05	[18].4	Trace
428	Farina, quick-cooking, enriched, cooked.	1 cup	245	89	105	3	Trace				22	147	[19].7	0	[19].12	[19].07	[19]1.0	0
	Macaroni, cooked: Enriched:																	
429	Cooked, firm stage (undergoes additional cooking in a food mixture).	1 cup	130	64	190	6	1				39	14	[19]1.4	0	[19].23	[19].14	[19]1.8	0
430	Cooked until tender.	1 cup	140	72	155	5	1				32	8	[19]1.3	0	[19].20	[19].11	[19]1.5	0
	Unenriched:																	
431	Cooked, firm stage (undergoes additional cooking in a food mixture).	1 cup	130	64	190	6	1				39	14	.7	0	.03	.03	.5	0
432	Cooked until tender.	1 cup	140	72	155	5	1				32	11	.6	0	.01	.01	.4	0
433	Macaroni (enriched) and cheese, baked.	1 cup	200	58	430	17	22	10	9	2	40	362	1.8	860	.20	.40	1.8	Trace
434	Canned.	1 cup	240	80	230	9	10	4	3	1	26	199	1.0	260	.12	.24	1.0	Trace
435	Muffins, with enriched white flour, muffin, 3-inch diameter.	1 muffin	40	38	120	3	4	1	2	1	17	42	.6	40	.07	.09	.6	Trace
	Noodles (egg noodles), cooked:																	
436	Enriched.	1 cup	160	70	200	7	2	1	1	Trace	37	16	[19]1.4	110	[19].22	[19].13	[19]1.9	0
437	Unenriched.	1 cup	160	70	200	7	2	1	1	Trace	37	16	1.0	110	.05	.03	.6	0
438	Oats (with or without corn) puffed, added nutrients.	1 cup	25	3	100	3	1				19	44	1.2	0	.24	.04	.5	0
439	Oatmeal or rolled oats, cooked.	1 cup	240	87	130	5	2	1	1	1	23	22	1.4	0	.19	.05	.2	0
	Pancakes, 4-inch diameter:																	
440	Wheat, enriched flour (home recipe).	1 cake	27	50	60	2	2	Trace	1	Trace	9	27	.4	30	.05	.06	.4	Trace
441	Buckwheat (made from mix with egg and milk).	1 cake	27	58	55	2	2	Trace	1	Trace	6	59	.4	60	.03	.04	.2	Trace
442	Plain or buttermilk (made from mix with egg and milk).	1 cake	27	51	60	2	2	Trace	1	Trace	9	58	.3	70	.04	.06	.2	Trace
	Pie (piecrust made with unenriched flour): Sector, 4-in., 1/7 of 9-in. diam. pie:																	
443	Apple (2-crust).	1 sector	135	48	350	3	15	4	7	3	51	11	.4	40	.03	.03	.5	1
444	Butterscotch (1-crust).	1 sector	130	45	350	6	14	5	6	2	50	98	1.2	340	.04	.13	.3	Trace
445	Cherry (2-crust).	1 sector	135	47	350	4	15	4	7	3	52	19	.4	590	.03	.03	.7	Trace
446	Custard (1-crust).	1 sector	130	58	285	8	14	5	6	2	30	125	.8	300	.07	.21	.4	0
447	Lemon meringue (1-crust).	1 sector	120	47	305	4	12	4	6	2	45	17	.6	200	.04	.10	.2	4

NUTRITIVE VALUES OF THE EDIBLE PART OF FOODS — Continued

[Dashes in the columns for nutrients show that no suitable value could be found although there is reason to believe that a measurable amount of the nutrient may be present]

FOOD, APPROXIMATE MEASURE, AND WEIGHT (IN GRAMS)		WATER	FOOD ENERGY	PRO-TEIN	FAT	FATTY ACIDS SATU-RATED (TOTAL)	UNSATURATED OLEIC	LIN-OLEIC	CARBO-HY-DRATE	CAL-CIUM	IRON	VITA-MIN A VALUE	THIA-MIN	RIBO-FLAVIN	NIACIN	ASCOR-BIC ACID
	Grams	Percent	Calories	Grams	Grams	Grams	Grams	Grams	Grams	Milli-grams	Milli-grams	Inter-national units	Milli-grams	Milli-grams	Milli-grams	Milli-grams
GRAIN PRODUCTS — Continued:																
Pie (Piecrust made with unenriched flour) — Continued:																
Sector, 4-in., ¹/₇ of 9-in. diam. pie:																
448 Mince (2-crust). 1 sector	135	43	365	3	16	4	8	3	56	38	1.4	Trace	.09	.05	.5	1
449 Pecan (1-crust). 1 sector	118	20	490	6	27	4	16	5	60	55	3.3	190	.19	.08	.4	Trace
450 Pineapple chiffon (1-crust). 1 sector	93	41	265	6	11	3	5	2	36	22	.8	320	.04	.08	.4	1
451 Pumpkin (1-crust). 1 sector	130	59	275	5	15	5	6	2	32	66	.7	3,210	.04	.13	.7	Trace
Piecrust, baked shell for pie made with:																
452 Enriched flour. 1 shell	180	15	900	11	60	16	28	12	79	25	3.1	0	.36	.25	3.2	0
453 Unenriched flour. 1 shell	180	15	900	11	60	16	28	12	79	25	.9	0	.05	.05	.9	0
Piecrust mix including stick form:																
454 Package, 10-oz., for double crust. 1 package	284	9	1,480	20	93	23	46	21	141	131	1.4	0	.11	.11	2.0	0
455 Pizza (cheese) 5½-in. sector; ⅛ of 14-in. diam. pie. 1 sector	75	45	185	7	6	2	3	Trace	27	107	.7	290	.04	.12	.7	4
Popcorn, popped:																
456 Plain, large kernel. 1 cup	6	4	25	1	Trace				5	1	.2			.01	.1	0
457 With oil and salt. 1 cup	9	3	40	1	2	1	Trace	Trace	5	1	.2			.01	.2	0
458 Sugar coated. 1 cup	35	4	135	2	1				30	2	.5			.02	.4	0
Pretzels:																
459 Dutch, twisted. 1 pretzel	16	5	60	2	1				12	4	.2	0	Trace	Trace	.1	0
460 Thin, twisted. 1 pretzel	6	5	25	1	Trace				5	1	.1	0	Trace	Trace	Trace	0
461 Stick, small, 2¼ inches. 10 sticks	3	5	10	Trace	Trace				2	1	Trace	0	Trace	Trace	Trace	0
462 Stick, regular, 3⅛ inches. 5 sticks	3	5	10	Trace	Trace				2	1	Trace	0	Trace	Trace	Trace	0
Rice, white: Enriched:																
463 Raw. 1 cup	185	12	670	12	1				149	44	[20] 5.4	0	[20] .81	[20] .06	[20] 6.5	0

No.	Food	Measure	Grams	Water (%)	Food energy	Protein (g)	Fat (g)	Saturated	Oleic	Linoleic	Carbohydrate (g)	Calcium	Iron	Vitamin A	Thiamin	Riboflavin	Niacin	Ascorbic acid
464	Cooked.	1 cup	205	73	225	4	Trace				50	21	[20] 1.8	0	[20] .23	[20] .02	[20] 2.1	0
465	Instant, ready-to-serve.	1 cup	165	73	180	4	Trace				40	5	[20] 1.3	0	[20] .21	[20] ...	[20] 1.7	0
466	Unenriched, cooked.	1 cup	205	73	225	4	Trace				50	21	.4	0	.04	.02	.8	0
467	Parboiled, cooked.	1 cup	175	73	185	4	Trace				41	33	[20] 1.4	0	[20] .19	[20] ...	[20] 2.1	0
468	Rice, puffed, added nutrients.	1 cup	15	4	60	1	Trace				13	3	.3	0	.07	.01	.7	0
	Rolls, enriched: Cloverleaf or pan:																	
469	Home recipe.	1 roll	35	26	120	3	3	1	1	1	20	16	.7	30	.09	.09	.8	Trace
470	Commercial.	1 roll	28	31	85	2	2	Trace	1	Trace	15	21	.5	Trace	.08	.05	.6	Trace
471	Frankfurter or hamburger.	1 roll	40	31	120	3	2	1	1	1	21	30	.8	Trace	.11	.07	.9	Trace
472	Hard, round or rectangular.	1 roll	50	25	155	5	2	Trace	1	Trace	30	24	1.2	Trace	.13	.12	1.4	Trace
473	Rye wafers, whole-grain, 1⅞ by 3½ inches.	2 wafers	13	6	45	2	Trace				10	7	.5	0	.04	.03	.2	0
474	Spaghetti, cooked, tender stage, enriched.	1 cup	140	72	155	5	1				32	11	[19] 1.3	0	[19] .20	[19] .11	[19] 1.5	0
	Spaghetti with meat balls, and tomato sauce:																	
475	Home recipe.	1 cup	248	70	330	19	12	4	6	1	39	124	3.7	1,590	.25	.30	4.0	22
476	Canned.	1 cup	250	78	260	12	10	2	3	4	28	53	3.3	1,000	.15	.18	2.3	5
	Spaghetti in tomato sauce with cheese:																	
477	Home recipe.	1 cup	250	77	260	9	9	2	5	1	37	80	2.3	1,080	.25	.18	2.3	13
478	Canned.	1 cup	250	80	190	6	2	1	1	1	38	40	2.8	930	.35	.28	4.5	10
479	Waffles, with enriched flour, 7-in. diam.	1 waffle	75	41	210	7	7	2	4	1	28	85	1.3	250	.13	.19	1.0	Trace
480	Waffles, made from mix, enriched, egg and milk added, 7-in. diam.	1 waffle	75	42	205	7	8	3	3	1	27	179	1.0	170	.11	.17	.7	Trace
481	Wheat, puffed, added nutrients.	1 cup	15	3	55	2	Trace				12	4	.6	0	.08	.03	1.2	0
482	Wheat, shredded, plain.	1 biscuit	25	7	90	2	1				20	11	.9	0	.06	.03	1.1	0
483	Wheat flakes, added nutrients.	1 cup	30	4	105	3	Trace				24	12	1.3	0	.19	.04	1.5	0
	Wheat flours:																	
484	Whole-wheat, from hard wheats, stirred.	1 cup	120	12	400	16	2	Trace	1	1	85	49	4.0	0	.66	.14	5.2	0
	All purpose or family flour, enriched:																	
485	Sifted.	1 cup	115	12	420	12	1				88	18	[19] 3.3	0	[19] .51	[19] .30	[19] 4.0	0
486	Unsifted.	1 cup	125	12	455	13	1				95	20	[19] 3.6	0	[19] .55	[19] .33	[19] 4.4	0
487	Self-rising, enriched.	1 cup	125	12	440	12	1				93	331	[19] 3.6	0	[19] .55	[19] .33	[19] 4.4	0
488	Caked or pastry flour, sifted.	1 cup	96	12	350	7	1				76	16	.5	0	.03	.03	.7	0

NUTRITIVE VALUES OF THE EDIBLE PART OF FOODS — Continued

[Dashes in the columns for nutrients show that no suitable value could be found although there is reason to believe that a measurable amount of the nutrient may be present]

Fats, Oils

	FOOD, APPROXIMATE MEASURE, AND WEIGHT (IN GRAMS)		WATER	FOOD ENERGY	PRO-TEIN	FAT	SATU-RATED (TOTAL)	UNSATURATED OLEIC	LIN-OLEIC	CARBO-HY-DRATE	CAL-CIUM	IRON	VITA-MIN A VALUE	THIA-MIN	RIBO-FLAVIN	NIACIN	ASCOR-BIC ACID
		Grams	Percent	Calories	Grams	Grams	Grams	Grams	Grams	Grams	Milli-grams	Milli-grams	Inter-national units	Milli-grams	Milli-grams	Milli-grams	Milli-grams
	Butter:																
	Regular, 4 sticks per pound:																
489	Stick. ½ cup	113	16	810	1	92	51	30	3	1	23	0	[2]3,750				0
490	Tablespoon (approx. ⅛ stick). 1 tablespoon	14	16	100	Trace	12	6	4	Trace	Trace	3	0	[2]470				0
491	Pat (1-in. sq. ⅓-in. high; 90 per lb.). 1 pat	5	16	35	Trace	4	2	1	Trace	Trace	1	0	[2]170				0
	Whipped, 6 sticks, or 2, 8-oz. containers per pound:																
492	Stick. ½ cup	76	16	540	1	61	34	20	2	Trace	15	0	[2]2,500				0
493	Tablespoon (approx. ⅛ stick). 1 tablespoon	9	16	65	Trace	8	4	3	Trace	Trace	2	0	[2]310				0
494	Pat (1¼-in. sq. ⅓-in. high; 120 per lb.). 1 pat	4	16	25	Trace	3	2	1	Trace	Trace	1	0	[2]130				0
	Fats, cooking:																
495	Lard. 1 cup	205	0	1,850	0	205	78	94	20	0	0	0	0	0	0	0	0
496	1 tablespoon	13	0	115	0	13	5	6	1	0	0	0	0	0	0	0	0
497	Vegetable fats. 1 cup	200	0	1,770	0	200	50	100	44	0	0	0		0	0	0	0
	1 tablespoon	13	0	110	0	13	3	6	3	0	0	0		0	0	0	0
	Margarine:																
	Regular, 4 sticks per pound:																
499	Stick. ½ cup	113	16	815	1	92	17	46	25	1	23	0	[2]3,750				0
500	Tablespoon (approx. ⅛ stick). 1 tablespoon	14	16	100	Trace	12	2	6	3	Trace	3	0	[2]470				0
501	Pat (1-in. sq. ⅓-in. high; 90 per lb.). 1 pat	5	16	35	Trace	4	1	2	1	Trace	1	0	[2]170				0

Item No.	Food, approximate measure	Grams	Water (%)	Food energy (cal)	Protein (g)	Fat (g)	Saturated (g)	Oleic (g)	Linoleic (g)	Carbohydrate (g)	Calcium (mg)	Iron (mg)	Vitamin A (IU)	Thiamin (mg)	Riboflavin (mg)	Niacin (mg)	Ascorbic acid (mg)
	Whipped, 6 sticks per pound:																
502	Stick, ½ cup	76	16	545	1	61	11	31	17	Trace	15	0	[22]2,500	—	—	—	0
	Soft, 2 8-oz. tubs per pound:																
503	Tub. 1 tub	227	16	1,635	1	184	34	68	68	1	45	0	[22]7,500	—	—	—	0
504	Tablespoon. 1 tablespoon	14	16	100	Trace	11	2	4	4	Trace	3	0	[22]470	—	—	—	0
	Oils, salad or cooking:																
505	Corn. 1 cup	220	0	1,945	0	220	22	62	117	0	0	0	—	0	0	0	0
506	1 tablespoon	14	0	125	0	14	1	4	7	0	0	0	—	0	0	0	0
507	Cottonseed. 1 cup	220	0	1,945	0	220	55	46	110	0	0	0	—	0	0	0	0
508	1 tablespoon	14	0	125	0	14	4	3	7	0	0	0	—	0	0	0	0
509	Olive. 1 cup	220	0	1,945	0	220	24	167	15	0	0	0	—	0	0	0	0
510	1 tablespoon	14	0	125	0	14	2	11	1	0	0	0	—	0	0	0	0
511	Peanut. 1 cup	220	0	1,945	0	220	40	103	64	0	0	0	—	0	0	0	0
512	1 tablespoon	14	0	125	0	14	3	7	4	0	0	0	—	0	0	0	0
513	Safflower. 1 cup	220	0	1,945	0	220	18	37	165	0	0	0	—	0	0	0	0
514	1 tablespoon	14	0	125	0	14	1	2	10	0	0	0	—	0	0	0	0
515	Soybean. 1 cup	220	0	1,945	0	220	33	44	114	0	0	0	—	0	0	0	0
516	1 tablespoon	14	0	125	0	14	2	3	7	0	0	0	—	0	0	0	0
	Salad dressings:																
517	Blue cheese. 1 tablespoon	15	32	75	1	8	2	2	4	1	12	Trace	30	Trace	0.02	Trace	Trace
	Commercial, mayonnaise type:																
518	Regular. 1 tablespoon	15	41	65	Trace	6	1	1	3	2	2	Trace	30	Trace	Trace	Trace	—
519	Special dietary, low-calorie. 1 tablespoon	16	81	20	Trace	2	Trace	Trace	1	2	3	Trace	40	Trace	Trace	Trace	—
	French:																
520	Regular. 1 tablespoon	16	39	65	Trace	6	1	1	3	3	2	.1	—	—	—	—	—
521	Special dietary, low-fat with artificial sweeteners. 1 tablespoon	15	95	Trace	Trace	Trace	—	—	—	7	2	.1	—	—	—	—	—
522	Home cooked, boiled. 1 tablespoon	16	68	25	1	2	Trace	1	Trace	2	14	.1	80	.01	.03	Trace	Trace
523	Mayonnaise. 1 tablespoon	14	15	100	Trace	11	2	2	6	Trace	3	.1	40	Trace	.01	Trace	Trace
524	Thousand island. 1 tablespoon	16	32	80	Trace	8	1	2	4	2	2	.1	50	Trace	Trace	Trace	Trace

Sugars, Sweets

Item No.	Food, approximate measure	Grams	Water (%)	Food energy (cal)	Protein (g)	Fat (g)	Saturated (g)	Oleic (g)	Linoleic (g)	Carbohydrate (g)	Calcium (mg)	Iron (mg)	Vitamin A (IU)	Thiamin (mg)	Riboflavin (mg)	Niacin (mg)	Ascorbic acid (mg)
	Cake icings:																
525	Cocolate made with milk and table fat. 1 cup	275	14	1,035	9	38	21	14	1	185	165	3.3	580	.06	.28	.6	1
526	Coconut (with boiled icing). 1 cup	166	15	605	3	13	11	1	Trace	124	10	.8	0	.02	.07	.3	0
527	Creamy fudge from mix with water only. 1 cup	245	15	830	7	16	5	8	3	183	96	2.7	Trace	.05	.20	.7	Trace
528	White, boiled. 1 cup	94	18	300	1	0	0	0	0	76	2	Trace	0	Trace	.03	Trace	0
	Candy:																
529	Caramels, plain or chocolate. 1 ounce	28	8	115	1	3	2	1	Trace	22	42	.4	Trace	.01	.05	.1	Trace

NUTRITIVE VALUES OF THE EDIBLE PART OF FOODS — Continued

[Dashes in the columns for nutrients show that no suitable value could be found although there is reason to believe that a measurable amount of the nutrient may be present]

FOOD, APPROXIMATE MEASURE, AND WEIGHT (IN GRAMS)		WATER	FOOD ENERGY	PRO-TEIN	FAT	FATTY ACIDS SATU-RATED (TOTAL)	UNSATURATED OLEIC	LIN-OLEIC	CARBO-HY-DRATE	CAL-CIUM	IRON	VITA-MIN A VALUE	THIA-MIN	RIBO-FLAVIN	NIACIN	ASCOR-BIC ACID
	Grams	Percent	Calories	Grams	Grams	Grams	Grams	Grams	Grams	Milli-grams	Milli-grams	Inter-national units	Milli-grams	Milli-grams	Milli-grams	Milli-grams

SUGARS, SWEETS — Continued:

FOOD, APPROXIMATE MEASURE, AND WEIGHT (IN GRAMS)	Grams	Water %	Food Energy Cal.	Protein g	Fat g	Sat. g	Oleic g	Linoleic g	Carb. g	Calcium mg	Iron mg	Vit. A IU	Thiamin mg	Riboflavin mg	Niacin mg	Ascorbic mg
Candy — Continued:																
530 Chocolate, milk, plain. 1 ounce	28	1	145	2	9	5	3	Trace	16	65	.3	80	.02	.10	.1	Trace
531 Chocolate-coated peanuts. 1 ounce	28	1	160	5	12	3	6	2	11	33	.4	Trace	.10	.05	2.1	Trace
532 Fondant; mints, uncoated; candy corn. 1 ounce	28	8	105	Trace	1				25	4	.3	0	Trace	Trace	Trace	0
533 Fudge, plain. 1 ounce	28	8	115	1	4	2	1	Trace	21	22	.3	Trace	.01	.03	.1	Trace
534 Gum drops. 1 ounce	28	12	100	Trace	Trace				25	2	.1	0	0	Trace	Trace	0
535 Hard. 1 ounce	28	1	110	0	Trace				28	6	.5	0	0	0	0	0
536 Marshmallows. 1 ounce	28	17	90	1	Trace				23	5	.5	0	0	Trace	Trace	0
Chocolate-flavored sirup or topping:																
537 Thin type. 1 fluid ounce	38	32	90	1	1	Trace	Trace	Trace	24	6	.6	Trace	.01	.03	.2	0
538 Fudge type. 1 fluid ounce	38	25	125	2	5	3	2	Trace	20	48	.5	60	.02	.08	.2	Trace
Chocolate-flavored beverage powder (approx. 4 heaping teaspoons per oz.):																
539 With nonfat dry milk. 1 ounce	28	2	100	5	1	Trace	Trace	Trace	20	167	.5	10	.04	.21	.2	1
540 Without nonfat dry milk. 1 ounce	28	1	100	1	1	Trace	Trace	Trace	25	9	.6	0	.01	.03	.1	0
541 Honey, strained or extracted. 1 tablespoon	21	17	65	Trace	0				17	1	.1	0	Trace	.01	.1	Trace
542 Jams and preserves. 1 tablespoon	20	29	55	Trace	Trace				14	4	.2	Trace	Trace	.01	Trace	Trace
543 Jellies. 1 tablespoon	18	29	50	Trace	Trace				13	4	.3	Trace	Trace	.01	Trace	1
Molasses, cane:																
544 Light (first extraction). 1 tablespoon	20	24	50	—	—				13	33	.9	—	.01	.01	Trace	—
545 Blackstrap (third extraction). 1 tablespoon	20	24	45	—	—				11	137	3.2	—	.02	.04	.4	—
Sirups:																
546 Sorghum. 1 tablespoon	21	23	55	0	—				14	35	2.6	—	Trace	.02	Trace	—
547 Table blends, chiefly corn, light and dark. 1 tablespoon	21	24	60	0	—				15	9	.8	—	0	0	0	0

Miscellaneous Items

No.	Food	Measure	Grams	Water (%)	Food energy (cal)	Protein (g)	Fat (g)	Saturated	Oleic	Linoleic	Carbohydrate (g)	Calcium (mg)	Iron (mg)	Vitamin A (IU)	Thiamin (mg)	Riboflavin (mg)	Niacin (mg)	Ascorbic acid (mg)
	Sugars:																	
548	Brown, firm packed.	1 cup	220	2	820	0	0				212	187	7.5	0	.02	.07	.4	0
	White:																	
549	Granulated.	1 cup	200	Trace	770	0	0				199	0	.2	0	0	0	0	0
550		1 tablespoon	11	Trace	40	0	0				11	0	Trace	0	0	0	0	0
551	Powdered, stirred before measuring.	1 cup	120	Trace	460	0	0				119	0	.1	0	0	0	0	0
552	Barbecue sauce.	1 cup	250	81	230	4	17	2	5	9	20	53	2.0	900	.03	.03	.8	13
	Beverages, alcoholic:																	
553	Beer.	12 fl. oz.	360	92	150	1	0				14	18	Trace		.01	.11	2.2	
	Gin, rum, vodka, whiskey:																	
554	80-proof.	1½ fl. oz. jigger	42	67	100						Trace							
555	86-proof.	1½ fl. oz. jigger	42	64	105						Trace							
556	90-proof.	1½ fl. oz. jigger	42	62	110						Trace							
557	94-proof.	1½ fl. oz. jigger	42	60	115						Trace							
558	100-proof.	1½ fl. oz. jigger	42	58	125						Trace							
	Wines:																	
559	Dessert.	3½ fl. oz. glass	103	77	140	Trace	0				8	8			.01	.02	.2	
560	Table.	3½ fl. oz. glass	102	86	85	Trace	0				4	9	.4		Trace	.01	.1	
	Beverages, carbonated, sweetened, nonalcoholic:																	
561	Carbonated water.	12 fl. oz.	366	92	115	0	0				29			0	0	0	0	0
562	Cola type.	12 fl. oz.	369	90	145	0	0				37			0	0	0	0	0
563	Fruit-flavored sodas and Tom Collins mixes.	12 fl. oz.	372	88	170	0	0				45			0				
564	Ginger ale.	12 fl. oz.	366	92	115	0	0				29			0	0	0	0	0
565	Root beer.	12 fl. oz.	370	90	150	0	0				39			0	0	0	0	0
566	Bouillon cubes, approx. ½ in.	1 cube	4	4	5	1	Trace				Trace							
	Chocolate:																	
567	Bitter or baking.	1 oz.	28	2	145	3	15	8	6	Trace	8	22	1.9	20	.01	.07	.4	0
568	Semi-sweet, small pieces.	1 cup	170	1	860	7	61	34	22	1	97	51	4.4	30	.02	.14	.9	0

NUTRITIVE VALUES OF THE EDIBLE PART OF FOODS — Continued

[Dashes in the columns for nutrients show that no suitable value could be found although there is reason to believe that a measurable amount of the nutrient may be present]

FOOD, APPROXIMATE MEASURE, AND WEIGHT (IN GRAMS)		WATER	FOOD ENERGY	PROTEIN	FAT	FATTY ACIDS			CARBO-HY-DRATE	CAL-CIUM	IRON	VITA-MIN A VALUE	THIA-MIN	RIBO-FLAVIN	NIACIN	ASCOR-BIC ACID
						SATU-RATED (TOTAL)	UNSATURATED									
							OLEIC	LIN-OLEIC								
	Grams	Percent	Calories	Grams	Grams	Grams	Grams	Grams	Grams	Milli-grams	Milli-grams	Inter-national units	Milli-grams	Milli-grams	Milli-grams	Milli-grams

MISCELLANEOUS ITEMS — Continued:

	FOOD, APPROXIMATE MEASURE, AND WEIGHT	Grams	WATER	FOOD ENERGY	PRO-TEIN	FAT	SATU-RATED (TOTAL)	OLEIC	LIN-OLEIC	CARBO-HY-DRATE	CAL-CIUM	IRON	VITA-MIN A VALUE	THIA-MIN	RIBO-FLAVIN	NIACIN	ASCOR-BIC ACID
	Gelatin:																
569	Plain, dry powder in envelope. 1 envelope	7	13	25	6	Trace				0							
570	Dessert powder, 3-oz. package. 1 package	85	2	315	8	0				75							
571	**Gelatin dessert, prepared with water.** 1 cup	240	84	140	4	0				34							
	Olives, pickled:																
572	Green. 4 medium or 3 extra large or 2 giant.	16	78	15	Trace	2	Trace	2	Trace	Trace	8	.2	40				
573	Ripe: Mission. 3 small or 2 large.	10	73	15	Trace	2	Trace	2	Trace	Trace	9	.1	10	Trace	Trace		
	Pickles, cucumber:																
574	Dill, medium, whole, 3¾ in. long, 1¼ in. diam. 1 pickle	65	93	10	1	Trace				1	17	.7	70	Trace	.01	Trace	4
575	Fresh, sliced, 1½ in. diam., ¼ in. thick. 2 slices	15	79	10	Trace	Trace				3	5	.3	20	Trace	Trace	Trace	1
576	Sweet, gherkin, small, whole, approx. 2½ in. long ¾ in. diam. 1 pickle	15	61	20	Trace	Trace				6	2	.2	10	Trace	Trace	Trace	1
577	Relish, finely chopped, sweet. 1 tablespoon	15	63	20	Trace	Trace				5	3	.1					
	Popcorn. See Grain Products.																
578	**Popsicle, 3 fl. oz. size.** 1 popsicle	95	80	70	0	0	0	0	0	18	.0	Trace	0	0	0	0	0
	Pudding, home recipe with starch base:																
579	Chocolate. 1 cup	260	66	385	8	12	7	4	Trace	67	250	1.3	390	.05	.36	.3	1
580	Vanilla (blanc mange). 1 cup	255	76	285	9	10	5	3	Trace	41	298	Trace	410	.08	.41	.3	2
581	**Pudding mix, dry form, 4-oz. package.** 1 package	113	2	410	3	2	1	1	Trace	103	23	1.8	Trace	.02	.08	.5	0

Item	Food	Measure	Grams	Water (%)	Food energy (cal.)	Protein (g)	Fat (g)	Saturated (g)	Oleic (g)	Linoleic (g)	Carbohydrate (g)	Calcium (mg)	Iron (mg)	Vitamin A (I.U.)	Thiamin (mg)	Riboflavin (mg)	Niacin (mg)	Ascorbic acid (mg)
582	Sherbet.	1 cup	193	67	260	2	2				59	31	Trace	120	.02	.06	Trace	4
	Soups:																	
	Canned, condensed, ready-to-serve:																	
	Prepared with an equal volume of milk:																	
583	Cream of chicken.	1 cup	245	85	180	7	10	3	3	3	15	172	.5	610	.05	.27	.7	2
584	Cream of mushroom.	1 cup	245	83	215	7	14	4	4	5	16	191	.5	250	.05	.34	.7	1
585	Tomato.	1 cup	250	84	175	7	7	3	2	1	23	168	.8	1,200	.10	.25	1.3	15
	Prepared with an equal volume of water:																	
586	Bean with pork.	1 cup	250	84	170	8	6	1	2	1	22	63	2.3	650	.13	.08	1.0	3
587	Beef broth, bouillon consomme.	1 cup	240	96	30	5	0				3	Trace	.5	Trace	Trace	.02	1.2	
588	Beef noodle.	1 cup	240	93	70	4	3	1	1	1	7	7	1.0	50	.05	.07	1.0	Trace
589	Clam chowder, Manhattan type (with tomatoes, without milk).	1 cup	245	92	80	2	3				12	34	1.0	880	.02	.02	1.0	
590	Cream of chicken.	1 cup	240	92	95	3	6	1	2	1	8	24	.5	410	.02	.05	.5	Trace
591	Cream of mushroom.	1 cup	240	90	135	2	10	2	3	5	10	41	.5	70	.02	.12	.7	Trace
592	Minestrone.	1 cup	245	90	105	5	3	1	1	Trace	14	37	1.0	2,350	.07	.05	1.0	
593	Split pea.	1 cup	245	85	145	9	3	1	2	Trace	21	29	1.5	440	.25	.15	1.5	1
594	Tomato.	1 cup	245	90	90	2	3	Trace	1	Trace	16	15	.7	1,000	.05	.05	1.2	12
595	Vegetable beef.	1 cup	245	92	80	5	2				10	12	.7	2,700	.05	.05	1.0	
596	Vegetarian.	1 cup	245	92	80	2	2				13	20	1.0	2,940	.05	.05	1.0	
	Dehydrated, dry form:																	
597	Chicken noodle (2 oz. package).	1 package	57	6	220	8	6				33	34	1.4	190	.30	.15	2.4	3
598	Onion mix (1½-oz. package).	1 package	43	3	150	6	5				23	42	.6	30	.05	.03	.3	6
599	Tomato vegetable with noodles (2½-oz. pkg.).	1 package	71	4	245	6	6				45	33	1.4	1,700	.21	.13	1.8	18
	Frozen, condensed:																	
	Clam chowder, New England type (with milk, without tomatoes):																	
600	Prepared with equal volume of milk.	1 cup	245	83	210	9	12				16	240	1.0	250	.07	.29	.5	Trace
601	Prepared with equal volume of water.	1 cup	240	89	130	4	8				11	91	1.0	50	.05	.10	.5	
	Cream of potato:																	
602	Prepared with equal volume of milk.	1 cup	245	83	185	8	10	5	3	Trace	18	208	1.0	590	.10	.27	.5	Trace
603	Prepared with equal volume of water.	1 cup	240	90	105	3	5	3	2	Trace	12	58	1.0	410	.05	.05	.5	
	Cream of shrimp:																	
604	Prepared with equal volume of milk.	1 cup	245	82	245	9	16				15	189	.5	290	.07	.27	.5	Trace
605	Prepared with equal volume of water.	1 cup	240	88	160	5	12				8	38	.5	120	.05	.05	.5	

NUTRITIVE VALUES OF THE EDIBLE PART OF FOODS — Continued

[Dashes in the columns for nutrients show that no suitable value could be found although there is reason to believe that a measurable amount of the nutrient may be present]

MISCELLANEOUS ITEMS — Continued:

FOOD, APPROXIMATE MEASURE, AND WEIGHT (IN GRAMS)			WATER	FOOD ENERGY	PROTEIN	FAT	FATTY ACIDS SATURATED (TOTAL)	UNSATURATED OLEIC	LINOLEIC	CARBOHYDRATE	CALCIUM	IRON	VITAMIN A VALUE	THIAMIN	RIBOFLAVIN	NIACIN	ASCORBIC ACID
		Grams	Percent	Calories	Grams	Grams	Grams	Grams	Grams	Grams	Milli-grams	Milli-grams	International units	Milli-grams	Milli-grams	Milli-grams	Milli-grams
Soups — Continued:																	
Oyster stew:																	
606 Prepared with equal volume of milk.	1 cup	240	83	200	10	12				14	305	1.4	410	.12	.41	.5	Trace
607 Prepared with equal volume of water.	1 cup	240	90	120	6	8				8	158	1.4	240	.07	.19	.5	....
608 Tapioca, dry, quickcooking.	1 cup	152	13	535	1	Trace				131	15	.6	0	0	0	0	0
Tapioca desserts:																	
609 Apple.	1 cup	250	70	295	1	Trace				74	8	.5	30	Trace	Trace	Trace	Trace
610 Cream pudding.	1 cup	165	72	220	8	8	4	3	Trace	28	173	.7	480	.07	.30	.2	2
611 Tartar sauce.	1 tablespoon	14	34	75	Trace	8	1	1	4	1	3	.1	30	Trace	Trace	Trace	Trace
612 Vinegar.	1 tablespoon	15	94	Trace	Trace	0				1	1	.1	....	....	....	....	....
613 White sauce, medium.	1 cup	250	73	405	10	31	16	10	1	22	288	.5	1,150	.10	.43	.5	2
Yeast:																	
614 Baker's, dry, active.	1 package	7	5	20	3	Trace				3	3	1.1	Trace	.16	.38	2.6	Trace
615 Brewer's, dry.	1 tablespoon	8	5	25	3	Trace				3	17	1.4	Trace	1.25	.34	3.0	Trace
Yogurt. See Milk, Cheese, Cream, imitation Cream.																	

Footnotes:

[1]Value applies to unfortified product: value for fortified low-density product would be 1500 I. U. and the fortified high-density product would be 2290 I. U.

[2]Contributed largely from beta-carotene used for coloring.

[3]Outer layer of fat on the cut was removed to within approximately ½ inch of the lean. Deposits of fat within the cut were not removed.

[4]If bones are discarded, value will be greatly reduced.

[5]Measure and weight apply to entire vegetable or fruit including parts not usually eaten.

[6]Based on yellow varieties. White varieties contain only a trace of cryptoxanthin and carotenes, the pigments in corn that have biologic activity.

[7]Year-round average. Samples marketed from November through May, average 20 milligrams per 200-gram tomato; from June through October, around 52 milligrams.

[8]This is the amount from the fruit. Additional ascorbic acid may be added by the manufacturer. Refer to the label for this information.

[9]Value for varieties with orange-colored flesh; value for varieties with green flesh would be about 540 I. U.

[10]Value listed is based on products with label stating 30 mg per 6-fl.-oz. serving.

[11]For white fleshed varieties, value is about 20 I. U. per cup, for red-fleshed varieties, 1,080 I. U. per cup.

[12]Present only if added by the manufacturer. Refer to the label for this information.

[13]Based on yellow-fleshed varieties; for white-fleshed varieties value is about 50 I. U. per 114-gm peach and 80 I. U. per cup of sliced peaches.

[14]This value includes ascorbic acid added by manufacturer.

[15]Values for iron, thiamin, riboflavin, and niacin per pound of unenriched white bread would be as follows:

	Iron	Thiamin	Riboflavin	Niacin
Soft crumb	3.2	.31	.39	5.0
Firm c	3.2	.32	.59	4.1

[16]Unenriched cake flour used unless otherwise specified.

[17]This value is based on product made from yellow varieties of corn; white varieties contain only a trace.

[18]Eased on product made with enriched flour. With unenriched flour, approximate values per doughnut are: iron, 0.2 mg; thiamin, 0.01 mg, riboflavin, 0.03 mg, niacin, 0.2 mg.

[19]Iron, thiamin, riboflavin, and niacin are based on the minimum levels of enrichment specified in standards of identity promulgated under the Federal Food, Drug, and Cosmetic Act.

[20]Iron, thiamin, and niacin are based on the minimum levels of enrichment specified in standards of identity promulgated under the Federal Food, Drug, and Cosmetic Act. Riboflavin is based on unenriched rice. When the minimum level of enrichment specified in the standards of identity becomes effective the value will be 0.12 mg per cup of parboiled rich and of white rice.

[21]Year-round average.

[22]Eased on the average vitamin A content of fortified margarine. Federal specifications for fortified margarine require a minimum of 15,000 I. U. of vitamin A per pound.

INDEX